BIOLOGY: BRAIN & BEHAVIOUR

# Neurobiology

**Springer**
*Berlin*
*Heidelberg*
*New York*
*Barcelona*
*Budapest*
*Hong Kong*
*London*
*Milan*
*Paris*
*Santa Clara*
*Singapore*
*Tokyo*

David Robinson (Ed.)

# Neurobiology

With 189 Figures

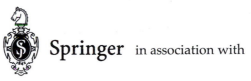 Springer in association with  The Open University

Unless otherwise stated, all contributors are (or were at the time this book was written) members of The Open University

## Academic Editor

David Robinson

## Authors

Sarah Bullock
Basiro Davey
Geoff Einon
David Robinson
Vicky Stirling
Alison Taylor

## External Assessors

Richard Andrew, School of Biological Sciences, University of Sussex
 (Series Assessor)
John O'Keefe, Anatomy Department, University College, London
 (Book Assessor)

*Biology: Brain & Behaviour* **series**

1 Behaviour and Evolution
**2 Neurobiology**
3 The Senses and Communication
4 Development and Flexibility
5 Control of Behaviour
6 Brain: Degeneration, Damage and Disorder

**Library of Congress Cataloging-in-Publication Data**
Neurobiology/David Robinson (ed.)
Includes bibliographical references and index.
 ISBN 3-540-63546-7 (pbk.)
 1. Neurobiology. I. Robinson, David, 1949-
QP355.2.N483 1997
573.8—dc21 97-37177 CIP

Published by Springer-Verlag, written and produced by The Open University

Cover design: *design & production* GmbH, Heidelberg

Printed and bound by Kyodo Printing Co (S'pore) Pte Ltd

ISBN 3-540-63546-7 Springer-Verlag Berlin Heidelberg New York

This text forms part of the Open University *Biology: Brain & Behaviour* series. The complete list of texts which make up this series can be found above. Details of Open University courses can be obtained from the Course Reservations and Sales Office, PO Box 724, The Open University, Milton Keynes MK7 6ZS, United Kingdom: tel. (00 44) 1908 653231. Alternatively, much useful course information can be obtained from the Open University's website: http://www.open.ac.uk

3.1

SPIN 10640674 #39/3137 – 5 4 3 2 1 0

# CONTENTS

# PREFACE

*Neurobiology,* like any other textbook, is designed to be read on its own, but it is also the second in a series of six books that form part of *SD206 Biology: Brain & Behaviour,* a course for Open University students. Associated with this book is a CD-ROM, *The Human Brain: An introduction to the human nervous system,* which explores the structure and function of the human brain using computer graphics and computer-generated 3-D models.

Each subject is introduced in a way that makes it readily accessible to readers without any previous knowledge of that area. Questions within the text, marked with a □, are designed to help readers understand and remember the topic under discussion. (Answers to in-text questions are marked with a ■.) The major learning objectives are listed at the end of each chapter, followed by questions (with answers given at the end of the book) which allow readers to assess how well they have achieved these objectives. Key terms are identified in bold type in the text; these are listed, with their definitions, in a glossary at the end of the book. Key references are given at the end of each chapter, where appropriate. A 'general further reading' list, of textbooks relevant to the whole book, is also included at the end.

The study of the brain and behaviour is an experimental science. This means that it involves the collection of observations, the formulation of specific hypotheses to explain those observations and the carrying out of experiments to test (confirm or falsify) those hypotheses. Throughout this book, these different aspects of the investigative process are emphasized, often through the use of in-text questions in which the reader is invited to engage in the process of deductive reasoning themselves. An understanding of the scientific method, as it applies to the behavioural and brain sciences, is an important aim of this book.

This book deals with animal nervous systems: what they consist of, how they work and how they are studied. This is a huge topic and this book does not set out to provide a complete and comprehensive coverage of the subject. The main intention of the book is to provide basic neurobiological knowledge, but it also aims to provide an interesting and informative account of an important area in biology, and one that is essential if a thorough understanding of behaviour is to be achieved.

The first chapter outlines very briefly the various approaches to studying nervous systems taken by the different disciplines and explains how it is possible to consider different levels of explanation for the properties of the nervous system. Chapter 2 describes the cells that make up the nervous system, the use of microscopy to study ultrastructure and how the cells interact with each other. In Chapter 3, the electrical properties of nerve cells are described in greater detail, concentrating on the properties that allow them to transmit information. The ionic movements that occur during the travel of an action potential along a neuron are described and related to the conditions that exist in the neuron in the resting state. This chapter includes details of how electrical events in the nervous system are observed and recorded.

The communication of information from one cell to another is considered in Chapter 4. A discussion of the structure and function of the synapse leads on to consideration of the neuron as an information processor. The chapter concludes with a survey of the classes of chemicals that act as neurotransmitters. Chapter 5 provides a basic description of the immune system and its links with the nervous system. The cells that defend vertebrates from infection have much in common with the cells of the nervous system and it is possible that they have a common evolutionary origin. The level of 'cross-talk' between immune and nervous system is such that the two systems could be viewed as parts of a single interactive network.

Chapter 6 describes the nervous systems of invertebrates and emphasizes the commonality of certain features of nervous systems across the whole range of animals. Invertebrates have provided experimental models for studying the function of nervous systems and a number of examples are given. Then, in the next chapter, Chapter 7, nervous systems and the control of behaviour are described, using invertebrate examples. A system that is well understood is the flight control system of the locust in which a central pattern generator produces the sequences of stimulating signals for the flight muscles. The locust exemplifies some general principles governing the control of behaviour by the nervous system and the generation of repetitive patterns. Chapter 8 introduces vertebrate nervous systems, concentrating on the mammalian system and particularly the human brain. The overview of the brain on the CD-ROM is particularly relevant to this chapter.

The senses and movement—the 'ins' and 'outs'—of the nervous system are considered in Chapter 9, while Chapter 10 looks at how reflex behaviour and adaptive behaviour are controlled by the nervous system. Finally, Chapter 11 discusses the relationship between the brain and the mind, cognition and consciousness.

Before you begin to read this book, there are some important points that you should bear in mind.

## 1  Experiments on animals

The use of living animals in research is a highly emotive, contentious and political issue. You are no doubt aware of the strong views held by animal liberationists. There is also considerable debate among scientists concerning what kinds of experiments and procedures are acceptable and what are not. Most scientists working with animals seek to minimize any suffering that animals may experience during experiments and each researcher makes his or her own judgement as to whether the suffering caused by an experiment is justified by the scientific value of the results that the experiment yields. The ethics of animal experimentation is not simply a matter of individual judgement, however, but is a matter of concern for society as a whole. In Britain and many other countries, all researchers work within strict guidelines enforced by government; for example, the Home Office licenses all animal experimentation in the UK. Some academic societies, such as the Association for the Study of Animal Behaviour, and many institutions, such as medical schools, have Ethical Committees that oversee animal-based research. In this book, a number of experiments are described; this in itself raises ethical issues because reporting the results of an experiment may be thought to be giving tacit approval to that experiment. This is not necessarily true and it should be pointed out that some of the experiments described were carried out several years ago and a number of them would not be carried out today, such has been the shift in opinion on these issues within the biological community. Paradoxically, certain experiments carried out many years ago, such as those on the effects of maternal deprivation on young monkeys, produced such strong and distressing effects on their subjects—results that were not generally anticipated—that they have had a substantial impact on the kind of experiments that are permitted today.

## 2   Latin names for species

A particular individual animal belongs to various categories. If you own a pet, it may, for example, be categorized as a bitch, a spaniel, a dog, a mammal, or an animal. Each category is defined by particular features that differentiate it from other, comparable categories. The most important level of categorization in biology is at the level of the species. When a particular species of animal is referred to in this book, its Latin name is also given, e.g. earthworm (*Lumbricus terrestris*).

# CHAPTER 1
## EXPLAINING THE BRAIN— THE NEUROSCIENCES

## 1.1 Introduction

Most animals have a nervous system. The nervous system contains cells that are specialized in the rapid passing of signals throughout the animal's body. The system coordinates the activity of the animal by controlling other cells such as the muscle cells that produce movement. It receives information about the outside world through sensory organs such as eyes and ears. The internal state of the animal (e.g. body temperature, fluid level, described in Book 1, Chapter 7) is also monitored by the nervous system. This flow of information into and out of the nervous system means that there are extensive interconnections within it. These can encode patterns of signals that control purposeful movements like feeding or reproductive behaviour. Learning can also occur because the circuitry can continually change during use. Nervous systems range in complexity from the relatively simple network found in sea anemones (Chapter 7 of this book) to that found in mammals where the brain is of a substantial size.

The human brain (Figure 1.1, *overleaf*) is composed of about 1400 g or so of a pink tissue enclosed within the skull with an extension called the spinal cord running down inside the backbone. The brain has an intricate and very beautiful structure. It is this structure that is one of the main subjects of this book—what it is and what it does.

The brain is continually at work even when the body's musculature is at rest and it has a continuous need for oxygen and sugar to fuel its activities. Its pink colour is given by its blood supply which terminates in a very fine network of capillaries extending throughout the brain, delivering oxygen to its many millions of  basic units—called nerve cells or **neurons**. Deprivation of oxygen for as little as four minutes can lead to irreversible damage to neurons and their death. Cells in other tissues in the body are replaced when they die, but there is no replacement of neurons.

The external appearance of the human brain is dominated by the massive pair of *cerebral hemispheres* that fold over and largely conceal the underlying structures to which they are also intimately connected. Each hemisphere is covered by a sheet of neurons a couple of millimetres thick, called the cerebral cortex. This sheet, which contains several thousand million neurons, is crumpled like a piece of tissue paper to fit into the skull, giving it a convoluted appearance. But, unlike crumpled tissue, the cerebral cortex folds in a very regular way so that individual valleys and peaks—called *sulci* (singular *sulcus*) and *gyri* (singular *gyrus*) respectively—can be used as named landmarks when identifying specific regions of the hemispheres (Figure 1.1).

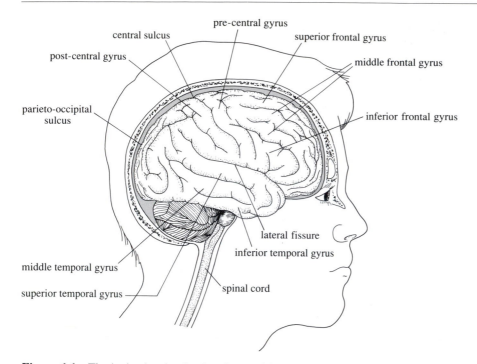

**Figure 1.1** The brain showing landmarks provided by the convolutions of the cerebral hemispheres. You are not expected to remember all the different names of the sulci and gyri.

As you read through this book, you will get an understanding of how the brain and other nervous system structures are built up from different types of neuron. From Chapters 2 and 3, you will see that, in one respect, neurons are little chemical 'factories' continually creating specialized substances, some of which are used to communicate with other neurons. These chemicals are formed from other chemicals ('raw materials') taken from the brain's blood supply. These chapters will also describe the way in which specific groupings of neurons contribute both to the brain's structure and to its functions in controlling behaviour. Throughout, there will be an emphasis on what the brain does—what can be said about the relationships between its structure and its functions in controlling behaviour.

This book will be concerned both with similarities and differences between species. Much of our understanding of the human nervous system has been gained by looking at the nervous systems of non-humans. For example, insight into the general properties of the neuron, applicable to any species, has been gained by looking at neurons of the squid. For reasons described in Chapter 3, the squid is simply the most convenient animal to study. Provided due caution is exercised, much is to be gained by such comparison between species. However, another important aspect of this book is to explore specialization. For example, Chapter 7 will look at how combinations of neurons serve such specialized functions as generating flight in locusts. So, throughout the book, keep in mind that neurons and combinations of neurons can in some cases carry out similar functions in different species but in other cases can also be highly specialized to serve particular functions peculiar to a particular species.

In Book 2 the term 'function' is used in a different sense from its usage in Book 1. In Book 2, questions about the function of a brain structure will be questions about how it 'works' and what it 'does', rather than how it increases fitness. Answers to questions about what parts of the brain do will generally be in terms of the way in which collections of neurons interact to process the information they convey or the way in which they act to modify the way that other structures work.

## 1.2    The neurosciences—disciplines and content

For centuries, the brain and nervous system have been a subject for exploration, study and conjecture. However, it is in the last quarter century, which has been marked by an explosion of activity in the neurosciences, that the greatest advances in understanding have taken place. Despite these advances, the nervous system of animals is probably the least understood of any system in the body. This is partly because of its inaccessibility—the brain and spinal cord in vertebrate animals is firmly encased within the skull and vertebral column—but, more importantly, the complexity of the system is substantially greater than that of any other system in the body.

A range of scientific disciplines contributes to work in the neurosciences: pharmacology, anatomy, physiology, physics, chemistry and psychology. However, as you will appreciate as you read this book, the neurosciences are also very dependent upon technological advance. The growth in neuroscience research has proceeded in parallel with the growth in technology along the same exponential curve. As a result of the collaborative efforts of neuroscientists, a lot is known about the way in which the nervous system develops, the way in which individual components function and the way in which groups of components work together to process sensory information and produce behaviour. Emerging from work in the last ten years has been the beginnings of an understanding of how the cognitive functions of the human brain (introduced in Book 1, Chapter 8) might map onto the brain's structure.

One of the first contributions from the neurosciences you will encounter comes from neuroanatomy. Here, naming the landmarks of the brain is the starting point for an explanation of how the brain works. The working hypothesis of the neuroanatomist is that differences in structure imply differences in function—and being able to name different structures is the starting point for questions about what the different structures do. So, the new names that appear in the early chapters are the pegs upon which explanations of the functions of different parts of the brain will be hung.

The work of the neuroanatomist in identifying, distinguishing and naming the different parts of the brain starts the journey towards functional explanations. The next step is the identification of the connections between brain structures—in the brain these are called pathways or tracts. A pathway will typically consist of many neurons. The identification of pathways between structures implies that the structures communicate—that is, the output of one region provides the input for another. The existence of pathways between brain structures implies a flow of information from one to the next. Here, neurophysiology comes into play.

The basic building block within the nervous system is the neuron. It is a specialized cell and Chapter 2 describes some of the similarities between this cell and a single-celled animal called *Amoeba*. Neurons are specialized in transmitting information along an extension of the cell, called an *axon*, from one point in the nervous system to another. Neurons also process information. Figure 1.2 gives an example of a function served by neurons. In this case it is simplified to show just two neurons. A sharp object impinges upon the skin. A neuron whose tip is at the skin is activated (or 'excited') by the presence of the object and conveys this activation along its axon towards the spinal cord. At the spinal cord, this neuron (neuron 1) passes the activation to a second neuron (neuron 2) which carries the activation up to the brain. Until it reaches the spinal cord, neuron 1 forms part of the **peripheral nervous system**. The brain and spinal cord together constitute the **central nervous system (CNS)**. Therefore neuron 1 enters the CNS and immediately makes contact with neuron 2 of the CNS. The brain interprets the pattern of activation in terms of a potentially damaging (or *noxious*) stimulus. In other words, *information* is conveyed from the periphery to the brain. The axon of neuron 2 is one of many axons forming a distinct pathway or tract in the spinal cord that carry noxious information from detector neurons (e.g. neuron 1) to the brain. In response to the activation in neuron 1, instigated by a noxious stimulus, local action would be effected; muscles would be recruited to remove the foot from the source of injury. Such defensive organization is described in Chapter 8. This example shows one of the functions of neurons, as detectors of threatening events, in this case potential damage to the tissues.

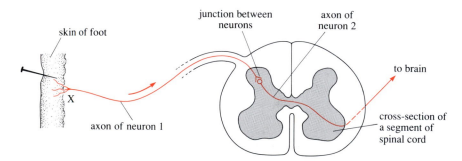

**Figure 1.2** Simplified schematic sketch of two neurons and their locations. At its tip (marked X) a specialized neuron (neuron 1) detects damage to body tissue. It conveys activation from the site of damage, along its axon, to the junction between neurons 1 and 2 within the spinal cord. At this point, neuron 2 conveys the activation (within the spinal cord) to the brain.

Traditionally in the neurosciences, neurons have been given an exclusive place in terms of detectors of what is happening in the world. However, in recent years, another system, the immune system, has been the focus of much interest. In much the same way as the nervous system monitors the world for such physical insults as tissue damage, so the immune system monitors the presence of foreign material such as viruses. These new ways of looking at parallels between the nervous and immune systems form the topic of Chapter 5.

Fortunately the world also contains benign events! Figure 1.3 shows an example of the detection of one such event, which is looked at in detail in Book 3. Light from an object reaches the eyes. Here the information is translated into activity in neurons. Pathways of millions of axons connect the eyes to the brain, transmitting visual information to the brain. (Here a point of ambiguity might trouble you. Neuroscientists speak of *the* optic nerve, which consists of millions of neuronal axons within that pathway that convey information from the eyes to the brain. For this reason, it is best to keep to the term 'neuron' to describe the individual nerve cell and to use 'nerve' only to describe pathways consisting of the axons of many neurons.) Suppose the subject is asked to touch the object in question. Neurons carry information from the brain out to the muscles in the arm, thereby controlling the hand's position. For simplicity only two such neurons have been shown. Note the junction between the two neurons in this pathway. Such junctions will form the focus of interest in Chapter 4.

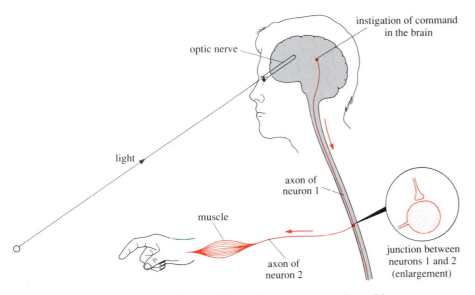

**Figure 1.3**   Pathway involved in moving a finger towards an object.

What does it mean to say that a neuron can be *activated* and thereby that it can convey *information*? To answer this, the electrical properties of cells need to be considered. This is the domain of neurophysiology and biophysics, as will be described in Chapter 3. The physical properties of the membrane (outer surface) of the neuron, as explored within biophysics, gives insight into how the neuron's electrical properties arise. If the electrical state of a neuron is probed, it will be found to exhibit a small voltage (like a miniature battery). If this voltage remains constant, the cell is said to be resting. Neurons have the property that they can suddenly change their voltage. They are then described as being active (or 'excited'). It is by this activity that information is transmitted. Figure 1.4 (*overleaf*) shows a record of the electrical activity of a neuron. The sudden, spike-like, change in activity is known as an **action potential**. The action potentials each last about a millisecond (a thousandth of a second, abbreviated as ms), which indicates how fast the nervous system operates. So, to refer back to Figure 1.2, the nail touching the foot initiates action potentials at point X in the neuron. Action potentials then travel along the axon. On arriving at the end of the axon of neuron 1, the action potentials initiate further action potentials in neuron 2; these travel along the axon of neuron 2, conveying the information to the brain.

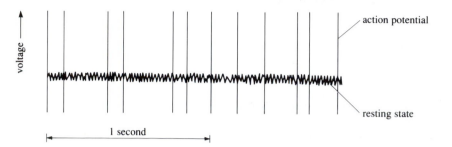

**Figure 1.4**  Record of activity in a neuron, showing periods of resting and a number of action potentials.

A neuron can exhibit action potentials at different rates, as shown in Figure 1.5. A high frequency (as shown in (c)) conveys different information from a low frequency (as shown in (a)). For example, a low frequency of action potentials in neuron 1 and thereby neuron 2 in Figure 1.3 would cause a slight muscular contraction whereas a higher frequency would cause a stronger muscular contraction.

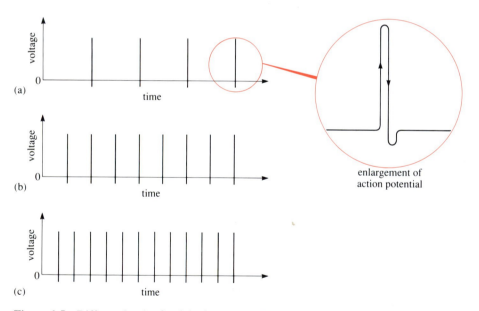

**Figure 1.5**  Different levels of activity in a neuron. Frequency of action potentials increases from (a) to (c).

Neurons not only transmit information from one part of the body to another, as shown in Figures 1.2 and 1.3, but, acting together in systems, they also process information. For example, decision making, described in Book 1, Chapter 7, has neurons at its physical base. An understanding of how information is processed in networks of neurons within brain structures is furthered by a neurochemical perspective, which unravels the way in which neurons are organized at a molecular level and how their behaviour is influenced by specific chemicals. For example, both Figures 1.2 and 1.3 show a small gap between neuron 1 and neuron 2. A chemical, manufactured in neuron 1, is secreted at this gap and, by means of this chemical, activity in neuron 1 causes increased activity in neuron 2.

☐   What does this increased activity consist of?

■   More frequently occurring action potentials.

In this case, neurochemists would say that there is **excitation** from neuron 1 to neuron 2. Neuron 1 *excites* neuron 2. However, in some cases, activity in one neuron will cause fewer action potentials to occur in another neuron than would be the case if the first neuron were inactive. In this case the first neuron exerts **inhibition** upon the second.

Neurochemists are concerned with how the functions of the neuron depend upon interactions between molecules within, and on the surface of, the neuron itself. This concerns questions of how action potentials are generated and how drugs and other chemical substances influence this generation. For example, whether activity in a neuron excites or inhibits another neuron depends upon such chemical interactions.

As you work through this book, you will encounter contributions made from neuroanatomy, neurophysiology, biochemistry and biophysics that help in understanding how the brain works. There is also the perspective of looking at the brain as a  producer of *behaviour* appropriate to its external environment. Here, there is input from disciplines concerned with the functions of brain structures in directing behaviour. These contributions come from physiological psychology and cognitive neuropsychology.

To some extent, physiological psychology shares with neurophysiology a concern with general explanations of behaviour, i.e. what bits of the brain do. Both capitalize on the fact that there is a high degree of similarity in the basic plan and organization of the brain between related species—particularly in mammals. In describing the roles of brain structures and brain systems, information has been gained from studying animals as diverse as rats, cats and monkeys. The difference between the two disciplines is in terms of (a) the kinds of concepts that are employed and (b) the framework in which explanation is given. Neurophysiologists' interest in behaviour usually stops at the point where muscles are activated to produce movement. Their explanations are based upon observable bits of the nervous system such as the properties of individual neurons. Physiological psychologists, on the other hand, though also wishing to associate behaviour with nervous system structures, are more interested in the function of the brain seen in a broader context. They are concerned with the way in which an organism's *interactions with its environment* are organized, involving psychological  concepts such as learning, memory and motivation. This perspective will be introduced in the later chapters of this book (Chapters 8, 10 and 11).

In contrast to both neurophysiologists and physiological psychologists, cognitive neuropsychologists are interested in the contributions of structures of the human brain to the uniquely human capability of being able to think, talk and reason using a high-level symbolic language. This perspective will be developed in Chapters 8–11 of this book and in Books 3 and 6.

The discussions and explanations made in this book lie within the broad framework provided by the neo-Darwinian explanation of the evolution of species (Introduction and Guide and Book 1). Here an important premise is that the mammalian species alive today show many similarities in their structures because they evolved from a common ancestor: the prototypic mammal that marked the deviation from other lines of vertebrate evolution. Acceptance of this premise lets the neurophysiologist draw up 'blueprints' of the general functions of brain structures and systems—such as involvement in motor (control over muscles), and sensory or motivational functions based on investigations in a wide range of laboratory-reared mammals such as rats and monkeys.

There exists an important corollary (implication) of the evolutionary perspective in the context of explanations of brain function, as follows. Differences seen between the brain structures of related species can be associated with the differences in their behavioural capacities. These behavioural differences, in turn, are related to the evolutionary pressures imposed by the animals' natural habitats. For example, the high degree of manual dexterity of the human in comparison with other primates can be seen to be paralleled by a development within the motor systems of the human brain. Similarly, the human use of symbolic language can be seen to be paralleled by developments within specific regions of the cortex and in other brain structures.

# 1.3   Levels of explanation and system properties

Often, the disciplines of the neurosciences are described as contributing different **levels of explanation**. (You first met this concept in the *Introduction and Guide*.) In such terms, of the disciplines discussed so far, biophysics provides the 'lowest' level. The term 'lowest' carries two meanings, neither of them implying that the discipline is less important. Biophysics and biochemistry study events at the smallest scale. Neurons are composed of chemicals and biophysicists look at nothing smaller than the properties of chemicals. The other meaning of 'lowest' is that the discipline of neurophysiology traditionally builds upon those of biophysics and biochemistry. Thus, neurophysiology is the next level up both in terms of size of the domain of interest and in terms of what is building upon what. Neurophysiology is followed by physiological psychology and cognitive neuropsychology. In this scheme, the role of neuroanatomy is to identify the structures to be investigated.

For several reasons, this idea of *levels* of explanation must be treated with care (one reason is that there are several different ways of looking at levels, only one of which is discussed here). By virtue of their level, some disciplines (e.g. biochemistry) appear to be more 'basic' than others. However, this does not mean that neurochemists have all the answers. It does not mean that ultimately all explanations of behaviour or neurophysiological processes will be *reduced* to explanations in terms of interactions between molecules. Neurochemistry, however, can provide coherent explanations of those aspects of neural processes which involve interactions between molecules. For example, the neurochemical 'fact' that the physical structure of some molecules enables them to interact by interlocking— in the way that a lock and key fit together—helps explain how neuron 1 in Figure 1.2 and 1.3 excites neuron 2 rather than inhibits it. It can help to explain why some drugs have a potent effect on the responses of neurons whereas others do not. Also, as you will see in later chapters, the 'fact' that some chemical structures can change shape helps explain how neurons are able to generate their action potentials. Fortunately, the biochemical facts and processes invoked to help explain how neurons 'work' do not require a working knowledge of chemistry in order to understand this—as you will see as you progress through the book.

The other reason why caution is needed in describing a hierarchy of levels is that you need to be aware that the process of explanation is a two-way street. Although traditionally researchers have tended to look to lower levels to provide explanations, it is now recognized that insight into lower-level events can sometimes be gained by looking at higher-level events. For example, study of the psychology of the whole animal can sometimes provide insights that facilitate explanations of events at the level of neurons and their interconnections.

Investigators working at one level are often able simply to 'take for granted' events at a lower level. In fact, one needs to do so in order to proceed. There is insufficient time to keep stopping to ask why things are as they are. For example, the neurophysiological level of explanation is an endeavour that takes for granted that neurochemical processes are taking place within the neuron. In his or her day-to-day research, the neurophysiologist need not be concerned with the biochemical basis for the difference between excitatory and inhibitory interaction between neurons. At this level of investigation, it is the fact that interactions can be excitatory or inhibitory that is important rather than how the differences are mediated at the chemical level. Here, the neurophysiologist is concerned with what a neuron is doing as a component of a neural circuit rather than how it is doing it. For the neurophysiologist, it is how the patterns of excitatory and inhibitory connections within a pathway transform the information being conveyed in the pathway that is important.

In considering levels of explanation, to some authors the concept of a **system property** proves useful. The meaning of this term is described as 'the whole is more than the sum of the parts'. Take a simple example. A central heating system is composed of such components as a heater, a detector of temperature and a dial on the wall. From the way in which these components are assembled, the property of temperature regulation arises. This property depends upon the properties of the components but is something that is not evident in the individual components. Rather it is a property of their interaction and can only be understood at the level of the whole *system*.

The neurophysiological explanations you will encounter in this book are attempts to explain functions of particular parts of the brain in terms of the properties that emerge from systems of neurons or systems of brain structures with specific patterns of connections and interconnections. One example that will be discussed later is how the pathways that start in receptors in the skin that are sensitive to deformation of the skin and end in a specific region of the cerebral cortex contribute to the sense of touch. The 'job' is one of decoding the interactions taking place between the neurons in the various relay stations *en route* from the skin to the cerebral hemispheres. Here, the neurophysiological contribution is more than just describing the patterns of inhibitory and excitatory connections that occur. Rather, it is concerned with the system properties of these neural circuits. For example, specific organizations of connections within the pathways conveying information about touch to the skin extract information about the size of a specific touch stimulus, others about direction of its movement. The neuroanatomist can identify the elements of a neuronal circuit and the way that they are 'wired' together. It is the neurophysiologist's contribution to explore the neural 'circuit' as a working system and determine its system properties.

So, to review the argument, a knowledge of biophysical and biochemical events is appropriate to understand how the neuron functions. However, when the behaviour of whole neurons is considered, it is found that new properties emerge that are not evident in the individual biophysical and biochemical events that underlie the activity of the neuron. The stock-in-trade of the neurophysiologist is therefore to be able to speak a language appropriate for the behaviour of the whole neuron, a language that describes these system properties. This use of levels of explanation and description does not deny that events at a neurochemical level influence the 'behaviour' of neural circuits or the behaviour of a whole animal. However, the language and concepts used to describe interactions at the neurochemical level are inappropriate to describe the properties that emerge from interactions between neurons. Also, the language and concepts used to describe interactions at a neurophysiological level are inappropriate to describe the properties of behaviour that emerge when an animal is responding to the contingencies of its environment. The problem is to find appropriate languages for relating events at the different levels.

Where does the psychologist's contribution come in? In the same way that the neurophysiologist provides the concepts for dealing with the system properties of local neural circuits, the psychologist provides the concepts for dealing with the system properties of the brain as a whole—learning, memory, motivation and perception are examples of psychological concepts which require specific expertise for their investigation. For example, one of the psychologist's inputs is to evaluate the effects of local changes in the biochemistry or physiology upon behaviour and to provide the explanatory framework within which such changes in behaviour are evaluated to establish the links between activity in particular brain systems and behaviour.

Complex conceptual problems can arise when a phenomenon or event at one level is used as an explanation of a phenomenon at a higher level. For example, when learning takes place (behavioural level), changes in the molecular structure of neurons in the central nervous system can be detected (biochemical level). So is memory reducible to changes in molecules that are observed when learning takes place? Even if biochemistry were to provide an exhaustive description of all the biochemical changes that accompany the storage of information in the brain, this would not constitute an explanation of memory that would *replace* descriptions provided by neurophysiology or psychology. Here, the problem is not just that scientists have not yet found a way of translating the language of psychology or physiology into the language of biochemistry or vice versa. It is inappropriate to attempt to explain behaviour at one level solely in terms of events at a lower level.

Perhaps the greatest challenge of all in the neurosciences is to obtain insight into how collections of neurons can give rise to the brain's property of exhibiting consciousness (Book 1, Chapter 8). Consciousness could be described as a system property arising from the interactions between the brain's neurons and it will be discussed in Chapters 10 and 11 of this book. As you will see as you work through this book, the endeavours of the neurosciences are complementary and aimed ultimately at a target that is perhaps the last real frontier of knowledge—an understanding of the human brain and how it exhibits consciousness.

# Objectives for Chapter 1

After reading this chapter, you should be able to:

1.1 Define and use, or recognize, definitions and applications of each of the terms printed in bold in the text. *(Question 1.1)*

1.2 Describe some of the disciplines that are involved in the neurosciences and their subject matter.

1.3 Describe how the ability of a neuron to transmit action potentials enables it to convey information. *(Question 1.2)*

1.4 Describe the relationship between the expressions 'levels of explanation' and 'system property'. *(Question 1.3)*

# Questions for Chapter 1

**Question 1.1** *(Objective 1.1)*
Insert the missing words in the following sentences.

The optic nerve is made up of millions of ..............., each of which is able to transmit ............... Each of these consists of a change in voltage across the ................ of the axon.

**Question 1.2** *(Objective 1.3)*
Activity in two neurons A and B influences activity in a third neuron C. C is normally inactive. When neuron A is active, C exhibits action potentials at a high rate but when both A and B are active the rate of action potential generation in C is relatively low. Complete the following sentence.

Neuron A ............... neuron C, whereas neuron B ............... it.

**Question 1.3** *(Objective 1.4)*
It is often argued that consciousness is a system property that arises from the interactions of millions of neurons. Does this mean that each individual neuron is slightly conscious?

# CHAPTER 2
# CELLS AND NERVOUS SYSTEMS

## 2.1 Introduction

Inside a human body there are a number of organs such as the heart, kidneys and brain. Each organ is a distinct structure that performs a particular task. The heart, for example, is an organ the function of which is to circulate the blood around the body; the kidney eliminates waste substances from the blood in the form of urine. Each organ is made up of tissue, which in turn is made up of individual *cells*. Whereas organs and tissues can vary greatly in size most cells are very small, of the order of a couple of hundredths of a millimetre in diameter. Tissues that perform similar tasks are remarkably similar in different animals: muscle tissue in human muscles is very like muscle tissue in a fish or even in a locust. This is because the cells in particular tissues have a structure and function that is suited to their task. Cells are the basic unit of structure of all living organisms and there is an even greater similarity in the structure of the components within cells across the animal kingdom.

A multicellular animal behaves as an integrated whole. The activities of all the separate cells in its body are coordinated and regulated. This regulation requires an efficient system of communication. There are three systems which provide this coordination: the nervous system, the endocrine system and the immune system.

As you should now know from reading Chapter 1, the nervous system is composed of cells, neurons, whose speciality is communication with one another. These neurons form a complex network of communication throughout the body. The cells of the nervous system are specialized to receive, analyse and transmit information from one part of the organism to another.

The endocrine system (Book 1, Section 2.9) consists of cells, some of which are neurons, which produce chemical messages called hormones that are carried in the blood to responding cells scattered throughout the body. The endocrine system regulates many functions of the body.

The **immune system** is a collection of cells responsible for protecting the body against invasion by **pathogens**, harmful organisms such as bacteria and parasites. The immune system of mammals and birds seems to be far more sophisticated than that in other animals, but all animals have some kind of system to protect them against pathogens.

This book is mostly concerned with the structure and function of the nervous system. Since neurons in all multicellular animals perform similar tasks, they are fundamentally similar in all animals from humans to sea anemones. This chapter describes what neurons are like and how they communicate with one another.

It will start with a description of a simple single-celled animal, an amoeba (plural: amoebae). The description of *Amoeba* (to give its Latin genus name) will illustrate how animals are able to interact with their environment and will also introduce you to the general structure of animal cells. In the second half of this chapter you will see how the special properties of cells in the nervous system in multicellular animals have evolved from those already present in amoebae.

## 2.2 *Amoeba*, a single-celled animal

Amoebae are single-celled animals that live in pond water (there are also pathogenic species of amoebae such as those that cause amoebic dysentery in humans). Most are only a couple of hundredths of a millimetre across and so are hardly visible to the unaided eye, but are easily observed using a microscope (see Box 2.1). A drop of pond water often contains many single-celled organisms, many of which move very quickly. Amoebae, however, move rather slowly, creeping over objects.

All animals, whether they are unicellular like amoebae or made up of many cells, need to find food to survive. An amoeba does this by engulfing smaller animals. Figure 2.1 shows a sequence of drawings of an amoeba trapping another smaller, single-celled animal. In order to examine what controls the behaviour of an amoeba you must first look at its structure.

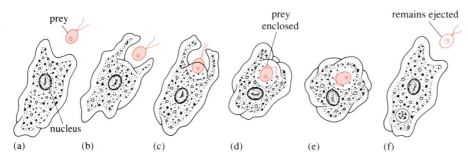

**Figure 2.1** *Amoeba* capturing prey.

## Box 2.1   The light microscope

Although some unicellular organisms can be seen with the aid of a magnifying lens, much higher magnification is necessary to see the structure of most cells. The microscope is a universally used magnification system and an invaluable tool for neuroanatomical investigations. It basically consists of a system of lenses.

The ordinary light microscope used in the laboratory is called a compound microscope and has three lenses. One of these, called the objective, is close to the object of interest (the specimen) and the second is close to the eye. These two lenses magnify the object in two steps. Figure 2.2 (*overleaf*) is a photograph of a compound light microscope. Because light is absorbed by both lenses, the light source must be concentrated through the object. This is done by another lens, called the condenser, beneath the specimen. The maximum magnification that can be achieved by the light microscope is about × 1 500. The light microscope can easily resolve (distinguish) individual cells in nervous tissue and much of their structure. However, the limit of resolution is 0.2 micrometres, abbreviated as 0.2 μm (1 μm is one-millionth of a metre) so the smaller structures inside cells are not visible (see Table 2.1). To examine them, greater magnification is required and a different tool, the electron microscope, is used (see Box 2.2, p. 22).

**Table 2.1**   A summary of sizes of structures in the central nervous system.

| Structure | Scale of measurement | Abbreviation |
|---|---|---|
| Central Nervous System (human) | metres | m |
| Groups of neurons | millimetres | mm |
| Single neurons | tens of micrometres | |
| Synapses | micrometres | μm |
| Synaptic cleft | nanometres | nm |
| Molecules | nanometres | nm |

*Notes*

1 millimetre = 0.001 m ($10^{-3}$ m)

1 micrometre = 0.001 mm ($10^{-6}$ m) (μ is the Greek letter *mu*. 1 μm is also called a *micron*); the diameter of a human hair is about 50 μm

1 nanometre = 0.001 μm ($10^{-9}$ m)

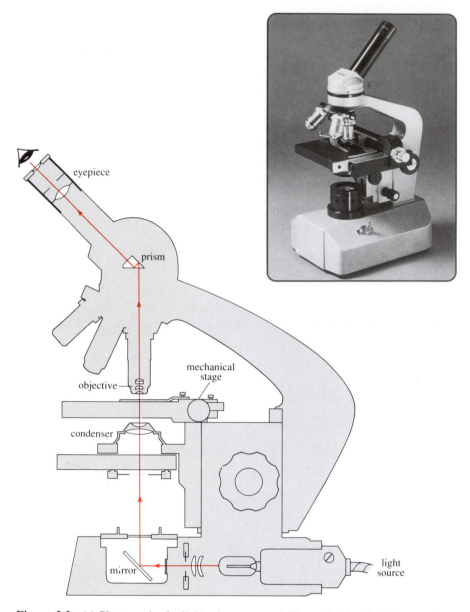

**Figure 2.2** (a) Photograph of a light microscope. (b) The path taken by light rays in a binocular microscope. The light from the bulb at the base is focused on the specimen by the condenser lens. To position the specimen accurately in the light path between the condenser and the objective lens, the specimen is held in a mechanical stage. Two gears at right angles to each other provide a means of making very fine adjustments to the position of the specimen.

## 2.2.1  The structure of an amoeba

Like all living cells, an amoeba is basically a bag containing the organic machinery necessary for life (Figure 2.3). This organic machinery is highly organized and consists of separate structures which perform particular tasks such as the breakdown of food molecules to produce energy and the synthesis of proteins which make up the structural components of the cell. As mentioned in Box 2.1, these structures are not visible with the light microscope, but they can be seen using an electron microscope (see Box 2.2, *overleaf*).

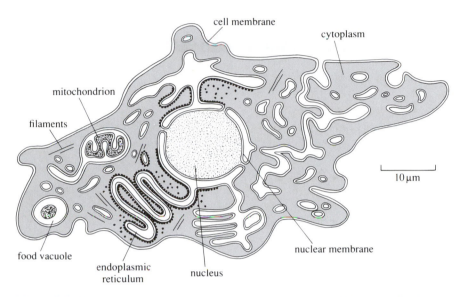

**Figure 2.3**  Diagram of an amoeba showing internal structures visible with the electron microscope. All animal cells contain these structures. The small bar you will see on many anatomical figures is called a calibration bar; it provides a measure of the actual size of the object. Most calibration units will be in mm or μm (see Table 2.1).

Within the cell, the structures are surrounded by the **cytoplasm**, a thick, protein-rich 'soup'. The cytoplasm contains innumerable molecules, many small particles and fibres of protein called filaments. These filaments provide the structural support of the cell and collectively they form what is called the cytoskeleton. The largest structure in the cell is the nucleus (Book 1, Chapter 3), which is usually visible with the light microscope. The nucleus contains the genetic material of the cell (the DNA) in the form of chromosomes. With the use of the electron microscope other smaller, oval-shaped objects become visible in the cytoplasm. These are the mitochondria (singular: mitochondrion), the 'powerhouses' of the cell. The mitochondria are responsible for generating the energy the cell needs to keep alive, from the breakdown of food molecules (mainly sugars and fats) in the presence of oxygen (this process is called respiration). There is also a complex network of tubes (the endoplasmic reticulum) studded with dense globules where the synthesis of the proteins which form the structure of the cell takes place. All living cells in both animals and plants contain these structures.

**Box 2.2  The electron microscope**

As mentioned in Box 2.1, the maximum degree of magnification that is possible is about × 1 500. Using extra, or stronger, lenses reveals nothing more and the details merely look bigger and vaguer. This is because it is physically impossible with a microscope which uses visible light to distinguish (or resolve) two points that are less than $0.2\,\mu m$ apart. The electron microscope uses electrons, which are much smaller than light particles (photons), to form the image and can achieve much greater magnification.

Figure 2.4 is a photograph of a typical electron microscope, with a diagram showing the pathways of the electrons. These are very similar to those of the light microscope. The beam of electrons, generated in a vacuum, is focused by using magnets as 'lenses'. The electrons pass through the specimen and are then focused onto a phosphor screen which glows at the points where the electrons hit it. As the electron beam passes through the specimen, dense components in the specimen cause deflection (scatter) of some of the electrons. If the deflection is great enough, those electrons will not reach the screen. Thus an image will be formed on the screen. Dark areas on the screen represent structures which have deflected electrons from the beam. Light areas indicate where the electrons have been able to pass through the specimen. To maximize the contrast between specific regions of the specimen in terms of electron scattering ability, specimens are stained before viewing (see Box 2.3). The electron microscope can achieve magnifications of up to half a million times or more, though a mere thirty thousand or so will reveal many intracellular structures. Electrons can only penetrate a small distance and therefore extremely thin tissue sections must be cut (around $0.1\,\mu m$ thick). To achieve this thickness, specimens are embedded in a plastic such as Araldite and sliced with a special diamond or glass knife (see Box 2.3).

The **cell membrane** forms the outer surface. It is the interface between the cytoplasm, the intracellular environment, and the external world, the extracellular environment. It is responsible for protecting the finely balanced machinery inside the cell from changes in the external environment. This is no simple matter: among other things, the membrane must allow food and oxygen in and waste products, e.g. carbon dioxide, out. The membrane is highly selective about which molecules and how many it lets through, and in which direction and when they are allowed through. One of the consequences of this selectivity (which requires energy) is that the composition within the cell (the intracellular fluid) is different from that outside the cell (the extracellular fluid), as will be explained more fully in Chapter 3. You have already come across the importance of maintaining the amount of water both intracellularly and extracellularly and how maintaining the balance can affect an animal's behaviour (Book 1, Chapter 7).

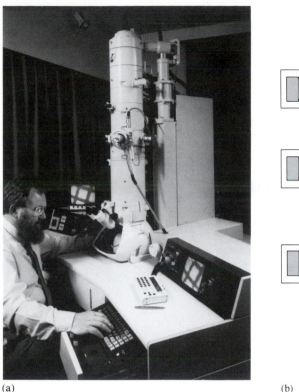

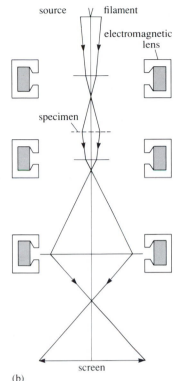

(a)                 (b)

**Figure 2.4**    (a) Photograph of a typical electron microscope. (b) Diagram showing the path of the electrons.

## 2.2.2 Behaviour of *Amoeba*

Figure 2.1 (Section 2.2) shows a sequence of drawings of *Amoeba* capturing prey. Let us look at the steps involved. First the animal must recognize the presence of nearby prey. Then its membrane must be able to signal to the rest of the animal to alter its movement. In the membrane are specialized receptor molecules which, when combined with a suitable signal molecule (released by the prey, for instance), cause a chain of activity in the cell leading to movement.

*Amoeba* moves towards such signal molecules because the membrane receptors closest to the source are most strongly activated. In the sequence of drawings in Figure 2.1, *Amoeba* first moves closer to the prey. It then changes its shape and engulfs the prey which is later digested. The sequence of activity leading to the actual capture of the prey is probably triggered by deformation of the membrane, either caused by touching the prey or by water currents generated by the movement of the prey. *Amoeba* does not always respond to another animal by engulfing it; if contact is made with a predator (another species of *Amoeba*, for instance) its response will be quite different. The response of *Amoeba* therefore depends upon the kinds of signals it receives. The cell membrane is able to respond selectively to different signals; it controls the behaviour of the animal. The membrane of animal cells is therefore a very active and complex entity. In Section 2.3 you will see how the basic properties of animal cell membranes have been harnessed for neuronal communication in multicellular animals.

After the prey has been surrounded by *Amoeba*, it becomes internalized (Figure 2.1c and d). This action is achieved by complex movements of the cell membrane. The prey becomes surrounded by cell membrane, inside the animal. The membrane-surrounded 'bubble' inside the animal is called a vacuole. Enzymes (Book 1, Section 3.2.2) are secreted into the vacuole and the prey is digested. After digestion, the remains of the meal are disposed of by reversing the process by which the vacuole was internalized, so that the unwanted contents of the vacuole are released into the extracellular environment (Figure 2.1f). The externalizing process is called exocytosis and is a property of all animal and plant cells. Exocytosis is particularly important because it is by this process that the chemical messages important in communication between neurons are released.

### 2.2.3 How does *Amoeba* move?

*Amoeba* moves by producing a finger-like extension of its cell membrane at one end, into which the cell contents—the cytoplasm—are pushed. The membrane is extended again and the cycle repeated (Figure 2.5). Movement results from the contraction of specialized structures made up of protein filaments lying close to the membrane. They work like miniature muscles; the molecules involved are very similar to those found in muscles. The animal will only move if part of the membrane is attached to a substrate, i.e. to something in the external environment. The attachment of the membrane to the substrate is achieved by receptors that establish anchoring points between the substrate and the network of filaments inside the cell. This creeping 'amoeboid' movement is also used by neurons when they establish connections with one another during development (this will be described in Book 4, Chapter 2).

In addition to enabling the whole *Amoeba* to move from one place to another, the filaments also provide a sort of active 'railway' for the transport of material from one part of the cell to another. As you will see in Section 2.3.1, this transport system is very important in the maintenance of the long extensions—the axons—of neurons.

# 2.3   From *Amoeba* to neurons

What is the connection between *Amoeba* and the nervous system? All multicellular animals are descended from single-celled animals. They are all composed of cells whose structure is basically the same: the cells all have an external membrane and contain the same types of intracellular structures. In multicellular animals, however, the cells in different organs are *specialized* to perform particular roles. The neurons in the nervous system are specialized for transmitting and interpreting information and communicating with one another and with other cells in the body. These abilities allow groups of neurons to act together in the coordination of the activities of the rest of the animal. The special properties of the membranes of neurons have evolved from the basic properties common to all animal cell membranes. Of course, the membrane of the neuron still has to perform its original function of maintaining the neuron's internal environment, in addition to its special role in communication.

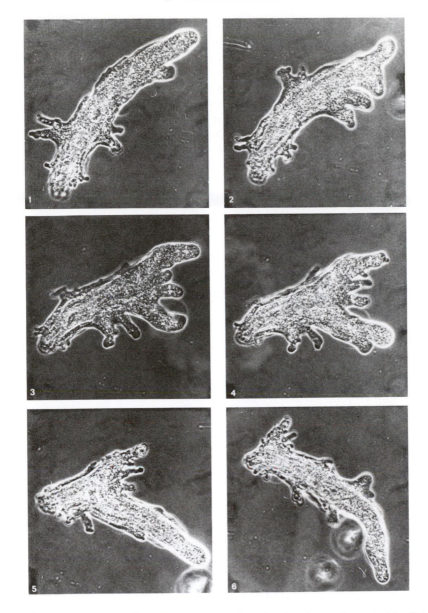

**Figure 2.5**   A series of photographs of a moving *Amoeba* taken 5 seconds apart with a light microscope. In frame 1 the animal is moving up and to the right, by frame 6 it has changed direction and is moving to the right and downwards. The granular appearance of the cytoplasm comes from the fact that it is full of proteins of different densities, but the structural detail is not resolvable at this magnification.

All animals interact with their external environment. In *Amoeba*, the cell membrane is responsible for signalling significant changes in the environment to the animal. In multicellular animals, the nervous system performs this role. The simplicity of *Amoeba* limits the nature of this interaction; a nervous system composed of many cells is capable of far more complex interactive behaviour.

## 2.3.1 Structure of neurons

Neurons, like most cells in the body, are too small to see with the unaided eye. Neuroanatomists use histological methods in conjunction with microscopes to study their structure. Histology is the art of staining tissue (colouring it by treating it with various chemicals) to reveal the structures of interest so that they are made visible when viewed with a microscope (see Box 2.3).

---

### Box 2.3 Preparing nervous system tissue for microscopical examination

In order to see the structure of neurons they must be made visible (Figure 2.8, p. 29). Since the illuminating light of the microscope must pass through the specimen, the specimen must be cut into slices, or sections, thin enough for light to pass through them. Prior to sectioning, the tissue is often treated with a chemical to hold the shape of the cells (a fixative) which also acts to stop the cells rotting (a preservative). The particular fixative chemical used depends on the subsequent staining procedure. Also, in order to make thin, even slices the tissue must be hardened in some way. Tissue can be hardened by freezing, by infiltrating it with paraffin wax or by embedding it in plastic.

The tissue is sliced on an instrument somewhat resembling a miniature bacon-slicer called a microtome. The resulting sections are generally 1–40 μm thick.

Choosing the appropriate staining method is important. There are thousands of different staining methods, each designed to reveal particular features of the cells such as their nuclei or their overall shape. One of the better known neuroanatomical staining techniques was developed by an Italian, Camillo Golgi, in the 1880s. This Golgi technique uses various silver salts under very precise conditions. This treatment stains only a very small proportion of cells, but stains them in their entirety. The technique marked a milestone in the development of neuroscience and it was used by the Spanish microscopist Santiago Ramon y Cajal to draw important conclusions about the basic principles of nervous system organization. The drawings of cells made by Cajal are so accurate that they are still used today, more than ninety years later, to illustrate standard neuroanatomy texts (Figure 2.6c).

---

Figure 2.6 shows some drawings of neurons from various parts of the vertebrate (animals with a backbone) nervous system. Figure 2.6c was made by Santiago Ramon y Cajal, who worked at the turn of the century. Cajal is regarded as the 'father of neuroanatomy' because of the enormous number of original observations he made on the structure of nervous systems. It was he who established that the nervous system is made up of separate neurons. He worked out how they might function as a communication system long before techniques for recording their activity had been developed.

Despite their differences in shape, all the neurons in Figure 2.6 have a common plan. From the cell body (which contains the nucleus, just like all animal cells) there extends one extra-long, thin tube called the **axon** and a collection of shorter, often highly branched extensions, or **dendrites**. The dendrites and cell body receive the inputs to the cell; the output from the cell is sent down the axon. Most axons are very fine ( less than 1 µm wide) and are often very long. For example, the axons that connect the neurons in the spinal cord (encased in the backbone) with the muscles and skin in your limbs, might be as much as a metre long. The axons between a giraffe's hip and its hoof are even longer! Because they are so long and thin, axons are often referred to as nerve fibres. Axons connect neurons together and are often branched: the axon of one neuron usually contacts many other cells. Contacts between axons and other neurons are found on the dendrites and the cell body. At these contact points, the axon forms a swelling, called the **axon terminal** (or terminal bouton), the largest of which are just visible with the light microscope. When viewed using an electron microscope, the structure of this special contact point, called the **synapse**, is seen to be rather complex (Figures 2.7, *overleaf*, and 2.8, p. 29). At the synapse, the membranes of the two neurons are very close together; the narrow gap between them, called the **synaptic cleft,** is only 20 nm wide (1 nanometre, abbreviated as nm, is one thousandth of 1 µm or $10^{-9}$ m). Inside the presynaptic terminal there are usually many small round structures called **synaptic vesicles**. For convenience, the membrane of the axon terminal is often referred to as the **presynaptic membrane**, and that of the neuron it connects with as the **postsynaptic membrane**.

The axon contains a well-ordered system of filaments (neurofilaments) and tube-like structures called tubules or microtubules, providing both support scaffolding and a transport system so that proteins synthesized in the cell body can be transported all the way down to the axon terminal. The region of the cell between the axon and the cell body is called the **axon hillock**.

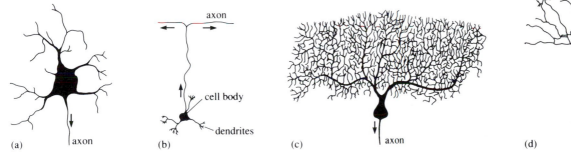

**Figure 2.6**   Some neurons from various regions of the mammalian nervous system showing variations in shape. (a) is found within, and close to the spinal cord; (b), (c) and (d) in different regions of the brain. These were all stained using the Golgi method (see Box 2.3).

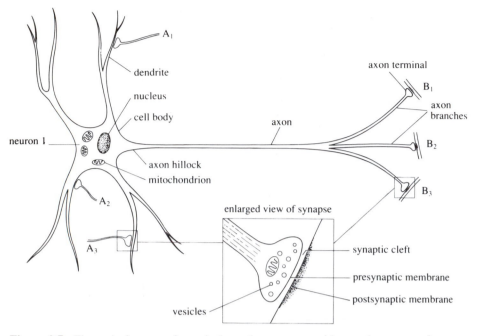

**Figure 2.7** The main features of a typical vertebrate neuron with an enlargement of an axon terminal showing the structure of the synapse. Remember that the cell body, dendrites, axons and axon terminals all contain mitochondria and some endoplasmic reticulum.

## 2.3.2 How neurons communicate: axon conduction

The neuron's membrane plays a very important role in transmitting and receiving information, which it does with small electrical signals called action potentials. Details of how action potentials are measured and recorded are given in Box 2.4. (p. 31). If the electrical signals are amplified and fed through a loudspeaker, action potentials sound like brief clicks. A series of action potentials is known as a 'train' of action potentials. (Neurophysiologists often describe a train of action potentials as a burst of 'spikes' because of its appearance on a paper chart recorder; see Figure 2.9, p. 30.)

So how does the neuron generate these action potentials? The answer lies in the membrane. Section 2.2.1 mentioned that the cell membrane requires energy to import some molecules while exporting others. The consequence of this active 'pumping' is that the *concentrations* of certain molecules are different on the two sides of the membrane. Many of these molecules are electrically charged, that is, they have either a positive or a negative charge associated with them, so there is also a difference in *charge* across the membrane—one side of the membrane is relatively more positive and the other side is relatively more negative. This difference in charge is called a **potential difference**, which is measured in units called volts. In just the same way, a battery has a voltage or potential difference across its two terminals, one of which is positive and one negative. Like a neuron, a battery also generates its voltage by means of a 'membrane' which separates two differently charged solutions.

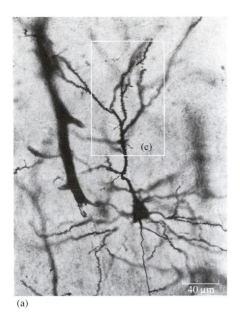

(a)

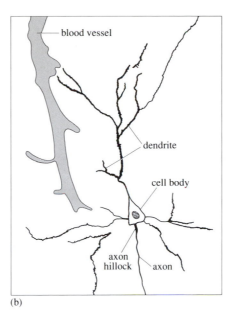

(b)

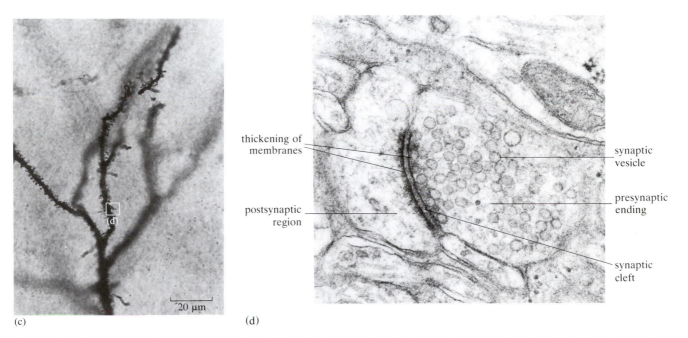

(c)

(d)

**Figure 2.8** The structure of a neuron in a section of the brain of a rat, stained by the Golgi technique (see Box 2.3). (a) A photograph of the specimen. (b) A labelled sketch. The cell body, dendrites and axon are filled with a dark substance. Many of the dendrites and the axon have been cut and are not included in the section. The large dark object to the left is a blood vessel which has also been stained. (c) An enlarged view of the area within the box in (a), showing a dendrite covered with small dendritic spines (the axon usually does not bear any spines). (d) Electron micrograph of an axon terminal contacting such a spine.

In the neuron, the potential difference across the membrane is usually called the **membrane potential**. If the permeability of the membrane to specific molecules changes, then the distribution of the charged molecules on either side will change. The membrane potential will also change as a result. A specific pattern of such changes in membrane potential constitutes the action potential recorded during the transmission of signals along axons (see Box 2.4). Thus changes in membrane potential underlie the ability of neurons to communicate with one another.

All neurons are able to show changes in membrane potential—they are electrically excitable. The generation of action potentials depends upon the cell membrane possessing particular types of pores, or *channels*, and pumps which control the movement of small charged molecules through the membrane. This will be described in more detail in Chapters 3 and 4.

Action potentials are initiated at the axon hillock. Once triggered there, the action potential travels along the entire length of the axon and into all its branches without any significant change in size. Since action potentials do not vary in size they are said to be conducted in an 'all or none' fashion. This transmission does not itself require energy but the 'recharging' of the membrane 'battery', upon which it depends, does.

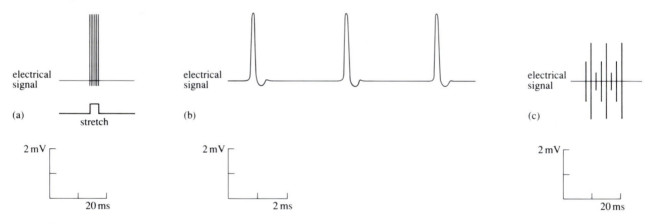

**Figure 2.9** (a) A burst of action potentials recorded from a single axon from a sensory receptor in a muscle when it is stretched. (b) In this record the paper speed is 10 times faster than in (a), as indicated in the calibration symbols below each trace. (c) A recording from a nerve containing several axons.

Note the calibration symbol at the bottom of each trace. This shows how much the pen is deflected vertically by a known potential and also how fast the paper is moving horizontally. This calibration can be used to measure the size of the signal and its time course.

## Box 2.4   Recording nerve activity

The electrical nature of neural activity was first demonstrated in the middle of the 18th century by Luigi Galvani. He observed that the frogs' legs he was dissecting on a zinc plate jumped when he touched the nerve with a metal object. (Incidentally, this observation also led to the invention of the battery.)

The electrical signals produced by neurons are very small (measured in millivolts (mv); 1 mv is a thousandth of a volt) and brief (measured in milliseconds (ms); 1 ms is one thousandth of a second). Monitoring the activity of neurons therefore requires sophisticated techniques of amplification and display that have only been developed in the last fifty years or so.

The simplest way to monitor or record action potentials is to lay a nerve (or in some special cases, part of an individual neuron) across two wires (called electrodes) and to measure the potential between the electrodes during the conduction of a nerve impulse produced either by natural stimulation (e.g. of sensory receptors) or by electrical stimulation. The potential is first amplified and then used to move a pen that draws a trace on a moving paper chart. You may have seen similar equipment used in hospitals to monitor brain or heart activity. The greater the signal, the greater the deflection of the pen. As the paper moves past the pen it will therefore draw a graph of the change in potential with time.

Figures 2.9a and 2.9b show some action potentials recorded at two paper speeds. Each action potential only lasts about a millisecond, so at the slower speed it appears as a simple line. At a much faster paper speed (ten times as fast) more details of how the potential changes with time can be resolved.

Nowadays many neurophysiologists do not use paper, but use a device called an oscilloscope to display nerve activity. In an oscilloscope the potential is displayed as the vertical deflection of an electron beam which hits a phosphor screen rather like a television or electron microscope screen. The electron beam moves across the screen at a constant rate which can be altered just like the paper speed in the chart recorder. Much higher speeds are possible using this method. Advances in microelectronics make it possible to measure the potentials and store and analyse the traces using computers.

The recording shown in Figure 2.9c was made from a nerve containing a number of axons. Although the action potentials in each axon are a constant size, the electrical signal picked up from axons close to the recording electrodes will be much larger than those further away.

## 2.3.3 How neurons communicate: synaptic transmission

The synapse (Figure 2.7, p. 28) is a protected environment specialized for neuron-to-neuron communication. When an action potential reaches the axon terminal it causes the release of packets of signalling molecules called **transmitters** or **neurotransmitters**. A single action potential will cause the release of a certain number of packets. A series of action potentials in rapid succession will cause the release of a greater number of packets. The packaging of the transmitters into little sacs or vesicles and the way these are released is very much like the process of exocytosis described in *Amoeba*. The transmitter molecules are not lost to the extracellular fluid because the synaptic cleft is so small. After they are released and have served their transmitter role, the molecules are either inactivated or reabsorbed by the presynaptic membrane and recycled. The postsynaptic cell can be another neuron, a muscle fibre, or a secretory cell like those found in glands. Most synapses can be recognized in electron micrographs by the presence of the vesicles in the presynaptic terminal and the definite thickening of the postsynaptic membrane (Figure 2.8d, p. 29).

As you might expect from the discussion of the membrane of *Amoeba*, the specialized postsynaptic membrane responds by virtue of receptors which combine with the transmitter molecules. The result of the receptor 'tasting' (like *Amoeba* detecting food) the right transmitter is a local change in the structure of the membrane. As a result of this change in structure, certain charged molecules can move more readily across the membrane and this produces a local change in the membrane potential called the **synaptic potential.**

The synaptic potential is quite different from the action potential: it is not conducted in an 'all-or-none' fashion, but rather it is a local change that travels away from the synapse in all directions, getting smaller the farther it goes. This passive spread of the electrical activity is rather like a ripple spreading out on a pool of water: the ripple gets smaller until eventually it disappears. Whereas action potentials last about 1 ms, synaptic potentials last about two to four times as long. There are two kinds of synaptic potential, those that *increase* the likelihood of the postsynaptic cell generating action potentials, called **Excitatory PostSynaptic Potentials (EPSPs)** and those that *decrease* the likelihood of the cell generating an action potential, called **Inhibitory PostSynaptic Potentials (IPSPs).**

Until recently it was assumed that the difference between synapses that excited cells and those that inhibited them depended upon the nature of the transmitter released at the presynaptic membrane. The transmitters were therefore classified as being either excitatory or inhibitory. During the 1980s, however, examples of transmitters were found that excite some neurons but inhibit others. The difference in the response is produced by differences in the nature of the membrane receptors in the postsynaptic membrane. It is more accurate therefore to describe synapses or receptors rather than transmitters as being excitatory or inhibitory.

An artist's impression of a neuron and its synapses is shown in Figure 2.10. Both the dendrites and cell body of the neuron are studded with literally thousands of synaptic terminals. Some are found on little protuberances on the dendrite called **dendritic spines** (Figure 2.8, p. 29), others terminate directly onto the dendrite or cell body. Some contain round vesicles, some flatter ones. Typically, neurons are contacted by hundreds if not thousands of terminals coming from many other neurons (Figure 2.10).

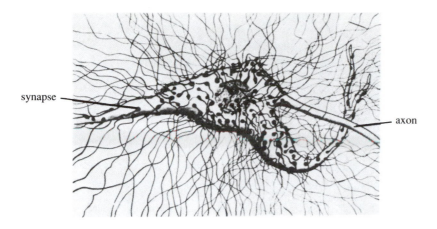

synapse

axon

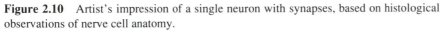

**Figure 2.10**   Artist's impression of a single neuron with synapses, based on histological observations of nerve cell anatomy.

If more than one excitatory synapse is activated at the same time, the EPSPs they produce will add together. If the combined EPSPs are large enough they will cause the membrane at the axon hillock to generate an action potential. The critical value of the membrane potential at which the neuron will generate an action potential is called the *threshold*. If the threshold value is maintained over time then a train of action potentials will be generated.

☐   Will the action potentials in the train differ in size, depending on the value of the membrane potential?

■   No, the action potentials will all be the same size, travelling in an all-or-none fashion along all the axon branches to the axon terminals.

Suppose that excitatory and inhibitory synapses are activated at the same time. In this case, whether or not an action potential is generated in a neuron will depend critically upon the balance between the EPSPs and IPSPs arriving at the synaptic terminals on that cell.

Notice that the synapse can only transmit in one direction. Thus action potentials in the presynaptic terminal excite the postsynaptic membrane, but *not* the other way round. As long as synapses actively generate EPSPs large enough to generate action potentials at the axon hillock, there will be a stream of such signals carried in the axon. There is a limit, however, to how rapidly action potentials can follow one another (in mammals the upper limit is about $1\,000\,\text{s}^{-1}$).

☐   What condition must be met for an action potential to be produced in a neuron?

■   The amount of excitation must exceed the inhibition by a large enough margin for the threshold to be reached at the axon hillock.

☐ From what has been said about the conduction of EPSPs and IPSPs, do they exhibit all-or-none conduction?

■ No. EPSPs and IPSPs decrease in size the further they travel away from the active synapse.

One effect of this decrease with distance is that the effectiveness of synaptic input will depend upon where on the cell the synapses are located. Those further away from the axon hillock will be less effective than those near to it. In general, inhibitory synapses (which contain flat rather than round vesicles) are usually found close to the cell body. The effectiveness of synapses also depends on the structure of the synaptic terminal. Some especially large and powerfully excitatory synapses have a very complex structure in which the postsynaptic cell sends 'fingers' into the enlarged axon terminal. From recordings made from the cells they contact, it is known that such synapses produce large EPSPs.

The output of a neuron therefore depends on the relative activity of excitatory and inhibitory synapses and also upon their spatial arrangement and patterns of temporal activity. Trains of action potentials arriving at terminals will produce longer and larger EPSPs or IPSPs in the postsynaptic neuron than individual ones.

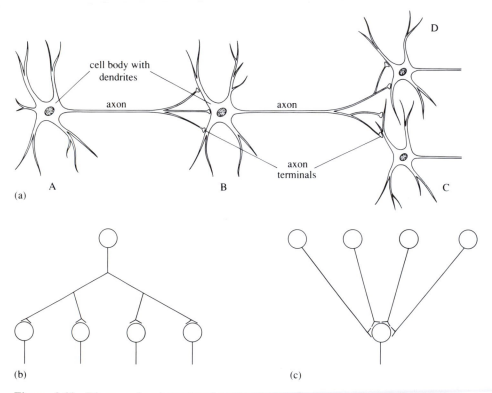

**Figure 2.11** Diagram showing several arrangements of neurons: (a) several neurons connected by synapses; (b) one neuron innervating (synapsing onto) many other neurons (divergent output); (c) one neuron receiving inputs from many neurons (convergent input).

☐  Figure 2.11a is a diagram of neurons connected by synapses. Which neurons influence which?

■  The axon of neuron A synapses with the dendrites and cell body of neuron B, therefore activity in neuron A will influence neuron B. Activity in neuron B will not affect neuron A although it will influence neurons C and D.

Some neurons have widely distributed axons, contacting maybe hundreds of other neurons in different parts of the nervous system (Figure 2.11b). Such neurons are said to have **divergent outputs**. Others may receive inputs from large numbers of neurons but only influence a few (Figure 2.11c). These neurons are described as receiving **convergent inputs**. In the nervous system as a whole, there are many divergent and convergent connections.

Many neurons do not generate action potentials until the excitatory synaptic input significantly exceeds the inhibitory input. In others there is always some background activity, a sort of 'ticking over' of action potentials. Any change in the relative levels of excitation and inhibition in these continuously active neurons results in a change in the *rate* of firing of the action potentials.

The nervous system is composed of many thousands of neurons. From this brief description you can see that each neuron is not a simple switching device that turns on or off, but is a complex computing device that weighs the balance between excitation and inhibition.

### 2.3.4  Neuronal communication: summary

In Section 2.2 the role of the membrane surrounding *Amoeba* in the detection of relevant changes in the external environment was described. The similarity between this membrane and that surrounding the neuron was then discussed.

☐  How do neurons receive inputs from other neurons?

■  With receptors on the dendrites and cell body. These are activated by molecules of transmitter.

☐  How do neurons communicate over long distances?

■  By action potentials that travel unchanged down the axon and all its branches.

☐  Will the arrival of an action potential at an axon terminal always result in the generation of an action potential in the postsynaptic cell?

■  No, an action potential will only arise at the axon hillock if the threshold is reached, i.e. if the excitation produced by the activity of many excitatory synapses exceeds by a certain amount the inhibition produced by activity at inhibitory synapses.

Figure 2.12 summarizes the structure and function of a neuron. It is obviously a very unrealistic simplification of the real state of affairs. Figures 2.8 (p. 29) and 2.10 (p. 33) showed how densely synapses are arranged on the dendrites and cell body. Some of these synapses will be excitatory and some inhibitory, while some are closer to the axon hillock than others. The response of the neuron will depend

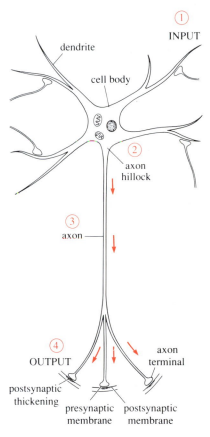

**Figure 2.12**  The structure and function of various parts of the neuron. Input at the dendrites (1) travels across the cell to the axon hillock (2) where an action potential will be initiated if the threshold is reached. The action potential travels unchanged down the axon (3) to all the axon terminals (4) where transmitter is released onto the next cell, or cells, in the chain.

critically upon the timing, identity and location of active synapses. It is the pattern, in time and space, of excitation and inhibition arriving at the dendrites and cell body of a neuron that determines whether or not it will send action potentials down its axon. Thus the neuron is not a simple switch that relays on and off messages: it is a complex computing device whose function is only just beginning to be unravelled.

☐ What would you expect to record from the axon if the level of excitation far exceeded the inhibitory input over a 2 second period?

■ A train of action potentials at a high frequency.

☐ Would you expect the size of the action potentials to change over time?

■ No, the action potentials within any one axon are always the same size.

Some neurons receive thousands of synapses, some of which are excitatory, some inhibitory. The response of a neuron depends upon the balance between excitation and inhibition.

# 2.4    Cells in nervous systems

Nervous systems are collections of neurons that act together in transmitting and processing information. Information is conveyed between neurons in the pattern (or time sequence) of action potentials, much as the pattern of drum beats or puffs of smoke in a smoke signal contains a message. The structure of nervous systems and the way in which neurons are connected together, is complex and will be described later in this book; here some common variations in cell structure that allow the nervous system to detect, analyse and respond to stimuli will be briefly reviewed.

## 2.4.1    The input cells, receptors: excitable cells that receive information

In Book 1, Chapter 2, you learnt something about the role of the sense organs in the causation of animal behaviour.

☐ What are the three categories of sensory receptor?

■ *Exteroceptors* provide the nervous system with information about the external world. The *enteroceptors* monitor aspects of the animal's internal state. The *proprioceptors* provide information about the position and movement of parts of the body.

Some sensory receptors respond to the presence of chemicals, perhaps produced by food or mates or even oxygen. Others are sensitive to, for example, vibration or light. A few are illustrated in Figure 2.13. Sensory cells act as **transducers**, converting whatever form of energy they are responsive to into electrical signals.

Remember how *Amoeba* responds to the presence of food molecules; sensory cells in multicellular animals work in a similar fashion. Some have a very special structure related to their function and details of how they work will be given in Book 3. Receptors are named after the kinds of energy they transduce. **Mechanoreceptors** are sensitive to mechanical deformation, **photoreceptors** to light energy, **chemoreceptors** to chemicals and **thermoreceptors** to temperature changes, for example.

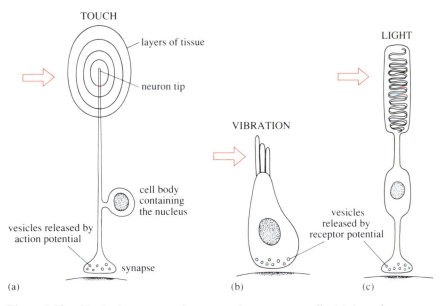

**Figure 2.13**   The basic structure of some vertebrate sensory cells. (a) A mechanoreceptor sensitive to touch in the skin. (b) A special mechanoreceptor sensitive to sound in the ear. (c) A photoreceptor in the eye. In all the drawings the arrow indicates where transduction takes place.

All sensory cells produce electrical potentials when excited by particular kinds of energy. These are called **receptor potentials**. Unlike the action potential, which is all-or-none in magnitude, receptor potentials can vary smoothly from their minimum to maximum values. They are therefore described as 'graded'.

☐   In what way are the receptor potentials similar to synaptic potentials?

■   Both are graded, rather than all-or-none.

In some cases, graded receptor potentials produce action potentials in the first neuron in the sequence itself. An example of this is the sensory neuron shown in Figure 2.13a. The tip of the neuron is embedded within several layers of concentrically arranged tissue. When this tissue is deformed by mechanical impact, i.e. touch, a receptor potential is produced at the embedded tip. If this potential is of sufficient magnitude, action potentials arise at the tip and travel towards the synapse.

☐   From the account of transmitter release given in Section 2.3.3, what would you suggest determines the rate at which transmitter is released at this synapse?

■ The rate at which action potentials arrive.

☐ Looking one stage earlier, what determines the frequency of these action potentials?

■ The magnitude and duration of the graded receptor potential produced at the tip of the neuron.

Figures 2.13b and c (p. 37) show neurons that operate in a somewhat different way. In the case of the neuron shown in Figure 2.13b, vibration generates a receptor potential. This graded potential does not initiate action potentials in the cell. Rather, the amount of transmitter released at the synapse depends upon the magnitude of the graded receptor potential within the cell responding to the vibration. The cell shown in Figure 2.13c works in a similar way. The absorption of light generates receptor potentials and the release of transmitter depends upon their magnitude. In each case (a–c), the second neuron, in turn, transmits the information further into the nervous system. In each case, the activity in the second neuron depends upon the rate at which transmitter is released at the synapse.

Enteroceptors, which monitor, for example, body temperature, blood sugar or oxygen levels, are very different in design from exteroceptors, like the ones shown in Figure 2.13, which monitor the external environment.

In general, animals respond to changes in their external or internal environment and so sensory receptors are especially sensitive to *changes* rather than to a steady state.

## 2.4.2 Output cells, effectors: excitable cells that move

Cells that bring about, or *effect*, action beyond the nervous system (e.g. muscle fibres) are termed **effector cells**. Muscle fibres are examples of excitable cells that enable multicellular animals to move. They contain a well-ordered system of contractile filaments of similar composition to those responsible for movement in *Amoeba* (Figures 2.14 and 2.15). A class of neurons called **motor neurons** (Figure 2.14) form synapses with muscle fibres. When an action potential arrives at the synapse between the motor neuron and the muscle fibre (also called the **neuromuscular junction**), transmitter is released onto the highly convoluted postsynaptic membrane, which is called the **end plate** (Figure 2.15). The end plate contains receptors that respond to the transmitter by producing an excitatory potential (the **end plate potential**). This potential causes an action potential in the muscle fibre similar to that found in the neuron. This muscle action potential spreads over the whole of the muscle fibre membrane and initiates a reaction between adjacent contractile filaments so that they contract, causing the muscle to shorten. Muscle contraction is described in more detail in Chapter 7.

There is a major difference between synaptic transmission at a dendrite (Section 2.3.3) and at the neuromuscular junction. The arrival of an action potential at the neuromuscular junction always causes a muscle action potential to be generated and the muscle to contract.

In vertebrates, all motor neurons are excitatory. The degree of contraction of the muscle depends upon the number of axons to the muscle that are active and the frequency of action potentials in each. In contrast, in some invertebrates such as

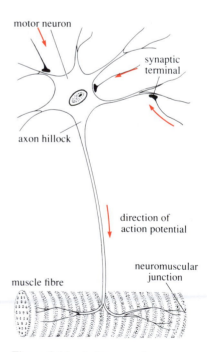

**Figure 2.14**  A diagram of a motor neuron contacting a muscle fibre which contains bundles of contractile filaments.

crabs and lobsters, some neuromuscular junctions are inhibitory on muscles while others are excitatory. In such animals, the degree of muscular contraction depends on the balance of activity between the two kinds of synapse.

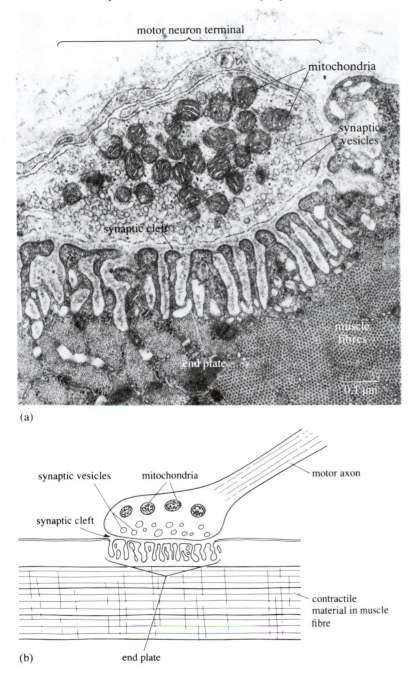

(a)

(b)

**Figure 2.15**   (a) Electron micrograph of a neuromuscular junction between a motor axon terminal and a skeletal muscle fibre of an adult mouse. Notice the complex array of filaments in the muscle fibre and the large number of mitochondria in the terminal. (b) Diagram of the junction to illustrate its main features.

There are many other kinds of effector cells besides muscle fibres. In all cases, synaptic activation of the cell produces some kind of work such as ejection of a liquid, pulses of light or movement. Glands contain effector cells that, when excited, cause the release of substances, such as digestive enzymes, sweat or hormones. Glow worms have effector cells that produce light when excited. Many animals such as frogs, chameleons and cuttlefish have special effector cells in the skin that are responsible for the animal's ability to change its colour.

### 2.4.3   Between input and output—some varieties of neurons

So there is input to the nervous system and output from it. What happens in between? Nervous systems consist of networks of interconnected neurons that are concerned with information processing. Within all nervous systems there is a variety of shapes and sizes of neurons (Figure 2.6, Section 2.3.1). One basic distinction is between neurons with very short axons (which influence local neurons) and those with long axons that convey information from one area to another.

Another distinction is between neurons that have predominantly inhibitory effects on other neurons and those that have predominantly excitatory effects. For many years it was thought that a particular neuron only produced one type of transmitter. However more and more examples are being found of neurons releasing several transmitters.

☐   Considering the various parts of the nervous system, does a particular transmitter type always have the same effect on postsynaptic cells?

■   No, as was discussed in Section 2.3.3, there are examples of one transmitter inhibiting one type of cell while exciting others.

☐   How is a given variety of transmitter able to cause an EPSP in one cell and an IPSP in another?

■   The effect that a transmitter will have on the postsynaptic cell will depend on the kinds of transmitter *receptors* in the postsynaptic membrane.

So it is feasible that a neuron might inhibit some of the cells it contacts while exciting others. This greatly increases the complexity of the task of understanding exactly how particular networks of neurons might operate.

### 2.4.4   Non-neural cells in the nervous system—the glial cells and others

Nervous systems do not contain only neurons; various types of other cells are also found there. In all nervous systems neurons are surrounded by glial cells or glia. Until quite recently these were regarded as just a kind of 'glue' holding the cells together. However, glial cells play a very important role in nervous activity; they are responsible for maintaining the environment around the neurons. The composition of the extracellular fluid around a neuron is critical in maintaining the membrane potential and therefore for generating action potentials. Some glial cells are in close contact with blood vessels; these control what substances can enter the environment of the neurons. Neurons and axons are surrounded by glial cells

(Figure 2.16). In vertebrates, special glial cells wrap themselves round and round axons like a Swiss roll to form a thick, whitish, insulating layer called **myelin**. Myelin acts as electrical insulation and speeds up the rate of transmission of the action potential enormously. Each cell only wraps around a small portion of the axon and the gaps between the glial cells are called **nodes of Ranvier** (see Figure 2.16). Some glial cells wrap individual axons while others wrap several. There are also axons which do not have myelin, called unmyelinated axons, though they are still surrounded by glial cells. It is very rare to find neurons or axons not in contact with glia.

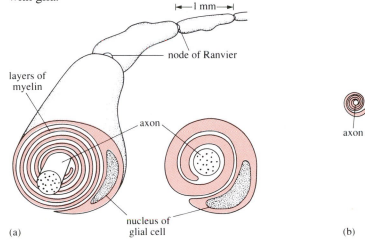

(a)

(b)

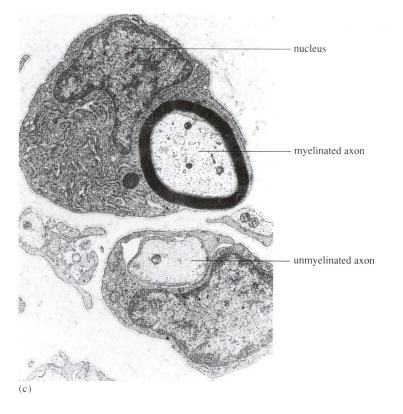

(c)

**Figure 2.16** Diagram showing how myelinating glial cells ensheath axons in (a) a peripheral nerve where one glial cell wraps round one axon and (b) the brain where one glial cell wraps around several axons. (c) An electron micrograph of a myelinated axon in young rat peripheral nerve; the centre of the axon is filled with neurofilaments and neurotubules.

The proper functioning of the nervous system depends critically upon the composition of the extracellular fluid. There are other special (non-glial) cells which form a protective barrier, called the **blood–brain barrier,** between the blood and brain tissue. The cells of the blood–brain barrier, together with the glial cells, regulate the composition of the fluid which bathes the neurons. The presence of the blood–brain barrier becomes important when considering how various drugs can influence neurons.

## Summary of Chapter 2

The description of *Amoeba* served to introduce you to some features of the structure and function of animal cells in general. The functions of the different structures are the same in *Amoeba* as in the cells of the human body. This account also illustrated how animals interact with their environment in order to survive. The cell membrane of *Amoeba* plays a vital role in the activity of the animal—it is responsible both for regulating the internal environment of the cell and for detecting relevant change in the external environment. It can be described as the information processing and control system of the cell. In animals like humans, which are made up of many cells, the nervous system performs and elaborates this role.

The second half of the chapter was devoted to a brief survey of the structure and function of the cells in the nervous system. The nervous system is a special, highly organized group of excitable cells that can receive, interpret and transmit information. Chapters 3 and 4 describe in rather more detail how neurons function.

The nervous system is responsible for directing the responses an animal makes to changes in its external and internal environment. The complex behaviour patterns you learnt about in Book 1 are generated by the nervous system. Neurons in all animals have a similar structure and function—what differs is the way in which they are connected with one another. A survey of the nervous systems in various groups of animals will be given in Chapters 6 and 8.

## Objectives for Chapter 2

When you have completed this chapter you should be able to:

2.1    Define and use, or recognize the definitions and applications of each of the terms printed in bold in the text. (*Question 2.1*)

2.2    Describe the role of the cell membrane in the behaviour of *Amoeba*. (*Question 2.2*)

2.3    Describe the basic appearance of vertebrate neurons and the function of the various intracellular structures. (*Question 2.3*)

2.4    Explain the significance of the membrane in the function of the neuron. (*Question 2.4*)

2.5     Explain the difference between an action potential and a synaptic potential and the significance of this difference. (*Question 2.5*)

2.6     Describe the role of receptor cells and effector cells in nervous system function. (*Question 2.6*)

2.7     Explain the importance of multiple synapses and synaptic action in nervous system function. (*Question 2.7*)

2.8     Describe the function of glial cells. (*Question 2.8*)

# Questions for Chapter 2

**Question 2.1** (*Objective 2.1*)
Complete each of (a)–(e) with one selection from 1–7.

(a)   The nucleus …

(b)   A mitochondrion …

(c)   An axon …

(d)   The endoplasmic reticulum …

(e)   A synapse …

1     … is the 'powerhouse' of the cell.

2     … is a long process extending from the cell body of a neuron.

3     … is the site of protein synthesis in a cell.

4     … is the junction between cells, comprising an area of the membrane of each.

5     …contains the genetic information of the cell.

6     …contains a number of myelin sheaths.

7     …forms a sheath around the neuron.

**Question 2.2** (*Objective 2.2*)
Describe the role of the cell membrane in detecting, engulfing and digesting prey in *Amoeba*.

**Question 2.3** (*Objective 2.3*)
Label the dendrites, axon, cell body, axon hillock, myelin sheath, node of Ranvier and neuromuscular junction in the diagram of the motor neuron in Figure 2.17.

**Question 2.4** (*Objective 2.4*)
Why is the electrical property of the cell membrane so important to neural function?

**Question 2.5** (*Objective 2.5*)
What is the principal difference between an action potential and a synaptic potential?

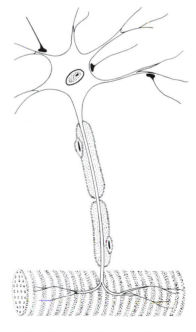

**Figure 2.17**   Diagram of a motor neuron contacting a muscle.

**Question 2.6** (*Objective 2.6*)

In what ways are membrane receptors and sensory receptors similar?

**Question 2.7** (*Objective 2.7*)

The nervous system has been likened to a complex series of wires and simple on-or-off switches which works rather like an old-fashioned telephone exchange. Is this an accurate description?

**Question 2.8** (*Objective 2.8*)

What are glial cells and what is their role in nervous system function?

# CHAPTER 3
# ELECTRICAL PROPERTIES OF NEURONS

## 3.1 Introduction

The neuron's function as an element in the nervous system—receiving, transforming and transmitting messages—depends upon its ability to convey action potentials, as you learnt in Chapters 1 and 2. A major success for the neurosciences over the period since the 1940s and 1950s has been in providing descriptions of the way in which the neuron carries out these functions. An understanding of how the neuron operates at the molecular level is doubly important because it also helps an appreciation of the ways that chemical substances such as hormones and drugs can change nervous system functions. This chapter will extend the discussions of Chapter 2 by looking at the neuron as an electrical device and at the molecular basis for the action potential. Chapter 4, will consider in more detail the way in which the neuron produces and responds to chemical transmitters.

When a neuron is not transmitting an action potential, it is described, electrically, as being at its resting potential. In order to understand the action potential it is thus necessary first to know about the electrical state that provides the background against which the action potential occurs. The explanations leading up to the description of the resting membrane potential may appear somewhat long-winded but each step is deliberately described very carefully in this chapter. In places, there is deliberate over-simplification to ensure that you follow these steps, even though this simplification has been achieved at the expense of precise rigour in terms of chemistry and physics.

The latter part of this chapter is devoted to a detailed explanation of the mechanisms involved in generating and propagating an action potential. How an action potential occurs in one small section of an axon is considered first, followed by a description of how the action potential is propagated along the axon. How a change in electrical potential in one region of a neuron influences the electrical potential of neighbouring regions is demonstrated. The ability of the neuron to transmit action potentials depends on particular properties of its membrane and something of the molecular bases of these properties are explained.

# 3.2 Properties of the neuron membrane: diffusion, equilibrium, ions and channels

## 3.2.1 Electrical properties of neurons

This section introduces explanations for the resting membrane potential and action potentials that have been provided by a branch of neuroscience called biophysics, which looks at the way that the neuron membrane is adapted so that the neuron has the vital property of excitability (that is, the ability to be electrically stimulated. The electrical properties exhibited by neurons are closely associated with the difference in chemical composition between the fluid inside the cell (the intracellular fluid) and that outside the cell (the extracellular fluid). First, you need to know what is meant by electrical voltage, current and conductance. This is most easily explained with the aid of an analogy. Consider the two cylinders of water shown in Figure 3.1a. When the tap is opened, water flows from left to right until the pressure (height) of water is equal on the two sides. There is, therefore, a current of water driven by a difference in pressure between the two sides. The aperture formed by turning the tap offers a certain resistance to the flow of current, for instance, the larger the aperture, the lower the resistance and the larger the current. The term 'conductance' is useful here. Conductance bears an inverse relation to resistance (which can be expressed mathematically as conductance = 1/resistance). This simply means that an aperture that has a high resistance has a low conductance (the current of water is small) and an aperture with low resistance has a high conductance (the current of water is large).

In Figure 3.1b, the pressure difference is reversed, and consequently the current flows in the opposite direction. Suppose that the difference in pressure or height of water between the two cylinders in Figure 3.1a were arbitrarily to be designated as 'positive'. That of Figure 3.1b would then be 'negative'. The direction of the current depends upon whether the pressure difference is positive or negative.

Electric current through a conducting medium (for example, a piece of metal or a salt solution) is crudely analogous to the flow of water, as shown in Figure 3.2. Just as water flows from a region of high pressure to a region of low pressure, electric current flows when there is a difference in charge (Section 2.3.2), or *potential*. Such a potential difference is measured in volts and so an alternative name for potential difference is 'voltage'. The 'resistance' of a material is a term that characterizes the difficulty that an electric current has in passing through it.

Voltages can be measured by an instrument called a voltmeter. For measuring voltages across the membranes of living cells (i.e. for measuring the difference in potential between the inside and outside of the cell), electrodes are used that are insulated except at the tip, which penetrates the cell. If any kind of cell is impaled by an electrode, a small voltage is usually observed between the cell's interior and exterior. The peculiarity of the neuron as a cell is that it employs the difference in chemical composition and the associated electrical potential between the two sides of the cell membrane for the function of communication. The action potential, the basis of communication, is a very rapid change in the voltage across the neuron membrane.

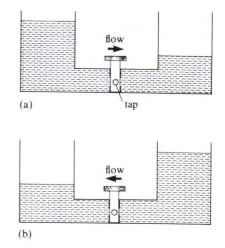

**Figure 3.1** Water pressure difference between two cylinders. (a) The pressure difference will cause water to flow from left to right. (b) The pressure difference will cause water to flow from right to left.

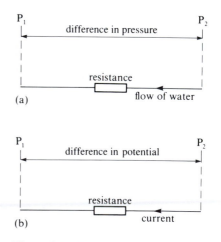

**Figure 3.2** Diagrams showing the analogy between electric current and the flow of water.

### 3.2.2 Diffusion and equilibrium

The cells of the body have an internal chemical composition that is different from that of the extracellular fluid that bathes them. In order to explain how cells maintain such a balance of different chemicals across the membrane, it is necessary to understand the process of diffusion.

A general property of molecules in solution is that they have a continuous random motion. As a result, dissolved substances tend to 'spread out' from a region of high concentration to regions of low concentration until they are evenly distributed. They are said to move down a **concentration gradient**. Similarly, water molecules move from a region of high water concentration to one of low water concentration. A good illustration of this phenomenon is to think of what happens when you drop a spot of ink into water. Initially, it appears as a dark area in the water but then, as the ink molecules and water molecules gradually mix, the fluid becomes a paler, but uniform, colour with the ink molecules being evenly distributed between the water molecules.

The process whereby substances in liquid or gas form attain uniform distribution is called *diffusion*. Unless something prevents the passage of the molecules, this phenomenon of diffusion ultimately produces a uniform mixture of molecules. In other words, the concentration of each component is the same throughout the medium.

Figure 3.3a shows a section through a tubular membrane that forms a semipermeable barrier between two fluids. A **semipermeable membrane** is one that readily allows certain molecules (e.g. water or glucose) through, but presents an obstacle to the movement of other molecules (e.g. large proteins). Figure 3.3a asks you to imagine an experiment in which on the outside of the membrane is placed one fluid, pure water, and on the inside a fluid of different composition, a substance dissolved in water. It is conventional to refer to the dissolved substance as the *solute* and the medium in which it is dissolved as the *solvent*. In our example, suppose that this particular solute is able to pass across the membrane only at pores, or channels, shown simply as holes in Figure 3.3a (for the sake of developing the argument, the fact that the membrane has some permeability to water will, for the moment, be ignored).

Because of their random motion, some solute molecules will be in a position to escape from the inside of the tube to the outside. Put another way, the solute's unequal distribution on either side of the membrane creates a *concentration gradient* across the membrane. Given enough time, solute will pass through the membrane until the concentration is equal on the two sides, reducing the gradient to zero. When this state prevails, the molecules are still moving about randomly but there are as many solute molecules leaving as entering. The system is said to be in **equilibrium**, because the number of molecules leaving balances the number entering. Therefore, the concentrations of solute on each side of the membrane do not change. Note that this is not a static equilibrium but a *dynamic* one; many molecules will be crossing all the time but there is no *net* movement in either direction.

Now refer to Figure 3.3b, where pure water is on the inside of the membrane, and water plus a different solute is on the outside. There will be a net movement of solute to the inside of the tube until equilibrium is reached. In Figure 3.3c the

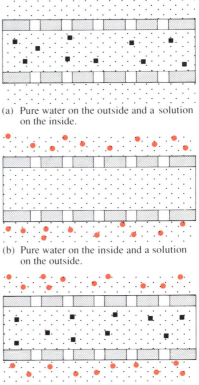

(a) Pure water on the outside and a solution on the inside.

(b) Pure water on the inside and a solution on the outside.

(c) Different solutions on either side.

**Figure 3.3** Development of simple models of features of the cell membrane, axoplasm and extracellular fluid. (a) Pure water on the outside and a solution on the inside. (b) Pure water on the inside and a solution on the outside. (c) Different solutions on either side, denoted by ● and ■.

situations shown in Figures 3.3a and 3.3b are combined. At the start there is a membrane and two distinct segregated solutions, one on the inside and one on the outside. There will be a simultaneous tendency for solute 1 to move to the outside and solute 2 to the inside. Ultimately, there will be an equal concentration of solute 1 on the two sides, the same being true for solute 2.

Though it is a gross simplification, used for the purpose of developing the explanation, think of Figure 3.3c as a primitive model of a section of neuronal axon. The membrane is now the cell membrane. The fluid on the inside is the intracellular fluid of the axon (termed the *axoplasm*). The fluid that bathes the outside of the membrane is the extracellular fluid. The extracellular fluid is a relatively massive volume of fluid consisting of all the fluid outside the cells of the body, including the fluid part of the blood.

Water is present on either side of the membrane, but different substances are dissolved in intracellular water (e.g. a high concentration of potassium) and extracellular water (e.g. a high concentration of sodium). Because of diffusion, there will be a tendency for these substances to become uniformly distributed. The fact that they are *not* equally distributed in living cells, but are well segregated, is due to additional mechanisms that are a function of the cell membrane. The substances sodium and potassium now become the focus of attention. They are examples of 'ions' and Section 3.2.3 discusses what is meant by this term.

### 3.2.3  Ions

Section 2.3.2 introduced the term 'charge'. An ion is an electrically charged particle that has either a positive charge (termed a cation, pronounced 'cat iron') or a negative charge (termed an anion, pronounced 'an iron'). Charges of the same sign—positive and positive or negative and negative—repel one another, whereas charges of the opposite sign attract one another. When there are equal numbers of positive and negative charges in a solution these, in effect, 'cancel' each other out (though the charges are still present—they do not disappear) and the solution as a whole carries no net charge. It is said to be electrically neutral.

The familiar chemical compound sodium chloride (common salt), which is essential for the normal functioning of neurons, is formed of molecules consisting of a positively charged sodium ion ($Na^+$) and a negatively charged chloride ion ($Cl^-$). When salt is in its white, crystalline form, each $Na^+$ ion is associated with a $Cl^-$ ion and so the solid has no overall charge. In a solution in water, the relatively weak electrical bond between the $Na^+$ ions (positive charge denoted by the + sign) and $Cl^-$ ions (negative charge denoted by the − sign) breaks down and the $Na^+$ and $Cl^-$ ions are in a dissociated state.

Figure 3.4 shows the important differences in the compositions of the intracellular and extracellular fluids of the giant axon in the squid (studied because it is so large and relatively easy to manipulate in a laboratory), detailing the concentrations of the major ion types: potassium ($K^+$), sodium ($Na^+$) and chloride ($Cl^-$). The units used to describe the concentrations of ions in Figure 3.4 are $mmol\,l^{-1}$ (millimoles per litre), a technical measurement, the details of which are not important for this discussion. The important feature of this form of measurement is that it allows a comparison to be made between the concentrations of a particular ion type inside and outside the axon and between concentrations of different types of ion.

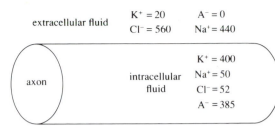

**Figure 3.4** Concentrations of ions inside and outside the giant axon of the squid. $K^+$ = potassium; $Na^+$ = sodium; $Cl^-$ = chloride; $A^-$ represents negatively charged organic ions. Units of concentration are mmol $l^{-1}$. Note that you cannot determine the potential across the membrane directly by adding up the figures for the concentrations of each ion. Not all the ions are shown, and factors in addition to concentration influence the final membrane potential.

Electrical charge is important for our discussion because, as you saw in Chapters 1 and 2, the neuron has an imbalance of electrical charge, i.e. a potential difference, between its inside and outside. Under certain circumstances this imbalance is used to provide the energy for some of the electrical phenomena that are about to be described—in much the same way that the voltage or potential difference of a battery provides the energy to power an electrical device, for example, a torch.

☐   Look at Figure 3.4—what are the important features of the distributions of ions across the squid giant axon membrane?

■   There are considerable differences in concentrations of the major ion types between the intracellular and extracellular fluids. Whereas there is a higher concentration of $K^+$ inside the cell, the concentrations of $Na^+$ and $Cl^-$ are much higher outside.

The neuron's excitability depends upon the movement of $Na^+$ and $K^+$ through its membrane, which in turn depends upon the $K^+$ and $Na^+$ concentration differences across the membrane. Also shown in Figure 3.4 is the relatively large concentration of negatively charged molecules given the generic label 'organic anions' ($A^-$) that are too big to move through the membrane.

In fact, neurons contain many more types of ion than are shown in Figure 3.4 but a good understanding of the resting membrane potential and the action potential can be obtained just in terms of the movement of the $Na^+$ and $K^+$ ions. To understand this movement across the membrane, it is necessary to look at the channels through which such movement occurs.

## 3.2.4   Channels

Ions move through the axon membrane or other regions of the neuron membrane at 'holes' or channels in the membrane. Embedded within the cell membrane are specialized complex protein molecules. These complex molecules have the capacity to change their shape under circumstances that will be described later. The specialized protein molecules form channels that, by opening and closing, alter the movement of ions and other substances across the membrane. Each type of ion has its own channel molecule, which, by virtue of the chemical structure of the molecule and diameter of the channel, excludes other types of ion. A membrane with open channels for a particular type of ion would be described as having a high conductance for that ion type, whereas a closed channel would have a low conductance.

Section 3.3 describes the electrical state of the resting membrane and shows the relevance of the conductance of the membrane and the difference in ion concentrations to this electrical state.

# 3.3   Resting membrane potential

As a first approximation, one can consider that, when an axon is resting, that is to say not transmitting an action potential, only the $Cl^-$ and $K^+$ channels are open. Hence, only the $K^+$ and $Cl^-$ ions are free to move in and out of the axon. Most of the $Na^+$ ions are confined to the outside of the axon and the large organic anions are trapped on the inside. Any ion type that is free to move has two forces acting on it. The first arises from the difference in concentration *of that particular ion* across the membrane. The second arises from the difference in electrical potential across the membrane; the inside is electrically negative with respect to the outside.

The difference in ion concentration for a particular ion type is associated with a concentration gradient for that ion. Assume that the channels for a particular ion are open to some extent. The ion will tend to move down its concentration gradient, in other words it will tend to migrate from a region of high concentration to a region of lower concentration. This arises from the principles of diffusion described in Section 3.2.2. The ink tended to move from a region of high ink concentration to one of low. Examine Figure 3.4 (p. 49).

☐   Is there a concentration gradient for $K^+$?

■   Yes, there is a higher concentration of $K^+$ on the inside of the membrane than on the outside.

☐   Are the channels for $K^+$ open to some extent in the resting state?

■   Yes, as indicated by the fact that there are $K^+$ ions on both sides of the membrane.

☐   What will $K^+$ ions tend to do as a result of the concentration gradient?

■   They will tend to move from the inside of the membrane to the outside, down the $K^+$ concentration gradient.

The other force tending to move ions across the membrane is the membrane potential: the *difference in charge* across the membrane. Note that it is meaningless to refer to a concentration gradient without specifying the substance in question, e.g. $Na^+$ concentration gradient or $K^+$ concentration gradient. The membrane potential is different. It arises from a difference in *total* charge across the membrane and all ion types contribute to this. So there is not a membrane potential for $Na^+$ that is different from that for $K^+$. In Chapter 1 and Chapter 2 (Section

2.3.2), you were introduced to the existence of a potential difference across the membrane of a neuron. In the resting state, this membrane potential is around −70 mV, the inside being negative with respect to the outside. The existence of a membrane potential provides a gradient that tends to move ions because positively charged ions tend to be attracted to areas that are more negative and negatively charged ions to areas that are more positive.

☐ Will the membrane potential tend to move $K^+$ ions across the membrane?

■ Yes, there is a surplus of negative charge on the inside, so it will tend to attract $K^+$ ions into the cell.

☐ Do the concentration gradient for $K^+$ and the membrane potential act in the same or opposite directions?

■ Opposite. The concentration gradient tends to expel $K^+$ ions from the axoplasm and the membrane potential tends to pull them back in.

At the *resting potential*, the concentration gradient is slightly stronger than the membrane potential.

☐ What will be the outcome of this?

■ A slight movement of $K^+$ ions out of the cell.

The fact that the cell maintains a high concentration of $K^+$ in spite of this 'leakage' requires an additional process, which is described in Section 3.4.

As said at the beginning of this section, as a first approximation, one can consider, at the resting potential, the membrane to be permeable only to $K^+$ and $Cl^-$. Strictly speaking, however, there is some permeability to $Na^+$. The resistance is not infinite. This very small permeability now needs to be considered.

☐ Is there a concentration gradient for $Na^+$?

■ Yes. The concentration of $Na^+$ is higher outside the neuron than inside.

☐ Will the concentration gradient tend to pull $Na^+$ ions into the cell?

■ Yes.

☐ Will the membrane potential tend to pull $Na^+$ ions into the cell?

■ Yes. The inside is negative with respect to the outside so this will attract $Na^+$ ions into the cell.

The fact that the membrane is almost impermeable to $Na^+$ means that rather little infiltrates the cell but none-the-less there is a very slight trickle in. What stops an accumulation of $Na^+$ ions on the inside and a depletion of $K^+$ ions is the topic of Section 3.4.

# 3.4 The sodium–potassium pump

Figure 3.5a shows a summary of the story developed so far. There is a concentration gradient of $K^+$ tending to move $K^+$ ions out of the cell. Acting in the opposite direction is the membrane potential tending to pull them in. The concentration gradient is larger than the membrane potential and so, were these to be the only two factors operating, there would be a slight trickle of $K^+$ ions out of the cell. Both the concentration gradient of $Na^+$ and the membrane potential act in the same direction to move $Na^+$ into the cell. Although the membrane offers a high resistance to the movement of $Na^+$, it is not infinite. Some $Na^+$ is able to leak through the membrane.

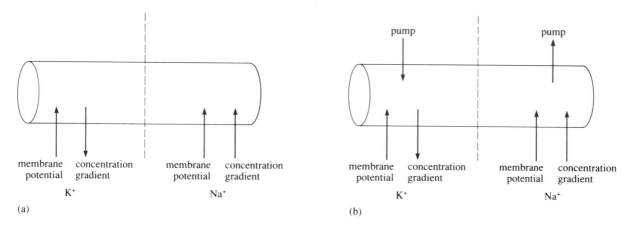

**Figure 3.5** Forces tending to move ions across the membrane. (a) The effects of membrane potential and concentration gradient on $K^+$ and $Na^+$. (b) Addition of the effect of the sodium–potassium pump on ion movements.

Figure 3.4 shows a marked segregation of $K^+$ ions (high concentration on the inside and low on the outside) and $Na^+$ ions (high concentration on the outside and low on the inside). The inevitable consequence of the forces shown in Figure 3.5a would be to break down this segregation, were it not for an additional factor, called a *pump*.

Neurons have a continuously acting pump mechanism that works to counteract the tendencies for $Na^+$ to leak in and $K^+$ to leak out, as represented in Figure 3.5b. The neuron cell body and axon membranes are able to expel $Na^+$ ions and retrieve $K^+$ ions at the same time. This **sodium–potassium pump** requires energy to move ions against the gradients tending to move them in the opposite direction.

By holding the ion concentrations almost constant on each side of the neuron's membrane, the sodium–potassium pump maintains a state of dynamic equilibrium. The number of $Na^+$ ions leaving the neuron equals the number entering. Similarly, the number of $K^+$ ions leaving equals the number entering. This account of the sodium–potassium pump completes the discussion of the bases of the resting potential. Section 3.5 looks at the measurement of both this potential and the action potential.

## 3.5  Observing electrical events

Figures 1.4 and 1.5 in Chapter 1 and Figure 2.9 in Chapter 2 introduced the form of the action potential: a movement of the membrane potential from its resting value of around −70 mV to a positive value of around +20 mV and then a return to the resting value. This section looks in more detail at how action potentials are measured and Section 3.6 looks at the explanation of the events that underlie the action potential.

Figure 3.6 shows an experimental set-up for recording the electrical activity from a neuron *preparation* (biological material that has been prepared in some way so that it can be studied). Here, because of its large size, the squid giant axon—which can be up to 1 mm in diameter—is the classic preparation for investigating the membrane mechanisms contributing to the neuron's function.

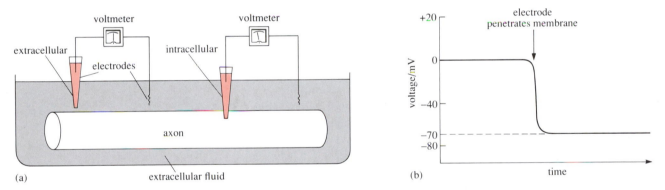

**Figure 3.6**  (a) Measurement of the membrane resting potential. On the left, the recording electrode is in the extracellular fluid. On the right, when the electrode has penetrated the axon and entered the intracellular fluid the voltmeter displays the membrane resting potential. (b) The change in potential as the electrode penetrates the membrane.

For these investigations a length of dissected squid giant axon (with its ends sealed to prevent leakage of intracellular fluid) is placed in a solution that closely approximates the composition of the extracellular fluid that normally bathes the outside of the axon and its 'parent' neuron body. Recordings of the electrical activity of the axon are made from a fine electrode connected to a sensitive meter that measures voltage (see Box 3.1, *overleaf*).

## Box 3.1   Microelectrodes: recording and stimulating neurons

Over a number of years, greatly refined experimental procedures for electrical recording from cells have been developed. Very fine electrodes made from glass tubing with a small bore (micropipettes), are now available. These then serve as microelectrodes, as shown in Figure 3.7.

In this way, it is possible to produce microelectrodes with tips so fine (about 0.1 µm) that they can penetrate the membranes of all but the smallest neurons without disturbing their function. Glass microelectrodes with larger tips (greater than 1 µm) are less prone to breakage, but these can only be used for extracellular recording. In this case, the electrode is moved close to the cell membrane to pick up its electrical activity. It is possible to record action potentials through both extracellular and intracellular microelectrodes. The resting membrane potential and fluctuations in membrane potentials (EPSPs and IPSPs, see Sections 2.3.3 and 3.9) can be recorded only with intracellular electrodes.

The microelectrode is filled with a concentrated ionic solution so that, at the exposed tip, it is in electrical contact with the recording site, but is electrically insulated elsewhere. A silver wire is normally inserted into the wide end of the electrode and this serves as a link between the fluid inside the microelectrode and the connections to the recording apparatus. A connection is also made to the fluid bathing the outside of the axon, so that the difference in potential across the membrane is recorded (Figure 3.7).

One might imagine that the impaling of an axon or cell body in this way, penetrating its membrane, would seriously disrupt those processes that one wishes to observe, but the evidence is that the disruption can be minimal. To stimulate the neuron, an external source of electrical current can be connected to the microelectrode to change the potential difference between the inside and outside of the cell.

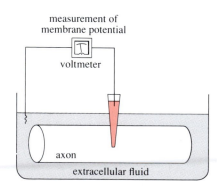

**Figure 3.7**   Microelectrode piercing an axon.

When the recording electrode is moved slowly from the fluid bathing the axon to penetrate its membrane and to come in contact with the intracellular fluid there is an abrupt change in the voltage measured. As the electrode enters the axon the voltage falls about 70 mV. That is, there is a voltage (or potential difference) of 70 mV between the inside and outside of the axon, with the inside being negative with respect to the outside.

This indicates that the inside of the axon (and also the neuron body itself) is electrically negative with respect to the outside when it is in the resting state. A negative membrane resting potential is a characteristic feature of neurons and other excitable cells such as sensory receptor and muscle cells.

Figure 3.8 shows a modification of the experiment represented in Figure 3.7 in which a stimulating electrode is placed at one end of the axon. The stimulating electrode is used to apply a brief pulse of electrical current to the axon. The recording electrode can be moved to record the membrane potential at different distances from the stimulating site.

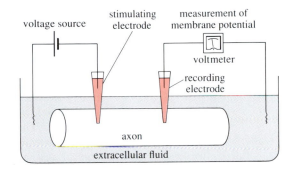

**Figure 3.8** Brief electrical pulses are delivered through the stimulating electrode fixed at one end of the axon. The recording electrode can be inserted at different places along the axon.

An experiment of the type outlined in Figure 3.8 shows that, when a brief electrical pulse is applied to one end of the axon, an electrical pulse about 90 mV in amplitude (size) can be detected some time later at any point on the axon, that is, a voltmeter connected to a recording electrode will show a change from about −70 mV to about +20 mV and back again (Figure 3.9). Here, two features are important:

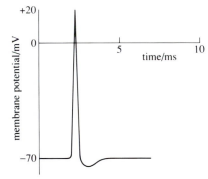

**Figure 3.9** The action potential.

1   With a recording electrode placed at any point along the length of the axon the measured change in voltage is always of the same size.

2   The further along the axon away from the stimulating electrode the recording electrode is placed, the longer it takes for the recording electrode to register any voltage change.

The interpretation of these observations is that the electrical stimulation triggers a wave of electrical activity that travels along the axon away from the point of stimulation. As the wave passes the recording electrode it appears on the voltmeter as an abrupt change in voltage, called an action potential. The constant size of the action potential indicates that it travels along the axon in an all-or-none rather than in a decremental fashion, as you will recall from Section 2.3.2. The *latency* is the time between the onset of the artificial electrical stimulation and the arrival of the action potential at the recording electrode. The increase in the latency as the recording electrode moves further away from the stimulating electrode shows that the action potential travels along the axon at a particular speed. This speed is much slower than that of electrical signals along metal wires.

# 3.6 Explaining the action potential

Figure 3.10 shows the sequence of events that constitute the action potential. In period 1, the axon is at the resting potential of $-70\,mV$. At time 2, a voltage is applied to the axon so as to make the membrane potential steadily less negative. In other words, the voltage *depolarizes* the membrane. Over the period marked 3, the effect of the applied voltage is straightforward: the membrane gradually becomes more depolarized. Then at the point in time marked 4, a sudden increase in depolarization occurs, not as a result of any sudden change in the stimulating voltage but as an intrinsic property of the axon. This sudden change takes the membrane potential to a positive value of around $20\,mV$.

When the voltage moves the membrane potential to a certain level of depolarization, to the level marked by the dotted line in Figure 3.10, a process intrinsic to the neuron membrane and the ions on either side is responsible for the swing to $+20\,mV$. The level of depolarization marked by the dotted line is the threshold, introduced in Section 2.3.3.

How can this sudden transition that occurs at the threshold be explained? The start of an action potential has been shown to coincide with the opening of channels for $Na^+$ ions. The voltage makes the membrane potential less negative and when the membrane potential reaches a certain level (the threshold), $Na^+$ channels in the membrane open. Channels that open at a particular voltage are described as **voltage-gated**.

☐  When $Na^+$ channels open, there are two forces acting on $Na^+$ ions which move them into the axon from the extracellular fluid. What are they?

■  Figure 3.4 shows that there is an $Na^+$ concentration gradient with a high concentration outside the cell and a low $Na^+$ concentration inside. So a concentration gradient for $Na^+$ will tend to move $Na^+$ ions into the cell. Also, since $Na^+$ ions are positively charged, they will be attracted by the excess negative charge inside the axon. In other words, the membrane potential will also tend to move $Na^+$ ions into the cell.

With the concentration gradient and membrane potential both acting to move $Na^+$ ions into the axon, given the opportunity of an open channel, $Na^+$ ions move in.

☐  What will be the effect on the membrane potential of $Na^+$ ions moving into the axon?

■  Positively charged $Na^+$ moving into the axon—a region which contains a predominance of negative ions—will make it less negative (i.e. more positive).

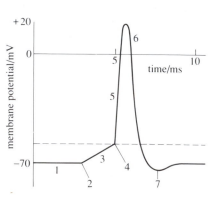

**Figure 3.10**   The action potential
1   Resting potential.
2   Depolarization starts to be applied.
3   Depolarization increases but is not yet sufficient to induce action potential.
4   Depolarization moves membrane potential to the threshold and action potential is triggered ($Na^+$ ions move in).
5   Membrane potential moves rapidly towards a positive value as $Na^+$ ions continue to move in.
6   $Na^+$ channels closed and $K^+$ channels open.
7   Membrane potential has hyperpolarized.

The potential of the inside of the axon becomes less negative with respect to the outside as positively charged $Na^+$ ions move from the extracellular fluid to the inside of the axon. The membrane potential therefore becomes smaller and eventually reverses to become a positive potential, as more and more $Na^+$ ions move in, as shown in Figure 3.10.

☐   As more $Na^+$ ions flow into the axon from the extracellular fluid what will be the effect on the membrane potential acting on the $Na^+$ ions?

■   At first it is reduced concurrently as the $Na^+$ ions move into the axon. After the membrane potential crosses the value of zero it reverses and becomes positive. As soon as the membrane potential becomes positive, the axon will tend to expel $Na^+$ ions rather than attract them in.

Strictly speaking, the movement of $Na^+$ ions into the axon will also lower the concentration gradient for $Na^+$ but the number of ions that move in is so small, as a percentage of those already present, that changes in this gradient are negligible and are usually ignored in describing the sequence.

That the membrane potential goes no further positive than $+20\,mV$ can only in part be explained by the fact that a positive membrane potential will tend to repel rather than attract $Na^+$ ions in. Calculations have shown that, even at $+20\,mV$, the $Na^+$ concentration gradient is still sufficiently strong, in spite of the reversed membrane potential, to attract $Na^+$ ions into the axon. So what stops the flow? The answer is to be found by looking at the voltage-gated channels in the membrane.

As just described, the fact that $Na^+$ ions are able to flow into the membrane is due to an opening of the $Na^+$ ion channels in the membrane as a result of the artificially induced depolarization. Such opening is short-lived; the peak of the action potential coincides with the closure of the ion channels. The conductance (Section 3.2.1) of the membrane is said to have changed. Conductance, when applied to excitable cells, is a term that provides a useful measure of the membrane permeability for an ion or ions.

☐   With reference to Figure 3.10, give an account of the $Na^+$ conductance of the membrane, starting at the resting potential and going to the peak.

■   At the resting potential, the conductance is very low. At the threshold, it increases sharply, then, at the peak, decreases to a low value.

Another factor is also involved. You might have reasoned that closing the $Na^+$ channels will stop the membrane potential moving any further in a positive direction but how can it be explained that it then immediately moves in a negative direction? (This process is termed **repolarization**.) The answer lies in a special population of $K^+$ channels in the membrane. This population is distinct from the permanently open $K^+$ channels mentioned in Section 3.3, which could be described as 'passive'.

The second population of $K^+$ channels are special in two ways:

1   They are voltage-gated. They open when the membrane potential, from being negative, approaches a zero voltage, whereas the $K^+$ channels that determine the resting membrane potential are passive (always open).

2   They have a relatively high conductance whereas the passive $K^+$ channels have a relatively low conductance.

☐   Examine both Figure 3.4 and Figure 3.10 at the point where membrane potential is at its most positive. What can you anticipate will be the consequence of the voltage-gated $K^+$ channels opening?

■   There is a higher concentration of $K^+$ ions inside than outside, i.e. a $K^+$ concentration gradient exists, so $K^+$ ions will move rapidly out of the cell.

During the very early phase of the action potential when only the low-conductance population of $K^+$ channels are open, $Na^+$ ions move into the axon, making it more positive. Because of the low conductance of the passive $K^+$ channels, relatively small numbers of $K^+$ ions flow out until the voltage-gated $K^+$ channels open. Also, unlike the $Na^+$ channels, the voltage-gated $K^+$ channels take a relatively long period to close.

When the voltage-gated $K^+$ channels are open, $K^+$ conductance is high for a period after the $Na^+$ channels have closed. This is shown in Figure 3.11. The movement of $K^+$ ions from the axon has the effect that the membrane potential briefly moves to a value more negative than the resting potential. This phase of the action potential is termed **hyperpolarization**. The resting potential is regained when the voltage-gated $K^+$ channels close.

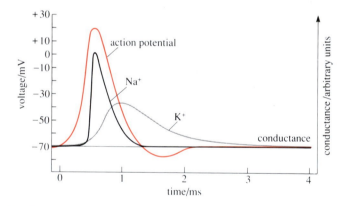

**Figure 3.11**   The $Na^+$ and $K^+$ ion flows during the action potential are shown by the membrane conductances of $Na^+$ and $K^+$ respectively.

To summarize, the time course of the action potential (as shown in Figure 3.10) can be divided into three phases:

1   Depolarization—the membrane potential becomes less negative or, in other words, more positive.

2   Repolarization—the membrane potential falls back towards membrane resting potential.

3   Hyperpolarization—the membrane potential 'undershoots' the membrane resting potential (that is, becomes more negative).

The descriptions of the ion flows across the axon membrane during the action potential may have given you the impression that, following a series of action potentials, the inward flows of $Na^+$ ions accompanied by the outward flows of $K^+$ ions would quickly deplete the $K^+$ ion population in the intracellular fluid and also saturate it with $Na^+$ ions. The effect of large and widespread changes in the ion concentrations would be to move the neuron to the point where no action potentials could be generated. In fact, the ion flows are quite local and in the context of the total ion population in the intracellular fluid, the changes in $Na^+$ and $K^+$ ion concentrations that they cause are relatively small.

As you saw in Section 3.4, neurons have a continuously active pump mechanism that works to counteract both $Na^+$ infiltration and $K^+$ loss. Under normal conditions this pump mechanism is sufficient to maintain the ion segregation even in the face of frequent action potentials. This pump operates at a relatively steady 'background' level; *over time* it is responsible for the expulsion of $Na^+$ ions from the cell and retrieval of $K^+$ such that no shift in concentration of ions occurs. Even following a number of action potentials, $Na^+$ does not normally accumulate in any large amount inside the cell. However, it is important not to make the all-too-common mistake of supposing that since depolarization is caused by a flow of $Na^+$ ions in, down their concentration gradient and membrane potential, repolarization is a result of the pump rapidly expelling $Na^+$ ions.

There have been several lines of experimental evidence that have led to the account of the action potential just given. That is to say, the evidence suggests that $Na^+$ ions constitute the inward movement of positive ions, measured as depolarization (which occurs because of a rapid but short-lived increase in the permeability of the cell membrane to $Na^+$). $K^+$ ions constitute the outward movement of positive ions, observed as repolarization and hyperpolarization (due to a slow but sustained increase in the permeability of the cell membrane to $K^+$). The ions responsible for these changes in polarity can be identified by changing their concentrations outside the axon. For example, if $Na^+$ is removed from the external fluid, the inward flow of positive ions, depolarization, is eliminated.

Such experiments show that, during depolarization, it is $Na^+$ permeability that increases. Experiments can also be carried out to demonstrate that the outward movement of positive ions, seen as repolarization and hyperpolarization, is constituted by $K^+$.

It is possible, by application of various chemical substances (whose names you should not try to remember), to distinguish the $Na^+$ and $K^+$ phases of ionic movement. Tetrodotoxin (TTX) is a poison obtained from some species of fish such as the puffer fishes (*Tetraodon*). It binds to the membrane $Na^+$ channel and blocks it. If an axon is bathed in TTX, there is no inward movement of positive ions following artificial depolarization but the delayed outward movement of $K^+$ is unaffected. If the interior of an axon is perfused with TTX, the inward movement of ions is not blocked, indicating that TTX must block $Na^+$ channels at the outside of the membrane. Whereas TTX selectively blocks the movement of $Na^+$, the substance tetraethylammonium (TEA) blocks $K^+$ movement across the membrane.

☐   What would you expect to see after applying TEA to an axon and then artificially depolarizing it?

■ The membrane $K^+$ channels would be blocked. The rising, $Na^+$-dependent phase of the action potential would be seen but not the repolarizing phase.

Such artificial dissection of the components of the action potential has enabled the natural sequence of events to be better understood.

A recently devised technique allows membrane potentials to be monitored by the use of voltage-sensitive dyes. These dyes change their optical properties according to the potential of the membrane to which they are bound and so can be used to follow the depolarization and hyperpolarization of neuronal membranes in brain slice preparations. Of course, the optical changes produced are very small, and very sophisticated equipment coupled with computerized enhancement techniques is required in order to observe them.

So much for the artificial stimulation of an action potential by applying an electrical voltage, but by now you might be wondering in what way this account can be related to how action potentials arise under natural conditions. Cast your mind back to the discussion of synaptic transmission in Section 2.3.3.

☐ What determines whether an action potential will arise at the axon hillock?

■ If the combined effect of the excitatory postsynaptic potentials (EPSPs) is sufficient to reach the threshold, an action potential will arise.

# 3.7 The action potential: overview

Now, you can think of the action potential in terms of a small number of concepts. Depolarization, if large enough to reach the threshold, opens $Na^+$ channels and an action potential occurs: the membrane potential moves from the resting potential of about $-70\,mV$ towards a potential of about $+20\,mV$ (Figure 3.10, p. 56). The $Na^+$ channels close after less than a millisecond, and the membrane voltage returns to the resting potential as a result of the voltage-gated $K^+$ channels opening.

☐ What features of the population of voltage-gated $K^+$ channels contribute to the explanation of the period of membrane hyperpolarization in the last phase of an action potential?

■ (a) They open later than the $Na^+$ channels as the membrane potential rises from $-70$ mV to zero.

(b) The $K^+$ ion conductance of the voltage-gated $K^+$ channels is greater than the passive $K^+$ channels.

(c) The voltage-gated $K^+$ ion channels stay open for a relatively long period after $Na^+$ ions have stopped flowing.

As a first approximation, such a sequence of events helps us understand what happens when an action potential is generated. The 'real-life' action potential is more complicated. But the description given so far is adequate for the needs of this course. It has highlighted the processes of channel opening and closure as vital factors in determining the state of a neuron. As well as contributing to an understanding of the action potential, an awareness of the effects of channel opening and closure can give insight into the ways that drugs and other chemicals can exert their influence upon the nervous system—by opening, closing or blocking channels for specific ion types.

## 3.8   Propagation of the action potential

The discussion so far has been concerned with the molecular events that cause a localized 'patch' of membrane to change its electrical potential in the form of an action potential. However, as you have seen already, the action potential travels along the axon. How does this occur?

Consider first the resting membrane and then imagine applying a local disturbance to the membrane potential so as to move it away from the resting potential at just one site. This localized disturbance will tend to affect neighbouring regions of membrane. A local change in membrane potential is 'broadcast' to surrounding regions of membrane but falls off rapidly with distance—it shows degradation. Figure 3.12 shows that local changes in membrane potential are broadcast but become diminished over distance.

☐   Where have you already met such a decrease in the magnitude of a change in membrane potential?

■   Receptor potentials and synaptic potentials discussed in Section 2.4.1, both show a similar decrease over distance.

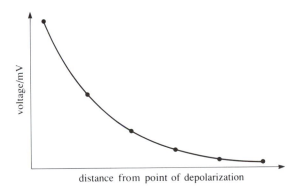

**Figure 3.12**   The effect of a local change in membrane potential falls off rapidly with distance.

☐   Figure 3.12 shows that the effects of a change in potential at one point in a membrane are 'broadcast' around that point. What are the logical implications of this for the transmission of action potentials?

■   The depolarization phase of the action potential will depolarize neighbouring regions of membrane. Depolarization opens $Na^+$ channels. Therefore, logically, the depolarization phase of an action potential might be expected to open voltage-gated receptors on either side of the point on the membrane undergoing the action potential.

Suppose that an action potential has been initiated at the axon hillock (see Figure 3.13). The membrane is rapidly depolarizing. This depolarization at the axon hillock will spread out and depolarize neighbouring regions. The axon contains voltage-gated $Na^+$ channels but the cell body does not. Depolarization at the axon hillock will cause depolarization to each side. Once this depolarization reaches the threshold level it will cause the voltage-gated $Na^+$ channels in the patch of axon membrane immediately adjacent to the axon hillock to open and $Na^+$ ions to move into the axon at this region.

☐  Imagine that the membrane just adjacent to the axon hillock (labelled X in Figure 3.13) has been depolarized by the action potential at the axon hillock. This depolarization reaches threshold at location X. What is the effect on membrane potential at X?

■  By depolarization reaching threshold at X, in effect, a new action potential is initiated at region X just adjacent to the axon hillock.

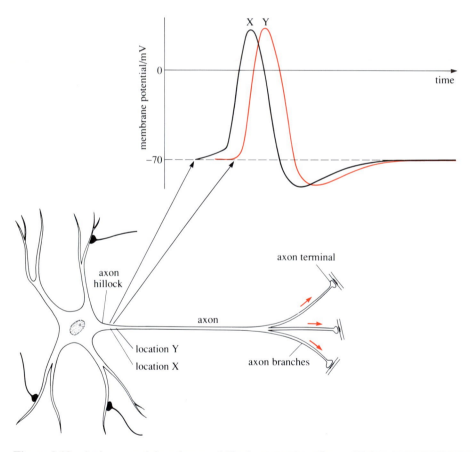

**Figure 3.13**   Action potentials at the axon hillock, at a region of axon (X) just to the right of the axon hillock and at a region of axon (Y) slightly farther away.

The newly created action potential at X will in turn induce depolarization at a region of axon slightly farther away from the axon hillock (location Y). At the point in time where an action potential arises at Y, the action potential is complete at the axon hillock. The action potential therefore moves along the axon. Events happening at small but discrete chunks of axon, X and Y, are used here as an aid to explanation. Whether you prefer to think in terms of such chunks or, more realistically, to consider a smooth transition of the action potential along the axon is a matter of personal taste and style of imagination.

In practice, an action potential only travels in one direction along an axon. For example, in Figure 3.13, it travels away from the axon hillock. Having got some way along an axon, the action potential keeps going! It does not double back to the axon hillock again. In sensory organs, the action potential simply travels away from the sensory organ to the central nervous system. However, if an axon is artificially stimulated at some point along its length to induce an action potential, an instant later *two* action potentials will be observed, one travelling in each direction away from the point of stimulation.

Why 'in real life' does an action potential travel in only one direction? In Figure 3.13 when the action potential has reached Y, why does it not induce a new action potential that travels to X and back to the axon hillock? The reason lies in a property of the voltage-gated $Na^+$ channels. These are normally closed, then they open, corresponding to the depolarization phase of the action potential. They then close again. Having closed, they are then unable to re-open for a while. They are said to be *refractory* and to be so for long enough to stop them being reactivated by an action potential travelling away from them. Imagine that in Figure 3.13, at the time the action potential has reached point Y, the channels in the membrane between the axon hillock and X are still refractory to opening.

The period after the $Na^+$ voltage-gated channels have opened and closed and during which they cannot be re-opened is called the **absolute refractory period**.

The speed at which an action potential travels along an axon, called the **conduction velocity**, depends on a number of factors. One determinant of conduction velocity is the diameter of the axon. Velocity is proportional to the diameter of the axon: the greater the diameter, the faster the conduction. Another determinant is whether or not the axons are sheathed with myelin (Section 2.4.4). In the peripheral nervous system, axons of sensory and motor neurons, and, in the central nervous system, axons which travel relatively long distances interconnecting different brain regions are sheathed with myelin, an insulating fatty substance. Myelin presents a barrier to the exchange of ions between the inside and outside of the membrane (see Figure 3.14, *overleaf*).

In the peripheral nervous system the myelin is made by cells called **Schwann cells** which wrap a myelin coating around the axon, as described in Section 2.4.4. In the central nervous system, myelin is provided by a different type of cell called an oligodendrocyte. The chemical characteristics of central and peripheral myelin differ. It has been suggested that this difference is one reason why peripheral axons recover from damage whereas central axons do not.

Examine Figure 3.14b. Note that the axon is coated by myelin-providing cells which sheathe it with a spiral of myelin layers. There is a small gap between the successive myelin sheaths. The gap is termed a node of Ranvier. Nodes of Ranvier occur every 1–2 mm and are about 2 μm in length. The myelin sheaths and nodes of Ranvier play a crucial role in the propagation of an action potential, as described below.

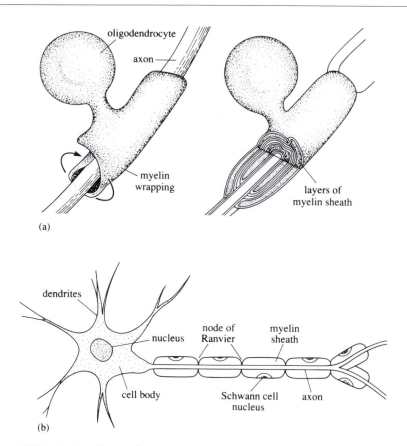

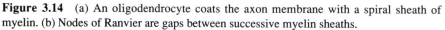

**Figure 3.14** (a) An oligodendrocyte coats the axon membrane with a spiral sheath of myelin. (b) Nodes of Ranvier are gaps between successive myelin sheaths.

The story that has just been developed, showing how an action potential travels smoothly along an axon, involved an axon lacking myelin. A neuron that has no myelin is said to be *unmyelinated*. The presence of myelin changes in one important respect the mode of transmission of the action potential, as follows.

Despite their small size, the membrane patches exposed at the nodes of Ranvier have a high density of voltage-gated $Na^+$ channels. The action potential is unable to progress along the region of axon covered by the insulating myelin. So, instead of smoothly invading each successive patch of membrane as in unmyelinated axons, in myelinated axons action potentials jump from one node of Ranvier to the next. This speeds up conduction velocity considerably compared with unmyelinated axons of the same diameter.

# 3.9 Receptor-gated channels: EPSPs and IPSPs

This account so far has described voltage-gated channels in the membrane and how they play a role in the action potential. It was introduced by considering the artificial stimulation of an action potential by application of an electric current. When the question of what triggers action potentials at the axon hillock under natural conditions was discussed, the summation of EPSPs was mentioned. EPSPs will be discussed in detail in Chapter 4. However, it is important to look at one aspect of them in the context of the account given of forces moving ions across the membrane and through ion channels in the membrane.

To do this and to complete the picture, a further class of channel—**receptor-gated channels**—must be introduced because these provide the major mechanism by which, under natural conditions, the neuron receives its input of information. One neuron releases transmitter and specialized receptors on a second neuron are activated. It is these receptors that are the subject of this section. These receptors are protein molecules the shape of which determines whether the channel is opened or closed.

Essentially, a receptor-gated channel is a membrane channel whose state of opening is dependent upon whether an associated receptor site is activated by its specific transmitter molecule. You should recall from Section 2.3.3 that these receptor sites are located on postsynaptic membranes. A neuron's information comes through the activation of receptors on its cell body or dendrites. Such activation consists of the opening or closing of ion channels. The effect of the transmitter being attached to its receptor is that the complex protein molecule forming the channel changes its shape. When the channel is open, ions, such as $Na^+$, are able to move across the membrane down their gradients. It is such flows of ions that are revealed as excitatory postsynaptic potentials.

You should recall from Section 3.6 that the voltage-gated channels found in the axon membrane, which play a crucial role in the generation of action potentials, are paths for specific ions. The specificity is determined partly by their size and partly by the chemical properties of the molecules that form the 'hole' through the membrane. The receptor-gated channels responsible for synaptic potentials—EPSPs and IPSPs—often show less specificity for the ions that flow through them. Some receptor-gated channels allow $Na^+$, $K^+$ and other ions all to flow through a single channel whereas others are specific to ions such as $Cl^-$ (chloride) or $Ca^{2+}$ (calcium—here the ion has a double positive charge, represented as $^{2+}$). Some receptor-gated channels have been demonstrated to close rather than open in response to the activation of their receptor site.

☐ Suppose that a population of receptor-gated channels in a particular region of membrane is specific to $Na^+$ ions. Activation of this population by transmitter opens $Na^+$ channels in the membrane. What will be the effect on ion flows at the region when transmitter attaches itself to the receptor?

■ $Na^+$ ions will move into the neuron at the local site. This is because both membrane potential and concentration gradient are in a direction to cause such movement.

□ Will this movement of Na$^+$ ions into the neuron have a local depolarizing or hyperpolarizing effect?

■ The movement will have a depolarizing effect. Positive charge moving into the neuron will make the inside less negative.

Opening of other channels can have a hyperpolarizing effect by, for example, allowing negative charge into the neuron or allowing K$^+$ to escape. The details of this need not concern you. However, in Chapter 4, when the discussion turns to EPSPs and IPSPs, you will be in a position to understand the basis of these changes of potential in terms of flows of ions across the membrane.

When a transmitter substance activates receptor-gated channels, it modifies the permeability of the membrane to a particular type of ion (or ions). Channel opening or closure will modify the membrane potential by causing it to move either towards the threshold or away from it. To describe the process simply, positive ions flowing into the cell will make the inside more positive (i.e. they will depolarize the cell), thereby taking the potential towards the threshold. In other words, they produce an EPSP. Negatively charged ions flowing into the cell will have the opposite effect; they will make the cell more negative (i.e. they will hyperpolarize the cell). In other words, they produce an IPSP.

# 3.10   The neuron: overview

The subject of this chapter has been the neuron's excitability—its capacity to generate and propagate action potentials. The chapter gave an explanation of the excitability of the neuron using a relatively small number of concepts. The specialized structures of the cell membrane, the voltage-gated channels and receptor-gated channels are central to this explanation. Under resting conditions, the membrane is largely impermeable to all ions except K$^+$ and Cl$^-$. At the resting value, the inside of the membrane is negative with respect to the outside, and the membrane potential is about $-70$ mV.

The effect of synaptic input to the cell, EPSPs and IPSPs, mediated by receptor-gated channels, is to change the membrane potential at the axon hillock. If the net effect of EPSPs is greater than that of IPSPs, this may activate voltage-gated Na$^+$ channels at the axon hillock sufficiently to initiate an action potential. The action potential has three phases. The first, depolarization, is dominated by the inward flow of Na$^+$ ions as the membrane potential moves in a positive direction. This first phase is terminated by the abrupt closure of the Na$^+$ channels. The second phase, repolarization, is dominated by K$^+$ outward flows through the voltage-gated K$^+$ channels. The third phase, hyperpolarization, is characterized by the membrane potential falling below the resting potential under the influence of the ion flows through the voltage-gated K$^+$ channels and then returning to the resting membrane potential as these voltage-gated channels close.

□ From the preceding discussions, can you think of a feature that distinguishes the membrane of the cell body and dendrites from the membrane of the axon?

■ The major difference is that the cell body and dendrites do not possess voltage-gated channels. The channels that are responsible for the generation of IPSPs and EPSPs are receptor-gated and their effects do not propagate across the dendrites and cell body at constant strength (unlike action potentials). Rather they influence the axon hillock by conduction of potentials in a way that falls off with distance (Section 2.3.3).

The converse is not true—axons have both voltage-gated channels and receptor-gated channels. The receptor-gated channels are usually sited close to the axon terminals, a topic of Chapter 4.

Figure 3.15 summarizes the electrical phenomena of the action potential and its transmission that this chapter set out to describe and explain. It does so by taking a slightly different perspective to that you have met already. The graph should look somewhat familiar as the action potential. However, this time it is different in one important respect. The action potentials shown earlier represented what happened at one particular location on the axon, the site of the recording electrode, and were shown as a function of time. Figure 3.15 shows electrical events over a wider section of axon at a particular instant of time. If the same imaginary photograph were to be taken a split second later, region 1 would be depolarized and region 2 hyperpolarized.

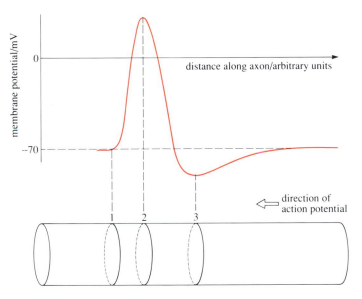

**Figure 3.15** Imaginary split-second photograph of the changes in membrane potential as an action potential passes. The action potential is moving from right to left. Region 1 of the membrane is still at the resting potential; region 2 is depolarized; and region 3 is hyperpolarized.

☐ What is the state of the voltage-gated channels at region 1 and to the left of it at the point in time illustrated in Figure 3.15?

■ They are closed since the membrane potential is at its resting value. However, unlike the region just to the right of 2, they are capable of being opened. An action potential has not just passed that section of axon.

☐ What effect does depolarization at region 2 have upon region 1?

■ Depolarization at region 2 induces depolarization at region 1. Voltage-gated $Na^+$ channels are opened at region 1.

☐ Given that the depolarization occurring at region 2 tends to depolarize the membrane by an equal amount on each side, why is it that the action potential only moves from right to left? Why is it that, when region 1 is depolarized, another action potential does not arise at location 2 on the membrane, i.e. going from left to right?

■ When region 1 is depolarized, region 2 will just have undergone an action potential. Even after it has returned to its resting potential, the $Na^+$ channels at region 2 will be refractory to further opening for a while. By the time they have regained their ability to open, the action potential will be way past to the left. It will have gone too far to exert sufficient depolarizing effect to induce a new action potential.

☐ What determines the speed with which the action potential moves along the axon?

■ (a) The axon's diameter—the larger this is, the faster the action potential—and (b) whether the axon is myelinated.

☐ From the account just given, is the axon in Figure 3.15 myelinated or unmyelinated?

■ Simply because no myelin is shown, you might reasonably have guessed that it is unmyelinated! However, the account was one of a smooth transition from right to left, rather than jumping from one node of Ranvier to another, which confirms it as an unmyelinated axon.

☐ Under resting conditions, there is a leakage of $Na^+$ ions into the cell and of $K^+$ ions out. With each action potential, additional $Na^+$ ions are introduced into the cell and $K^+$ ions escape. Long-term maintenance of ion segregation requires what?

■ A sodium–potassium pump that expels $Na^+$ ions and retrieves $K^+$ ions.

# Summary of Chapter 3

The electrical properties of neurons result from the ability of ions to move in and out of the cells. Such movement takes place through selective ion channels in the cell membrane.

The resting potential of a neuron membrane, that is, when it is not transmitting action potentials, is about $-70\,mV$. This resting potential is maintained in part by the activity of the sodium–potassium pump. The pump consists of specialized types of ion channels that help to maintain the membrane potential. The membrane pump moves ions across the cell membrane against the gradients that tend to move them the other way and therefore requires a supply of energy in order to operate. The sodium–potassium pump moves $Na^+$ ions out of the cell and $K^+$ ions in.

Ion channels that open only transiently in response to a specific stimulus are called gated channels. Voltage-gated channels open in response to specific changes in the membrane potential. Receptor-gated channels open or close as a result of transmitter occupying the receptor site associated with the channel.

An action potential is a sudden reversal of the resting potential across the neuronal membrane. Action potentials arise due to the ability of neurons to change their membrane ion permeability rapidly. If the axon membrane is depolarized and if this depolarization exceeds the threshold value, an action potential results. Action potentials operate on the all-or-none principle, that is, whatever the size of the applied stimulus, as long as it depolarizes the membrane beyond the threshold value, exactly the same size of action potential results.

The refractory period follows an action potential. It means that, under normal physiological conditions, an action potential passes along an axon in one direction only.

Axons may be myelinated or unmyelinated. In unmyelinated axons, the action potential travels smoothly along the axon. In myelinated axons, the action potential jumps from one node of Ranvier to the next. For a given diameter of axon, the action potential travels faster along a myelinated axon than along an unmyelinated axon.

# Objectives for Chapter 3

When you have completed this chapter, you should be able to:

3.1 Define and use, or recognize, definitions and applications of each of the terms printed in bold in the text. (*Question 3.1*)

3.2 Describe the principal differences in ion concentrations between the inside and outside of a neuron. (*Question 3.1*)

3.3 Describe how concentration gradients and the membrane potential are relevant to understanding movements of ions across the neuron membrane. (*Questions 3.1 and 3.2*)

3.4 Explain briefly the role of the sodium–potassium pump in maintaining the resting state of a neuron. (*Question 3.2*)

3.5 Explain how an action potential arises in terms of membrane potential and membrane ion permeability. (*Questions 3.3 and 3.5*)

3.6 Describe how an action potential travels along an axon and what influences its speed. (*Question 3.6*)

3.7 Describe the refractory period and explain why it is responsible for the one-way transmission of action potentials. (*Question 3.7*)

# Questions for Chapter 3

### Question 3.1 (*Objectives 3.1, 3.2 and 3.3*)
Which of the descriptions (a)–(c) gives an accurate representation of the differences in ion concentration across the neuron membrane?

Description (a)

| Ion | Inside | Outside |
|-----|--------|---------|
| $Na^+$ | high | low |
| $K^+$ | high | low |
| $Cl^-$ | low | high |

Description (b)

| Ion | Inside | Outside |
|-----|--------|---------|
| $Na^+$ | low | high |
| $K^+$ | high | low |
| $Cl^-$ | high | low |

Description (c)

| Ion | Inside | Outside |
|-----|--------|---------|
| $Na^+$ | low | high |
| $K^+$ | high | low |
| $Cl^-$ | low | high |

### Question 3.2 (*Objectives 3.3 and 3.4*)
Which of the following statements are true?

(a) In the resting neuron, the tendency for the concentration gradient of $K^+$ to move $K^+$ ions out of the cell is slightly stronger than the tendency of the membrane potential to pull them in.

(b) In the resting neuron, as far as $Na^+$ ions are concerned, the membrane potential and concentration gradient act in the same direction.

(c) A sodium–potassium pump expels $Na^+$ ions from the inside of the neuron and retrieves $K^+$ ions from the outside.

(d) Both $Na^+$ and $K^+$ ions carry a positive charge.

### Question 3.3 (*Objective 3.5*)
Which of the following statements are true?

(a) The initial rising phase of the action potential (depolarization) is due to the opening of voltage-gated $Na^+$ channels.

(b)  The initial rising phase of the action potential is due to the closure of K$^+$ channels.

(c)  The end of the rising phase of the action potential is due in part to the closure of the Na$^+$ channels.

(d)  The repolarizing phase of the action potential is due to K$^+$ ions being expelled from the cell by the sodium–potassium pump.

(e)  The hyperpolarizing phase of the action potential is due to a delay in closure of voltage-gated K$^+$ channels.

## Question 3.4 (*Objectives 3.3 and 3.5*)
Which of the following statements are true?

(a)  An EPSP is a move by the local membrane potential away from the resting potential (about −70 mV) to a less negative value.

(b)  An IPSP is a move of the local membrane potential away from the resting potential to a more negative value.

(c)  An EPSP could be caused by an opening of receptor-gated channels that allows an increased flow of positive ions into the cell.

(d)  An EPSP could be caused by an opening of receptor-gated channels that allows an increased flow of negative ions out of the cell.

(e)  An EPSP could be caused by an opening of receptor-gated channels that allows an increased flow of negative ions into the cell.

(f)  An IPSP could be caused by an opening of receptor-gated channels that allows an increased flow of positive ions out of the cell.

## Question 3.5 (*Objective 3.5*)
The following is an account of the events underlying the action potential given by a hypothetical SD206 student. Where has the student gone wrong?

An artificial stimulus is applied to depolarize the membrane. When the threshold is reached, a sudden swing in a positive direction occurs. Voltage-gated Na$^+$ channels in the membrane open and Na$^+$ ions move into the cell. This is the depolarization phase of the action potential, in other words, a move of membrane potential from a negative value to a less negative (or more positive value). This move in a positive direction is halted when the Na$^+$ channels close and the K$^+$ channels open. The sodium–potassium pump is then responsible for very rapidly moving Na$^+$ ions out of the cell and this underlies the repolarization phase of the action potential.

## Question 3.6 (*Objective 3.6*)
Which of the following influence the speed at which an action potential is transmitted along an axon?

(a)  Whether or not an action potential has recently been generated in the neuron.

(b)  The diameter of the axon.

(c)     Whether or not the axon is myelinated.

(d)     The rate at which $Na^+$ is being pumped out of the cell at the instant of passage of the action potential.

(e)     The length of the axon.

(f)     The balance of EPSPs and IPSPs that initiated the action potential in the first place.

## Question 3.7 (*Objective 3.7*)

The reason given for why an action potential normally only travels one way along an axon is to do with the refractory period. However, if an axon is artificially stimulated at a point somewhere between its two ends, two action potentials can be observed, one moving in each direction away from the point of stimulation. Is it possible to reconcile these two phenomena in terms of an account involving the refractory period?

# CHAPTER 4
# THE NEURON: SYNAPTIC TRANSMISSION

## 4.1  Introduction

Chapter 3 looked in detail at the transmission of information *within* a neuron, carried by action potentials. This chapter considers the junction *between* neurons, the point at which activity in one neuron influences the activity of another, i.e. the synapse. As you saw in Chapters 1 and 2, individual neurons and collections of neurons serve as processors of information. To understand how information is processed, it is necessary to look closely at the properties of the point of contact between neurons.

So how does the electrical activity in one neuron influence the activity in another? Nervous systems employ two means for doing this, the relatively simple but uncommon electrical synapse and the more complex but ubiquitous chemical synapse, which has been discussed already in this book. At the electrical synapse, the presynaptic membrane makes direct contact with the postsynaptic membrane. There is no gap and no storage or release of chemicals. Depolarization in the presynaptic neuron simply causes depolarization in the postsynaptic neuron. As you saw in Section 2.3.1, at the chemical synapse, chemical transmitter is released from one neuron and influences another at receptors on the postsynaptic membrane. This might seem a cumbersome way for one neuron to affect another when the electrical synapse seems so simple. So how can the rareness of electrical synapses be explained? The electrical synapse is a simple and highly effective way for action potentials in one neuron to induce them in another. However, the nervous system does much more than simply pass on action potentials from one neuron to another. Systems of neurons can do much more in the way of processing information by employing chemical synapses. As you saw in Chapter 2, at a given neuron, activation of one type of receptor by transmitter from one neuron will excite the cell whereas activation of another type by transmitter from another neuron will inhibit it.

An example from earlier in the course can illustrate how this property is needed in order to process information. The discussion of drinking in Book 1, Chapter 7, concluded with a diagram similar to that shown in Figure 4.1a. Drinking motivation is assumed to be determined by both excitatory factors (dehydration of intracellular and extracellular fluids) and inhibitory factors (e.g. a stomach full of water, the passage of water through the mouth for a period of time). This clearly requires the processing of different items of information by the brain. How do some events increase drinking motivation and others lower it? The answer is most probably by means of a system of neurons. The most simple way of envisaging this kind of processing is shown in Figure 4.1b. A neuron has both excitatory and inhibitory inputs at chemical synapses. The activity of the neuron depends upon the balance between excitation and inhibition.

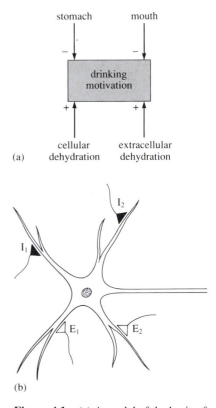

**Figure 4.1**  (a) A model of the basis of the determination of drinking motivation, and (b) suggested way in which neurons could process this kind of information. Excitatory inputs are made at $E_1$ and $E_2$; inhibitory inputs at $I_1$ and $I_2$.

This chapter will extend the discussions in Chapters 2 and 3 by looking in detail at the neuron as a chemical device, that is, at the way it responds to and produces the chemical messages called transmitters. The synapse is where the activity of one neuron can influence that of another, either to depolarize or hyperpolarize it, as described in Section 3.9.

This chapter examines the variety of chemical transmitters, synaptic structures and synaptic transmission within the nervous system from the point of view of how information is processed by neurons. Its aim is to show you that insight into the chemical events at the synapse is necessary in order to understand the interactions that take place within the nervous system and the properties of the system that emerge from these interactions.

# 4.2 Transmitters and receptors: chemical locks and keys

The process of chemical transmission is summarized in schematic form in Figure 4.2. At the synapse, the frequency of all-or-none action potentials arriving at the presynaptic terminal is translated into a graded release of transmitter chemical. When the action potential reaches the terminal of the axon, this depolarization causes the opening of voltage-gated *calcium* channels in the presynaptic membrane. (These $Ca^{2+}$ channels are similar to those described for sodium in Chapter 3.) $Ca^{2+}$ diffuses into the presynaptic terminal, which triggers the release of chemical transmitter at the synapse.

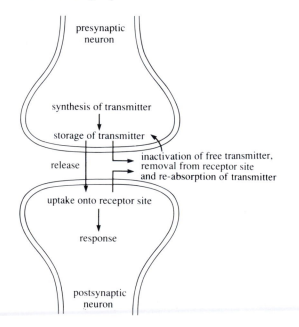

**Figure 4.2** Schematic representation of the processes involved in synaptic transmission.

Transmitter molecules move across the synaptic cleft (the gap separating the presynaptic and postsynaptic neurons) by diffusion and attach to specific receptors at the postsynaptic site. The rest of this section will examine the mechanisms by which transmitter release is triggered, taking the neuromuscular junction as a model, and discuss the binding of transmitter molecules to their postsynaptic receptors. Vertebrate and invertebrate synapses are very similar both morphologically, that is, structurally, and electrophysiologically, that is, functionally. It is thought that the similarities also extend to the biochemical events underlying transmitter release.

## 4.2.1 Transmitter release mechanisms

As explained in Chapter 2, chemical synapses are unidirectional, that is, they transmit information in one direction only. Such information travels from one neuron to another or from one neuron to a muscle fibre. By definition, it is always the case that activity of the presynaptic cell influences the activity of the postsynaptic cell. The arrival of an action potential at the terminal of the presynaptic neuron causes the release of a chemical transmitter from that terminal (see Figure 4.3). The transmitter chemical rapidly diffuses across the synaptic cleft and then influences the postsynaptic cell.

One feature that distinguishes chemical from electrical synapses is that, in chemical synapses, there is a delay between the arrival of an action potential at the presynaptic terminal and any effect that this brings about in the postsynaptic cell. This is due to the time it takes for transmitter to be released and diffuse across the synaptic cleft. This **synaptic delay**, as it is called, is generally of the order of about 0.5 ms.

Chemical transmitters are released from specific areas of the presynaptic cells which appear with the use of the electron microscope like swellings and are called axon terminals or terminal boutons (Section 2.3.1). Transmitter chemicals are both synthesized and stored within neurons. When a transmitter is released from the presynaptic site, it moves across the synaptic cleft and attaches to a receptor site on the postsynaptic cell membrane. This binding to the receptor changes the permeability of the postsynaptic membrane by opening or closing ion channels and this in turn changes the membrane potential of that cell. If the postsynaptic membrane becomes *depolarized* it is said to be excited and action potentials are more likely to occur. If, however, the postsynaptic membrane becomes *hyperpolarized*, it is said to be inhibited and action potentials are less likely to occur than when the neuron is unstimulated.

## 4.2.2 Cholinergic function

Probably the most extensively studied and well understood of all the chemical transmitters is acetylcholine, often abbreviated to ACh. Synapses where the transmitter released at the axon terminal is ACh are called **cholinergic**. The following sections will therefore refer most frequently to the cholinergic synapse. The principles arising from this discussion, however, are more generally applicable.

ACh is important in both neuronal and neuromuscular transmission. It is the chemical most commonly referred to in descriptions and discussions of synaptic transmission and its release at the neuromuscular junction will be described in

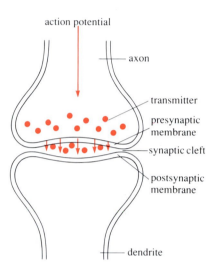

**Figure 4.3** A simplified diagram of chemical transmission. An action potential arriving at the presynaptic membrane triggers the release of chemical transmitter through the membrane. The transmitter diffuses across the synaptic cleft and influences the postsynaptic membrane.

Section 4.2.4. However, it should be borne in mind that ACh is only one of many different transmitter chemicals that occur in the nervous system. At present, about forty different kinds of chemical transmitter are known to exist (e.g. dopamine, noradrenalin, $\gamma$ (gamma)-amino-butyric acid, this last abbreviated to GABA) and it is likely that many more remain to be discovered. (The roles of these particular transmitters and others are discussed in Sections 4.2.5 and 4.5.)

It used to be thought that any given presynaptic cell is capable of releasing only one specific kind of transmitter molecule from its various axon terminals. Nowadays more and more research papers are being published showing that many neurons can release a variety of transmitters, depending upon the state of the cell and the nature of the action potentials that it receives. When a transmitter is released, it causes the postsynaptic cell, whose receptors it binds with, to alter its membrane permeability to specific ions. As an excitatory transmitter at the neuromuscular junction, ACh produces a large increase in the permeability of the postsynaptic cell membrane to positively charged ions (cations) but does not affect its permeability to negatively charged ions (anions). Although each transmitter molecule only binds to one channel receptor, a very small amount of transmitter can greatly alter the permeability of the postsynaptic cell membrane and this fact illustrates one of the most important properties of chemical transmitters—they provide the potential for *amplification* of the signal that they are transmitting.

## 4.2.3 Synaptic vesicles

Neurotransmitter molecules are synthesized within neurons and are then stored at the terminal (i.e. just before the presynaptic membrane) in 'packets' called synaptic vesicles.

How is the release of a transmitter triggered and what is the role of these vesicles? When an action potential travels down an axon and reaches the presynaptic terminal, this causes voltage-gated calcium ion ($Ca^{2+}$) channels in the presynaptic neuron to open. Normally, the extracellular calcium concentration far exceeds the intracellular concentration and so, once the channels are open, $Ca^{2+}$ enters the cell.

☐   How does $Ca^{2+}$ enter the cell?

■   It moves down both potential and concentration gradients. (Sections 3.2.2 and 3.3).

As with $Na^+$ channels, it is a change in the shape of the $Ca^{2+}$ channel proteins that opens up the pores through the membrane. The resulting local increase in $Ca^{2+}$ concentration inside the cell at the terminal triggers the release of neurotransmitter molecules by exocytosis (Section 2.2.2). Exocytosis is a process by which the synaptic vesicles fuse with the presynaptic membrane and their contents, the neurotransmitter molecules, then diffuse out into the synaptic cleft. This is illustrated in Figure 4.4. Exocytosis can be followed morphologically using the electron microscope but the molecular details of exactly how it occurs are still not well understood. Transmitter molecules are thus released in 'vesicles-full' or discrete amounts called quanta, each vesicle containing several thousand molecules of neurotransmitter chemical. The number of quanta that are released depends on how many action potentials arrive.

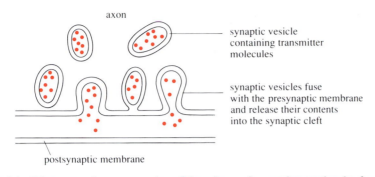

**Figure 4.4**   Diagrammatic representation of the release of transmitter molecules from the presynaptic membrane by exocytosis.

As soon as transmitter begins to be released into the synaptic cleft, it also begins to be removed. This removal may be by enzymic breakdown of the transmitter molecules or by their being taken up again into the presynaptic cell or into non-neuronal glial cells by **endocytosis**, a process which is the reverse of exocytosis. Re-uptake mechanisms can enable transmitter molecules to be released, recaptured and reused many times over. Another consequence of transmitter breakdown or re-uptake is that the postsynaptic cell receives a sharp signal which is in proportion to the electrical stimulus that triggered it, rather than a long and diffuse signal. Were it not for such mechanisms of removal of transmitter, then any transmitter released by activity in the presynaptic cell would 'hang around' for some time. Thus it would prove impossible for the presynaptic cell to effect a sharp change in activity of the postsynaptic cell.

☐   Given that there is a process of removal of transmitter, under what conditions will there be sustained activity in the postsynaptic cell (neuron or muscle)?

■   This will occur in response to *sustained* activity in the presynaptic neuron.

Obviously, a train of action potentials will produce a greater release of transmitter than a single action potential. This larger amount of transmitter translates into a larger and more sustained signal to the postsynaptic cell. In this way, the frequency of electrical impulses determines the size and duration of the chemical signal that is transmitted.

## 4.2.4   Acetylcholine release at the neuromuscular junction

Acetylcholine (ACh) can transmit signals between neurons and between neurons and muscle cells. Its action at the neuromuscular junction (Section 2.4.2) has been extensively studied and will be described here as a model of neurotransmitter release. But you should remember that the neuromuscular junction represents a specialized kind of synapse and also that ACh is only one of many different chemical transmitters.

Very small amounts of ACh are continuously being released at the neuromuscular junction, even when the presynaptic neuron terminal is at resting potential. This can be shown experimentally by measuring the small fluctuations in postsynaptic membrane potential, of the order of 0.5 to 1 mV, that occur even when the presynaptic membrane is not receiving any action potentials. Such small fluctuations are termed miniature postsynaptic potentials and occur in discrete multiples, or quanta, for example, 0.5 mV, 1 mV, 1.5 mV, etc. This means that they can be of a particular strength, twice that strength, three times that strength, etc. These findings led to the realization that synaptic vesicles release neurotransmitter molecules in quanta. The presynaptic vesicles that contain ACh can be seen with the electron microscope. In 1956, J. del Castillo and B. Katz put forward the hypothesis that these vesicles are in constant random motion within the axon at its terminal. This motion means that every so often a vesicle will come into contact with the presynaptic membrane. Such contact initiates exocytosis, ACh is released into the synaptic cleft, and a miniature postsynaptic potential results. When an action potential arrives at the presynaptic membrane, the voltage-activated $Ca^{2+}$ channels open and $Ca^{2+}$ enters the cell. This is thought to increase greatly the numbers of vesicle collisions with the membrane. Consequently much more ACh is released, with greater depolarization of the postsynaptic cell membrane.

Electron microscopic studies have shown that the numbers of vesicles in the presynaptic cells are greatly reduced following the passage of an action potential. Following an extensive train of action potentials, the release of ACh at the neuromuscular junction declines, often quite rapidly. It seems that only a relatively small pool of ACh is readily available for release, and once this pool has been used up, the axon terminal can no longer release transmitter in response to an action potential. The rate of renewal of ACh depends on the rate of synthesis of new ACh molecules by the presynaptic cell and also the rate of recycling of already existing molecules (Section 4.2.3).

## 4.2.5  Transmitter receptors

So far, the way in which chemical transmitters are stored at and released from the presynaptic terminal and the means by which they cross the synaptic cleft. have been considered. What is the mechanism by which a transmitter molecule arriving at the postsynaptic membrane alters the ion permeability of that membrane?

Experimental investigations of ACh receptors have been enormously helped by the discovery that snake venom toxins contain chemicals that attach, or bind, specifically and strongly to them. One of the most useful of these chemicals has been α (alpha)-bungarotoxin, obtained from the venom of a snake called the krait (*Bungarus*). α-bungarotoxin has been used to isolate and identify ACh receptors.

The areas of the postsynaptic membranes that are highly sensitive to a particular transmitter have a specialized structure that can be seen with the electron microscope. The postsynaptic membrane contains receptor molecules which, by virtue of their shape, bind specifically to a particular transmitter with a complementary shape. Much neurochemical research is devoted to identifying and studying these cell-surface receptors. When ACh binds to the neuromuscular junction ACh receptors, this binding induces a change in the shape of the receptors. Their changed shape causes the opening of specific ion channels in the membrane. Thus the transmitter may be thought of as a key which, by virtue of its shape fitting a particular lock, the receptor, opens a door, the ion channel. If the shape of the transmitter molecule does not fit the shape of the postsynaptic membrane receptors, it will not be able to influence that particular cell. At a given synapse, when many transmitter 'keys' fit many receptor 'locks', then many channels are opened. Enough ions can move across the membrane to change the voltage across it significantly.(Figure 4.5).

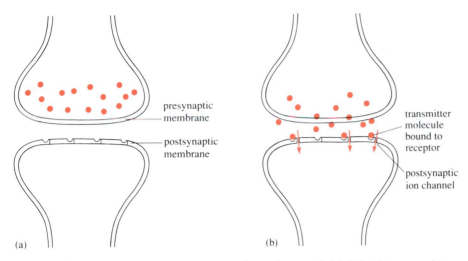

**Figure 4.5**   The synapse (a) prior to transmitter release and (b) following transmitter release, showing the action of transmitter molecules on postsynaptic membranes.

There are basically two types of postsynaptic receptor which are distinguished by how they deal with the incoming transmitter signal. Some receptor molecules are themselves ion channels which open when a transmitter binds to them and changes their shape. This opening leads to a change in the postsynaptic membrane potential, which produces excitation or inhibition of the initiation of action potentials in the postsynaptic cell. As an example of this, the ACh receptor channels mentioned previously are ion channels which mediate the effect of ACh on skeletal muscle.

The second type of receptor molecule passes the transmitted signal across the postsynaptic membrane and stimulates the production of a **second messenger** which then acts directly or indirectly to open or close ion channels in the membrane. In the brain, ACh can act on both types of receptor. Thus the effect of transmitter binding to postsynaptic receptor channels can be either direct or, via second messengers, indirect. Both types of transmitter binding ultimately control the permeability of the membrane to ions. Furthermore, the outcome of receptor binding can be either excitatory, in which case the membrane is depolarized, or inhibitory, in which case the membrane is hyperpolarized. This depends on the type of ion channel that is opened by the binding of transmitter. Transmitters activating an inhibitory synapse either prevent depolarization or decrease the magnitude of depolarization of the postsynaptic membrane by an excitatory transmitter.

At any given synapse, a particular transmitter is either excitatory *or* inhibitory, never both. However the same transmitter chemical can have opposing actions at different postsynaptic receptor sites. When released from the presynaptic terminals at neuromuscular junctions of skeletal muscles, ACh has an excitatory effect on the muscle receptors, first causing depolarization of the membrane and then causing opening of ion channels which in turn leads to muscle contraction. But at cardiac muscle receptors it has an inhibitory effect, causing the heart rate to be slowed. Within the brain, glutamate is regarded as the most important transmitter at excitatory synapses and GABA as the most important transmitter at inhibitory synapses. There also exist different kinds of receptor for the same transmitter. When bound to these different subtypes of receptor, the transmitter can activate different biochemical pathways within the cell or mediate subsequent effects on different classes of cell.

Receptor subtypes have been distinguished experimentally by their binding of pharmacological substances which affect the synapse by occupying receptor sites. Such substances are termed **agonists** and **antagonists**. Agonists are substances which mimic the effect of the natural transmitter molecule on the receptor whereas antagonists inhibit the action of the natural transmitter.

Binding of transmitter to a receptor leads to the opening or closing of membrane ion channels and changes in the membrane potential by either the direct or indirect (second messenger) mechanisms described. The change in membrane potential is called a postsynaptic potential or, in the case of muscle cells, end-plate potential. Transmitter binding to an excitatory receptor produces an excitatory postsynaptic potential (EPSP) whereas transmitter binding to an inhibitory receptor produces an inhibitory postsynaptic potential (IPSP) (See Figure 4.6). This confers the ability upon neurons to act as processors of information, which will be discussed in Section 4.3.

☐ Are the EPSP and IPSP moves towards or away from the threshold for action potential initiation?

■ The EPSP is a move towards the threshold, whereas the IPSP is a move away from it.

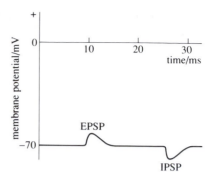

**Figure 4.6**  Excitatory and inhibitory postsynaptic potentials.

# 4.3   The neuron as an information processor

The Introduction to this chapter described a relatively simple example of the neuron as information processor. This section looks more closely at this role.

To start with, consider a neuron which is activated by a group of excitatory synapses. If enough EPSPs are produced within a limited time, the axon hillock depolarizes to the threshold level and an action potential results. In terms of processing information, this represents addition or 'summation' of the inputs to the neuron. Two kinds of such summation are distinguished, as follows.

**Temporal summation** is the term used to describe the integration within the dimension of *time* of incoming signals by the postsynaptic cell. Figure 4.7 shows an example of this. Activation of an excitatory synapse by an action potential causes an EPSP. If another action potential arrives sufficiently soon after the first, there will be an addition of the EPSPs with the result that the magnitude of depolarization is greater than that produced by a single action potential.

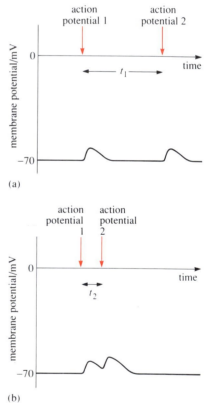

**Figure 4.7**  Temporal summation. (a) Triggering action potentials are time $t_1$ apart and two distinct EPSPs are seen. (b) Action potentials are closer together in time ($t_2$) and the EPSP produced by the first has not decayed to zero at the time the second occurs. Summation results.

**Spatial summation** is the process whereby a neuron integrates effects of synapses at different *locations* in the cell and the principle is the same as for temporal summation. Whether or not an action potential arises in the receiving neuron depends on the total amount of depolarization. Figure 4.8 represents spatial summation. Neurons 1 and 2 both make excitatory synapses upon neuron 3. Note the size of the EPSP caused by an action potential arriving at the terminal of neuron 1 or neuron 2.

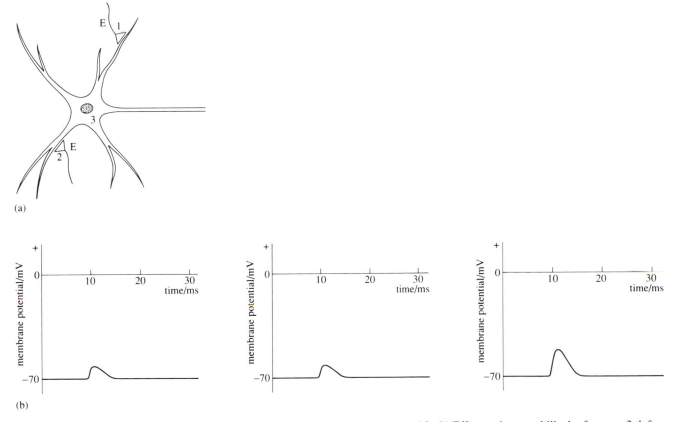

**Figure 4.8**   (a) A neuron (3) with two excitatory synapses made with neurons 1 and 2. (b) Effect at the axon hillock of neuron 3: left trace: of action potential arriving in neuron 1; middle trace: of action potential arriving in neuron 2; right trace: of action potentials arriving simultaneously at 1 and 2.

☐   What is the effect of action potentials arriving at both 1 and 2 simultaneously?

■   An additive effect on the size of the EPSP.

Temporal summation and spatial summation take place at the axon hillock.

Figure 4.9 (*overleaf*) shows a neuron with both excitatory and inhibitory synapses and the effect of action potentials arriving at each input both separately and simultaneously.

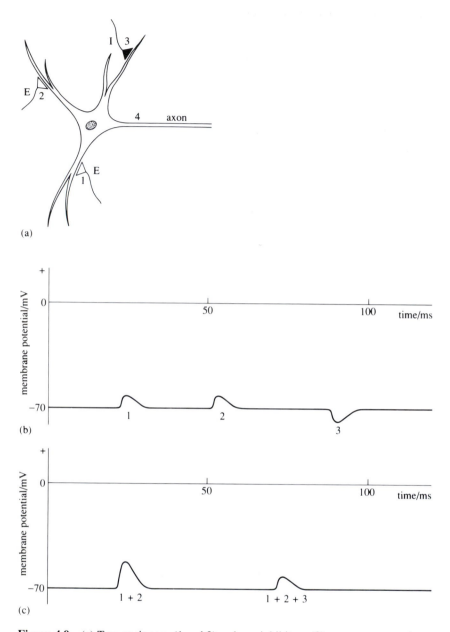

**Figure 4.9** (a) Two excitatory (1 and 2) and one inhibitory (3) synapses are made upon a neuron (4). (b) The change in membrane potential caused by stimulating each presynaptic neuron in turn. (c) The effect of stimulating 1 and 2 simultaneously and then 1, 2 and 3 simultaneously.

☐ What is the effect of the simultaneous arrival of action potentials at 1 and 2?

■ An EPSP that is greater than either 1 or 2 individually.

☐ What is the effect of action potentials arriving simultaneously at the excitatory synapses 1 and 2 and the inhibitory synapse 3?

■   An EPSP that is less than when 3 is inactive. Activity in 3 acts in the opposite direction to activity in 1 and 2.

A neuron might have many excitatory and inhibitory synapses activated simultaneously.

☐   What determines the magnitude of depolarization?

■   It is determined by the balance of activity of excitatory and inhibitory presynaptic neurons. The number of inputs is important: depolarization is more likely the larger the number of excitatory inputs and the fewer the number of inhibitory inputs.

As well as the number of inputs, the distance of each excitatory or inhibitory synapse from the axon hillock is important. For the sake of simplicity, the examples of spatial summation shown in Figures 4.8 and 4.9 assumed that all the inputs produced depolarization or hyperpolarization of about the same magnitude. As you should remember from Section 2.3.3, however, a synapse near to the axon hillock will have a greater effect on the overall amount of depolarization at the axon hillock.

To return to the simple example given in Figure 4.9, it can be seen that the magnitude of depolarization is the outcome of a balance between activity at the excitatory and inhibitory synapses. This is a simple example of the processing of information.

☐   A large depolarization in neuron 4 conveys what information?

■   A predominantly excitatory input: neurons 1 and 2 active but 3 inactive.

It has also been shown that, as well as producing immediate effects within the postsynaptic cell, neurotransmitters can also cause long-term changes such as modifying the transmission or receptor properties of that cell.

In Figure 4.9, activity in neuron 3 inhibits the effects of excitatory inputs no matter which excitatory input is active. Another type of inhibition, known as **presynaptic inhibition**, acts in a different way. In this case, activity in one neuron inhibits the effect of a *particular* excitatory input. In Figure 4.10, for example, neurons 2, 3 and 4 all excite neuron 5. Activity in neuron 1 will inhibit the effect of action potentials arriving at the terminal of neuron 2, i.e. the excitatory effects of neuron 2 will be reduced when neuron 1 is active..

☐   Suppose only neurons 3 and 4 are active. A certain level of depolarization is recorded in neuron 5. Then neuron 1 is active. What effect is seen on neuron 5?

■   None, since 1 can only inhibit the effect of 2 and 2 is not active.

An example of presynaptic inhibition is seen in the crustacean neuromuscular junction. J. Dudel and S. W. Kuffler demonstrated in the early 1960s that the amount of neurotransmitter released was decreased following electrical activity in a neuron (comparable to neuron 1 in Figure 4.10) that synapses onto the

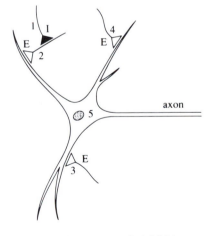

**Figure 4.10**  Presynaptic inhibition. Neurons 2, 3 and 4 form excitatory synapses on neuron 5. Presynaptic inhibition is exerted by 1 upon 2 but this inhibition is unable to influence excitation arising from 3 or 4.

presynaptic terminal. This inhibitory neuron releases GABA, triggered by the arrival at the presynaptic membrane of an action potential. In order to achieve its maximum effect, an action potential in the inhibitory neuron must reach the presynaptic terminal a few milliseconds before that in the excitatory neuron. The relative importance of presynaptic and postsynaptic inhibition (as in Figure 4.9) within the nervous system has yet to be established.

Having now read a discussion of synaptic transmission, storage, release, activation of receptors and removal of transmitter from the synapse, you are now in a position to consider the criteria for deciding whether a particular chemical is in fact a transmitter.

# 4.4   Identification of a transmitter chemical

The classical demonstration of chemical transmission was given in 1921 by Otto Loewi, a German physiologist, who bathed a frog's heart *in situ* (i.e. in place) with a saline solution similar to that which would normally bathe the heart, while electrically stimulating the vagus nerve of the frog. The vagus nerve acts to make the heart beat more slowly. Loewi collected the bathing fluid from the stimulated frog and used it to bathe the heart of a second, unstimulated frog. The unstimulated heart also beat more slowly when bathed in the fluid. He concluded that some chemical had been taken into solution in the bathing fluid that caused the unstimulated heart to respond as if its vagus nerve had been electrically stimulated. The active chemical was later shown to be ACh. Although the idea of chemical transmission between neurons and between motor neurons and muscle had been proposed towards the end of the 19th century, it was, for some time, actively discouraged by leading physiologists, who believed that all transmission was electrical in nature. Loewi gave the first convincing demonstration of the chemical nature of synaptic transmission.

The discovery of a chemical substance within a neuron is necessary for, but not conclusive proof of, the identification of that substance as a transmitter. Substances within neurons may have other functions, such as the maintenance of the basic metabolism of the cell. The following four criteria are minimal requirements for the identification of a substance as a transmitter chemical:

1   It must be synthesized within neurons and stored in their terminals.

2   It must be released into the synaptic cleft when the neuron is stimulated.

3   Receptors must be present on the postsynaptic membrane that are capable of being activated by the transmitter substance.

4   A specific inactivation process must exist to eliminate the transmitter from the synaptic cleft. For example, at the neuromuscular junction ACh is removed by being broken down by the enzyme acetylcholinesterase.

Each criterion relates to a process implicated in synaptic transmission. (These processes were represented schematically in Figure 4.2; Section 4.2.)

## Summary of Sections 4.1 to 4.4

Neurotransmitter molecules are synthesized within neurons and stored in membrane-bound synaptic vesicles. The depolarization of the action potential opens voltage-gated $Ca^{2+}$ channels at the axon terminal of the presynaptic neuron. This leads to a local increase in $Ca^{2+}$ concentration on the inside of the axon at its terminal. An increase in intracellular $Ca^{2+}$ concentration triggers the release of neurotransmitter by exocytosis of the synaptic vesicles. At the synapse, the frequency of all-or-none action potentials is translated into a graded release of neurotransmitter chemical.

There are two basic types of postsynaptic receptor for chemical transmitter molecules. Some receptors are themselves ion channels, whereas others pass the transmitted signal across the postsynaptic membrane in order to influence the release of second messenger molecules within the postsynaptic cell. These in turn affect ion channels in the postsynaptic membrane.

Binding of transmitter to an excitatory postsynaptic receptor produces an EPSP whereas binding to an inhibitory postsynaptic receptor produces an IPSP. Temporal and spatial summation refer to the integration of incoming EPSPs and IPSPs by the postsynaptic cell. Inhibition can be either postsynaptic or presynaptic. There are four criteria for deciding whether a chemical acts as a transmitter.

# 4.5   Chemical transmission and pathways in the nervous system

## 4.5.1   Introduction

The remainder of this chapter will be concerned mainly with discussing to what extent it is possible to deduce the function of the brain as a whole, in terms of physiological and behavioural responses, from knowledge of the structure and function of its component parts. In Sections 4.1 and 4.2 you learnt something about the functioning of individual neurons and how, by means of synaptic connections, they both influence and are influenced by, other neurons. This section will introduce the topic of how systems of neurons operate in a coordinated manner that depends both on the properties of the individual neurons in that system and on the way that the neurons are interconnected. It will also investigate how these properties and interconnections of neurons can be understood by looking at events at the molecular level.

To gain such understanding may seem an almost impossible task, given the enormous complexity of the nervous system. However, over the past twenty years or so, much progress has been made in understanding the mode of action of neuronal systems. Particularly valuable contributions have come from research involving the examination of organisms with relatively simple nervous systems in terms of relating neuronal function to their resulting behaviour. The understanding of simpler nervous systems provides a basis for unravelling the complexities of organization and function of vertebrate brains, including those of humans. It seems that the principles of neuronal structure and function vary remarkably little from the simplest to the most complex of nervous systems.

In Chapters 6 and 7 the term 'pathway' will be used in an anatomical sense to describe connections between different regions of the brain. This section looks at another criterion for distinguishing such pathways within the nervous system which is in terms of the transmitter chemicals that are used by systems of neurons. Advances in neurochemical techniques have enabled the identification of the transmitter substances found within specific regions of the brain. Groups of neurons that use a common transmitter substance have been identified. Within larger bundles of neurons, modern techniques permit the identification of components of the bundle that use different transmitter substances.

Having looked in Section 4.4 at the means by which it is decided whether a particular chemical really is a transmitter, the following sections will consider the distribution and properties of a few of the well-established nervous system transmitters. A variety of chemical transmitters and the brain systems that use them will be described. However, the transmitters detailed in this section by no means form a complete catalogue of those that exist in the nervous system; only a flavour of the wide range of chemicals that can perform the task of synaptic transmission is given. You should not make an effort to memorize the details in Sections 4.5.2–4.5.6. The principles (given in the Summary and the Objectives) are what is important. Several of the examples given will reoccur later and thereby gradually the more common names of transmitters will become familiar to you. Others mentioned will serve as a source of reference if you read other material outside this course.

## 4.5.2 Catecholamines

Because of certain common properties, three different neurotransmitters, dopamine, noradrenalin and adrenalin, are referred to by the generic name *catecholamines*. Neurons that use catecholamine neurotransmitters are called catecholaminergic neurons. Catecholamines have a similar basic structure and are produced from the same chemical substrate. Protein molecules are broken down by digestion in the gut into subunits called amino acids (see Book 1, Section 3.2.2). Two of these amino acids are called tyrosine and phenylalanine and Figure 4.11 shows how dopamine, noradrenalin and adrenalin are produced from tyrosine and phenylalanine. Tyrosine enters a catecholaminergic cell directly from the bloodstream or it can be made from phenylalanine by enzymes within the cell. (In phenylketonuria, an inherited lack of the enzymes needed for this conversion leads to accumulation of phenylalanine and retardation of normal development; see Book 1, Chapter 3.) Inside the cell, tyrosine is converted into dihydroxy-phenylalanine (abbreviated to dopa) and then into dopamine. Dopaminergic cells (i.e. those that release dopamine) transport the newly synthesized dopamine molecules to their synaptic terminals to be stored in synaptic vesicles. Noradrenergic cells, that is, those that release noradrenalin, convert dopamine into noradrenalin, and cells that release adrenalin go one step further and convert noradrenalin into adrenalin.

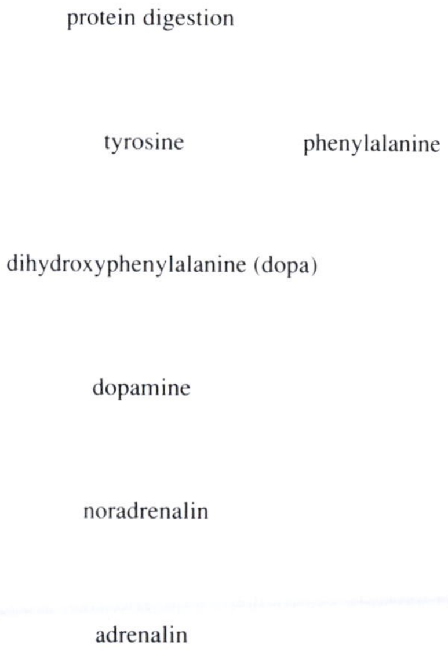

protein digestion

tyrosine          phenylalanine

dihydroxyphenylalanine (dopa)

dopamine

noradrenalin

adrenalin

**Figure 4.11** Synthesis of catecholamines from tyrosine and phenylalanine. Arrows represent the various stages of conversion.

Dopamine occurs in pathways essential for sensory and motor performance. It has been shown that in laboratory rats the release of dopamine is associated with behaviour such as licking, sniffing and gnawing. Various subtypes of dopamine receptor exist and the transmitter is known to be involved in processes of motivation (Book 1, Chapter 7) and positive reinforcement (Book 1, Chapter 6), and in such functions as temperature regulation, hormone release and vomiting.

Although it is believed that only a relatively few neurons actually synthesize this transmitter, it is found in many regions of the brain. A deficiency of dopamine leads to the loss of motor control seen as Parkinson's disease. Partial relief is afforded to sufferers by treatment with the dopamine precursor dopa (see Figure 4.11). (A precursor is a substance from which another is constructed.) Dopa, like nutrients and other essential materials, is delivered to the brain by cerebral blood vessels that run over its surface. However, there exists a blood–brain barrier (Section 2.4.4) formed by tight seals between the cells that line the blood vessels and this prevents the entry of many substances from blood into the brain.

☐   Patients with Parkinson's disease are given dopa by mouth. Dopamine will not work if administered in this way. Why might this be so?

■   Dopamine cannot cross the blood–brain barrier to enter the brain but dopa can.

Noradrenalin is one of the most important neurotransmitters in determining the capacity of the body to exhibit 'fight or flight' behaviour in the face of danger (Book 1, Section 2.9). It is released by neurons in internal organs such as the heart, spleen and gut. Noradrenalin has both excitatory and inhibitory effects in the central nervous system. In the brain, noradrenalin is synthesized by a few, highly-branched neurons and is involved in many aspects of brain function. It has been shown that noradrenalin is extremely important in the normal development of the visual system. Overstimulation of noradrenergic receptors leads to symptoms of mania and the transmitter is also known to be important in feeding and drinking.

Adrenalin is synthesized by cells in the brain and by a gland that will be described in Book 5, the adrenal gland. When secreted from the adrenal gland it acts as a circulating hormone often known as the 'fight or flight' hormone. As a neurotransmitter in the nervous system, it can have either excitatory or inhibitory effects. It is known to be involved in the regulation of body temperature, blood pressure and respiratory rate.

## 4.5.3   Acetylcholine (ACh)

Acetylcholine (ACh) was the first neurotransmitter to be discovered and, as discussed in Section 4.2.4, has an excitatory effect at skeletal neuromuscular junctions. In the central nervous system, ACh occurs throughout the brain and modifies the actions of other neurotransmitters. ACh release from neurons is involved in various aspects of behaviour, including arousal, motivation and emotion. There is strong evidence for its involvement in processes of learning and memory formation and some evidence for its involvement in depression and mania. Sufferers from Alzheimer's disease (senile dementia, which will be discussed in Book 6, Chapter 3) show reduced brain cholinergic function, and malfunction of the cholinergic system is also associated with Parkinson's disease.

In the inherited disease called Huntington's disease, ACh metabolism is known to be disrupted and to affect motor control and coordination (Book 6).

### 4.5.4 γ-amino-butyric acid (GABA) and glycine

γ-amino-butyric acid (GABA) was first discovered in 1950. It is the major transmitter at inhibitory neuromuscular junctions in invertebrates and at inhibitory synapses in the central nervous system of mammals. GABA produces its inhibitory effect by hyperpolarizing postsynaptic membranes, and acts via both $Cl^-$ ion channel receptors (Section 3.9) and second-messenger system receptors. Substances that block the action of GABA produce convulsions and these effects tie in with the fact that lack of GABA activity has been implicated in the occurrence of epileptic fits.

Glycine is another central nervous system transmitter occurring at inhibitory synapses. It has been widely studied and has been found in the brain and spinal cord. Its major function appears to be to regulate the action of another transmitter, L-glutamate. In addition, it is now thought that some receptors which were originally thought to be acted upon by GABA are in fact glycine receptors. GABA and glycine seem to have many very similar effects and thus it has proved difficult to identify their respective receptor neurons. Pharmacological agents such as strychnine, which blocks glycine receptors, and bicuculline, which blocks GABA receptors, have been used in attempts to distinguish their respective pathways.

### 4.5.5 Serotonin (5-hydroxytryptamine or 5-HT)

Serotonin, also known as 5-hydroxytryptamine (5-HT), is produced within the central nervous system by a few highly-branched neurons and binds to receptors with second messenger systems. Serotonin occurs in vertebrates and invertebrates and is found in particularly high concentration in many snake venoms. In the brain, serotonin plays a role in systems that mediate alertness and pain perception. It also occurs in the peripheral nervous system, where it activates the muscle of the intestines.

### 4.5.6 Peptides

Peptides are involved in the signalling of mood and pain. In some neurons, they are synthesized in the presynaptic cell (in which case, they can serve as neurotransmitters in the way described so far). However, they are often synthesized elsewhere, even outside the brain in glands such as the pancreas, or in the heart or the gut. They enter the brain in the bloodstream and then diffuse into groups of neurons. Acting in this way, they can affect large numbers of neurons simultaneously. Such an effect is therefore rather different from that of neurotransmitters where activity in a particular neuron causes a specific local change at the neuron or neurons with which it connects. Rather, this role of peptides is to cause changes in the sensitivity or reactivity of whole populations of neurons, to make them easier or more difficult to activate by neurotransmitters released at synapses. For this reason peptides are often called **neuromodulators**. Studies of neuromodulators have greatly increased our understanding of brain function. They can alter the transmission of signals across synapses in a variety of ways, by increasing or decreasing the release of neurotransmitter, or by changing the properties of the postsynaptic receptors. One such peptide, atrial natriuretic factor, has been shown to have its effect in brain regions concerned with regulating the cardiovascular system (the heart and blood vessels).

It is now known that many neurons synthesize peptide transmitters in addition to one or other of the 'classic' neurotransmitters described above. Peptides acting as hormones in non-neural tissue have been known for a long time but it was not until the 1970s that some of the same substances began to be found in the brain. Their specific localizations and functions are still not well understood. It is thought that within the brain some peptides act primarily as neurotransmitters whereas others act primarily as neuromodulators. Some peptides may also perform both functions. The transmitter called substance P and the enkephalins and endorphins are among those peptides that are thought to act as neurotransmitters in the accepted sense in that they are synthesized and released by cells at synapses.

**Enkephalins** and **endorphins** belong to a class of peptide transmitters called endogenous opioids. The term 'endogenous' refers to the fact that they are synthesized naturally within the body. They are synthesized in the central nervous system and elsewhere. Opioids act on opiate receptors, which can also be stimulated artificially by both legal and illegal means. Narcotic opiate drugs produce their analgesic and euphoria-inducing effects by acting at these same receptor sites. The term *analgesia* refers to a capacity to reduce the sensation of pain. Morphine is one of the better known examples of a drug in this class and is prescribed to reduce severe pain. Endorphins were discovered in 1975 and the molecules show some similarity to morphine.

Stimulation of regions of the brain that are rich in opioid-containing neurons produces analgesia, an effect that can be reversed by the administration of naloxone, a drug that blocks opiate receptors.

☐   Is naloxone acting as an agonist or an antagonist of opiates here?

■   Naloxone is acting as an *antagonist* to opiates because it inhibits the action of the natural transmitter.

Much research effort is being directed towards trying to produce artificial endorphin derivatives with the same effects as morphine but without its addictive properties. ß (beta)-endorphin is a transmitter released in the brain, the pituitary gland and the placenta. Its function is still not clear, though, when injected into rats, it produces analgesia and paralysis. ß-endorphin has been shown to be released from the pituitary gland in response to stress. Enkephalins are destroyed almost as soon as they are released in the brain and this fact has made investigations of their mode of action and effects very difficult. Attempts to produce analgesic drugs based on the action of endorphin and enkephalin neuromodulators and which have no undesirable effects have so far been unsuccessful.

Tissue damage is detected by **nociceptive** sensory receptors in the skin and internal tissues and is perceived as pain. These are not the same receptors as those involved in sensing pressure or touch. The transmitter employed by nociceptors (at the synapse shown in Figure 1.2; Section 1.2) is the peptide substance P which was discovered in 1931. Substance P also occurs as a transmitter in the gut where it causes muscle contraction. However, its function is still not fully understood.

### 4.5.7   Interactions between neurotransmitters

Sections 4.5.2–4.5.6 have given you a flavour of the multiplicity of neurotransmitters that exist in the nervous system, and the wide-ranging effects that they produce. However, it is very important to realize that few of these chemicals act in isolation. In general, the final effect of their release depends upon the interaction of different transmitters on the same or different groups of neurons. It was first realized in the mid-1960s that neurotransmitters interact with each other, both in the peripheral and in the central nervous systems. When their regional distributions are mapped out, many neurotransmitters overlap with each other.

The best understood neurotransmitter interactions are those that take place between ACh and dopamine in a part of the brain that you will meet in Chapter 8, termed the basal ganglia. They have been studied extensively because of their believed involvement in Parkinson's disease. In 1971, O. Hornykiewicz described their activity as *heterosynaptic interaction*. He used this term to describe the situation in which neurons using different neurotransmitters synapse onto a common postsynaptic output cell, or pathway, which mediates a particular behaviour pattern. In Figures 4.1b and 4.9 the transmitter activating the excitatory synapses might well be different from that activating the inhibitory synapses, in which case this would be an example of heterosynaptic interaction.

Another type of interaction is described as in-series interaction. This describes the situation in which different neurotransmitter chemicals are released by each member in a line, or series, of neurons. Alteration of the activity of any one of these cells modifies the function of the others. A situation in which one transmitter modulates the release of another transmitter within the same neuron is called sequential mediation. These interactions are shown in Figure 4.12.

The interactions that occur between neurotransmitters offer an explanation for the widespread effects of neurologically active drugs. Because most neurologically active drugs act at synapses, they involve many different neurotransmitters and produce many different behavioural results.

□   Why should this present a problem for people trying to develop new drugs that affect the nervous system?

■   When predicting the action of a particular drug, it is necessary to take into account all the potential involvement of different transmitters within the many complex pathways of the nervous system. Consequently, most drugs in present use as neuromodulators are characterized by a pronounced lack of specificity.

Section 4.5.8 will consider drug action in more detail.

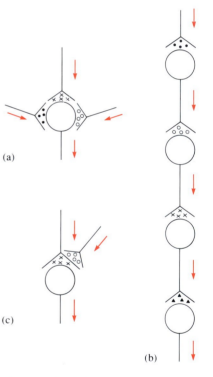

**Figure 4.12**   Schematic representation of (a) heterosynaptic interaction, (b) in-series interaction, and (c) sequential mediation. ●, ○, × and ▲ represent different transmitter chemicals.

## 4.5.8  Interfering with the synapse

You have already met examples of artificial interference with the ability of a synapse to convey information. The effect of morphine in stimulating opiate receptors was described in Section 4.5.6. Section 4.2.5 described agonists and antagonists, substances that act in the same way as, or oppose, respectively, the action of a neurotransmitter on the receptors. This section looks more broadly at changing the transmission properties of synapses.

Changes in synaptic transmission can, in effect, be brought about by anything that interferes with the release of transmitter molecules from the presynaptic membrane, their diffusion across the synaptic cleft, their binding to the postsynaptic receptors, or their subsequent removal from the receptors and destruction. *Blocker* is the term generally employed when the substance can completely prevent the action of the neurotransmitter (a particularly effective kind of antagonist), and the blocker is in turn called a poison when its action can lead to the death of the organism.

Many of the drugs used to treat depression and other mental illnesses have an effect on neurotransmission. They can be divided into three broad classes of compound: sedatives, tranquillizers and antidepressants. Despite the fact that they can cause physiological addiction, barbiturates are still occasionally used as sedatives. They induce sleep by depressing the activity of parts of the brain (e.g. the cerebral cortex). Drugs with tranquillizing effects include the benzodiazepines, such as the well-known and over-prescribed tranquilliser Valium (chemical name diazepam).

Changes in levels of catecholamines such as dopamine and noradrenalin appear to be implicated in depression. Antidepressants, such as amphetamines, are stimulants that generate alertness and feelings of confidence. They affect certain parts of the brain by increasing the release of catecholamines from presynaptic terminals and they also increase heart rate. Now that their other effects, such as addiction, are more widely appreciated, amphetamines are no longer prescribed by doctors in the United Kingdom as antidepressants. They have been replaced by a class of antidepressant drugs called the monoamine oxidase (MAO) inhibitors. Monoamine oxidase is found in the presynaptic cell and acts to break down such transmitters as dopamine, noradrenalin and 5-HT (see criterion number 4 in the list of criteria for identifying neurotransmitters in Section 4.4). Therefore, a monoamine oxidase inhibitor is something which acts against the substance that breaks down these transmitters.

☐  What then would you expect to be the effect at the synaptic level of treating someone with monoamine oxidase inhibitors?

■  The breakdown of dopamine, noradrenalin and 5-HT would be reduced and therefore the levels of these substances at the postsynaptic membranes of neurons having receptors for these substances would be increased.

Hallucinogens are psychotropic, or mood-altering, agents such as cannabis, cocaine and LSD (lysergic acid diethylamide) and these drugs have also been shown to interfere with chemical transmission. Cannabis lowers body temperature and stimulates appetite while at the same time reducing nausea. LSD increases heart-rate and blood pressure and also distorts perceptions of vision, touch and taste.

Curare is a chemical extracted from the bark of the cinchona tree; it was used by South American Indians to coat the tips of their poison arrows. Curare binds to the postsynaptic ACh receptors but does not activate them and so prevents the effects of ACh at the neuromuscular junction. This leads to paralysis of the muscles, including those used in breathing. Nicotine is another ACh receptor blocking agent. Release of ACh from the presynaptic terminals is inhibited by botulinum toxin, found in food contaminated with the bacterium *Clostridium botulinum*. This toxin produces severe food poisoning (botulism) which can end in death since it prevents ACh reaching the muscles used in breathing. Thus curare, nicotine and botulinum toxin all block ACh transmission but, whereas the effects of curare and nicotine are postsynaptic, that of botulinum toxin is presynaptic. By contrast, venom from the black widow spider causes ACh to be continuously secreted into the synaptic cleft and causes muscles to become permanently contracted (they go into *spasm)*.

A different effect on ACh receptors is displayed by the 'nerve gases'. These were first developed in Germany before World War II. These nerve gases inactivate acetylcholinesterase, the enzyme responsible for breaking down the ACh molecule.

☐  What effect would this have on the neuromuscular junction?

■  ACh is *not* removed from the postsynaptic membrane receptors, with the result that muscles go into spasm.

Since that time, the V-agent nerve gases have been produced at the government research establishment at Porton Down; these are even more deadly derivatives of the original compounds. A compound that inactivates insect nervous system acetylcholinesterase, but not the mammalian enzyme, has been used as an insecticide because it is not toxic to vertebrates.

## Summary of Section 4.5

Dopamine, noradrenalin and adrenalin belong to the catecholamine family of neurotransmitters and all have widespread activity in the brain. ACh has an excitatory effect on neuromuscular junctions. GABA is the main neurotransmitter at invertebrate inhibitory neuromuscular junctions and at inhibitory synapses in mammalian central nervous systems. Peptides can serve as neurotransmitters but can also affect large numbers of neurons simultaneously. In the latter capacity, they are often called neuromodulators. Many neurons synthesize peptide transmitters in addition to one or more 'classical' neurotransmitters.

Any observed behaviour must be regarded as the outcome of the action of more than one neurotransmitter. Transmitter interactions include heterosynaptic interactions, in-series interactions and sequential mediation. The main classes of drugs that affect neurotransmission are the sedatives, tranquillizers and anti-depressants.

# Summary of Chapter 4

Messages are passed across synapses by chemical transmitter molecules, except in the case of electrical synapses. The arrival of an impulse at the presynaptic terminal causes the intracellular $Ca^{2+}$ concentration to increase locally and this in turn triggers the release of neurotransmitter molecules from the synaptic vesicles where they are stored, by a process called exocytosis. Re-uptake mechanisms allow transmitter molecules to be recaptured and thereby released and reused many times over.

The postsynaptic membrane contains receptor molecules which, by virtue of their shape are specific for a particular transmitter with a complementary shape. Binding of transmitter to a postsynaptic receptor opens ion channels in the postsynaptic membrane. Some receptor molecules are themselves ion channels but others stimulate the production of second messengers within the postsynaptic cell. Receptors can be distinguished by their binding of pharmacological agonists or antagonists. Agonists mimic the effect of the natural transmitter molecule whereas antagonists inhibit the effect of the natural transmitter. Transmitter binding to an excitatory receptor produces an EPSP whereas transmitter binding to an inhibitory receptor produces an IPSP. Temporal and spatial summation are the mechanisms by which the postsynaptic cell integrates all the various incoming signals. Systems of neurons operate in a coordinated manner that depends both on the properties of individual neurons in that system and on the way that the neurons are interconnected.

Peptides are often called neuromodulators because they can influence large numbers of neurons simultaneously. Many neurons synthesize peptides in addition to one or more of the 'classical' neurotransmitters. The ways in which different neurotransmitters influence each other include heterosynaptic interactions, in-series interaction and sequential mediation.

Changes in synaptic transmission may be due to effects on the release of transmitter molecules from the presynaptic membrane, on their diffusion across the synaptic cleft, on their binding to postsynaptic receptors, or on subsequent removal from the receptors and breakdown.

# Objectives for Chapter 4

When you have completed this Chapter, you should be able to:

4.1   Define and use, or recognize, definitions and applications of each of the terms printed in bold in the text.

4.2   Explain the role of the synapse in the communication and processing of information. (*Questions 4.1 and 4.2*)

4.3 Describe the sequence of events by which a signal is transmitted across a chemical synapse. (*Questions 4.2 and 4.3*)

4.4 Explain the relevance of EPSPs and IPSPs in the initiation of action potentials. (*Question 4.4*)

4.5 Recognize or describe criteria that a substance must satisfy in order to be called a transmitter. (*Question 4.5*)

4.6 Explain the different effects of agonists, antagonists, blockers and poisons at the synapse. (*Question 4.6*)

# Questions for Chapter 4

### Question 4.1 (*Objective 4.2*)
The electrical synapse differs from the chemical synapse in which of the following ways?

(a) There is a wider synaptic cleft at electrical synapses.

(b) More varied signals can cross the electrical synapse, thereby increasing its capacity to process information.

(c) Electrical synapses have a longer synaptic delay than chemical synapses.

(d) Transmission across an electrical synapse is much faster than across a chemical synapse, transmission being virtually instantaneous.

### Question 4.2 (*Objectives 4.2 and 4.3*)
Identify the numbered parts (1–6) of the chemical synapse represented in Figure 4.13.

### Question 4.3 (*Objectives 4.2 and 4.3*)
Give a brief description of how a signal is transmitted across a chemical synapse.

### Question 4.4 (*Objective 4.4*)
In Figure 4.9 (Section 4.3), what would be the predicted effect on neuron 4 of action potentials in neurons 1 and 3 arriving simultaneously?

### Question 4.5 (*Objective 4.5*)
What four criteria must a substance satisfy in order to be recognized as a chemical transmitter?

### Question 4.6 (*Objective 4.6*)
Curare causes paralysis by preventing the binding of which of the following transmitters to its receptors?

(a) Dopamine

(b) GABA

(c) ACh

(d) Noradrenalin

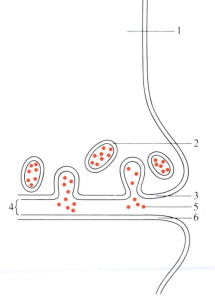

**Figure 4.13** Diagram of a chemical synapse.

# CHAPTER 5
# IMMUNITY AND THE NERVOUS SYSTEM

## 5.1 Towards a wider view of control and regulation

All animals, whether they are single-celled organisms like *Amoeba* or enormously complex creatures such as ourselves, must organize their behaviour and regulate their body chemistry in order to survive. Book 1, Chapter 7 introduced the notion of regulation of the internal environment of the body. In response to a challenge to the internal state, by, for example, being exposed to a dangerously cold environment, humans and other mammals take action to regulate their body temperature. Such control action involves both the internal physiology of the body (e.g. shivering) and behaviour (e.g. moving to a warmer environment). Such actions are organized by the nervous system.

Animals must interact in a controlled manner with the external environment which contains food, shelter, mates and so forth, while maintaining their internal environment in an optimum state. The larger and more complex the animal, the more complicated become the mechanisms for performing these two vital functions. Control and regulation are the prime functions of the nervous system, even in humans, where a love of jazz or the ability to imagine other worlds or write advertising slogans for washing powder is also a product of our complex brains. However, control and regulation are not solely under the direction of the nervous system and the task of this short chapter is to introduce you to the workings of another system of sensory and effector activity in the body, the immune system.

The cells that defend vertebrates from infection have much in common with neurons and may even have evolved from common ancestral cells in animals that were alive millions of years ago. In some modern-day species of insects, worms and snails, cells exist which simultaneously display some of the properties of neurons and some of the defence mechanisms present in the immune system of mammals. In years to come, it may be recognized that the traditional academic division between these two regulatory systems has arisen largely as an artefact of the ways in which they have been studied. The pioneers of neurophysiology and immunology had very different areas of interest which have tended to dominate the direction of subsequent research. Neurophysiologists were originally concerned with the effects of electrical stimulation of nervous tissue, whereas immunologists began by grafting tissue from one animal to another and documenting the graft rejection. Immunologists and brain scientists went entirely separate ways until their research programmes began to bump into one another in the early 1980s. As information piles up about the extent of 'cross-talk' between neurons and cells of the immune system, it is becoming necessary to face the probability that both are part of a single interactive network, with common evolutionary origins and common cellular and chemical methods of communication.

# 5.2 The mobile brain?

The sensory apparatus of the nervous system is adapted to detect and relay certain kinds of information about the internal and external world of the organism, information such as sounds, visual images, odours, tastes, temperature, light intensity, touch, and so on. These incoming sensory stimuli are processed into meaningful relationships by the central nervous system. Despite this immense sensory capability, there is a huge and varied category of stimuli that the nervous system is incapable either of detecting or of responding to, that nonetheless must be dealt with rapidly and specifically in order to maintain life.

☐ Can you suggest what these stimuli might be?

■ They are the many millions of different infectious or parasitic organisms that may invade the body of larger creatures, and the toxic molecules that these organisms produce. The immune system has evolved to detect these potentially harmful stimuli to which the nervous system is 'blind'.

The immune system of an adult human consists of at least $10^9$ million **white cells** (or leukocytes), of several different morphological and functional types. White cells are highly mobile and penetrate almost every part of the body, including the brain. They circulate in the lymphoid system (see Figure 5.1) and in body fluids (blood, lymph, tissue fluids in the spaces between cells and fluid in cavities in the brain and spinal canal). They are packed into the lymphoid organs such as the spleen, tonsils and lymph nodes, where you may become aware of swelling during certain types of infection (e.g. the swollen 'glands' in the armpits and groin that characterize glandular fever are actually lymph nodes enlarged by a huge proliferation of white cells fighting the infection). Some types of white cell have the ability to migrate through tissues by squeezing between cells and in and out through the walls of blood vessels. They can even penetrate into the brain. In this way, virtually every part of the body is 'patrolled'. Each of the millions of mobile white cells is able to recognize just one type of *pathogen* (a collective term for any infectious organism or toxic foreign molecule), and between them they are capable of detecting any pathogen that might enter the body. Viewed from this perspective, the immune system should be seen first and foremost as a huge dispersed and circulating sensory organ—or, as it has been dubbed, a sort of 'mobile brain'.

## 5.2.1 Precision and localization

The term 'mobile brain' is not as fanciful as it might seem at first. Like the nervous system, the immune system is routinely capable of pinpoint accuracy in detecting and identifying incoming stimuli. The response against the intruding organism is equally precise and locally directed, mirroring in some sense the localization of response by the nervous system to stimuli directed at a specific part of the body.

Imagine for a moment the extent of the sensory task facing an organism in a world where contact with numerous different kinds of bacteria, viruses, fungi and parasites cannot be avoided. Although many kinds of bacteria and fungi are harmless or beneficial, some are pathogenic (disease-causing), as are most viruses and parasites. Even bacteria are subject to infection by certain viruses, reminding

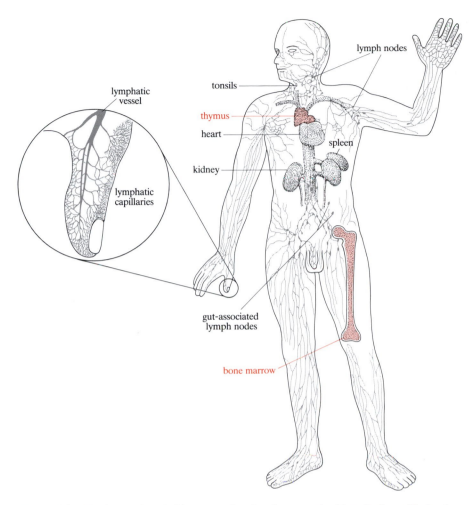

**Figure 5.1**   The human lymphoid system, showing the network of lymphatic capillaries that extends throughout the body, and the major lymphoid organs, including the bone marrow where all white cells originate. The lymphatic capillaries are filled with a pale nutrient fluid, called lymph, in which white cells circulate. They also circulate in the bloodstream and other body fluids and migrate through the tissues.

one of the famous line about bigger fleas having little fleas upon their backs to bite them. An effective sensory apparatus for detecting an infection before it takes hold must be capable of precise and localized recognition of all the millions of different pathogenic organisms and their toxic products that exist today, and any that might evolve in the future as a result of mutation. Each kind of pathogen has evolved a unique body structure, composed of distinctive arrangements of molecules. Many of these organisms also secrete toxic molecules with a unique chemical structure. The white cells of the immune system must recognize each of these 'foreign' chemical patterns and then mount a swift and highly specific attack on any that they encounter. Any cell or molecule that contains foreign chemical patterns in its structure is referred to by immunologists as an **antigen**.

☐   Why is precise recognition of antigens in the body absolutely vital?

■ There are two reasons:

(i) Antigens usually signify the presence of pathogenic organisms and unrecognized pathogens may prove to be lethal.

(ii) Inaccurate recognition of antigens may result in an immune attack being directed against cells or molecules that are part of the *normal* body tissues of the responding animal.

The nervous system is not able to fulfil these complex tasks: neurons are not able to recognize or destroy pathogens, the peripheral network of nerves does not reach every cell, nor does it penetrate the fluid-filled spaces in the body which form such good breeding grounds for pathogenic organisms. The immune system has evolved to perform these vital sensory and effector functions.

## 5.2.2 Immunological memory

The immune systems of most vertebrate animals (mammals, birds, amphibians, some fish and some reptiles) have another capacity in common with the nervous system, which you may be able to deduce from personal experience.

☐ Infections such as German measles (rubella), chickenpox and mumps are commonly termed 'childhood diseases' because they rarely re-infect an adult who has recovered from an episode of the illness in childhood. The person is referred to as being *immune* to that infection. However, immunity to (say) chickenpox gives no protection against any other infection. In what way does this capacity of the immune system resemble that of the nervous system?

■ The immune system is capable of a form of memory. It behaves as though it 'remembers' any infectious organism that it has met before, reacting much more quickly and effectively to eradicate the infection on subsequent meetings than it was able to do the first time around.

**Immunological memory** is central to the sharp decrease in susceptibility to any infection from which an animal has recovered, and to the protective effect of immunization against specific diseases. The process cannot be equated with cognitive learning, but it is simple to demonstrate that the immune system of most vertebrate species adapts in a specific way each time it encounters a new strain of infectious or parasitic organism. The 'memory' of each type of infectious organism is unique and specific, analogous to the precise memory that humans form of each face that they meet. The immune system 'greets' its previous acquaintances with a rapid barrage of cellular and biochemical defences, but approaches newcomers with a slow response that often allows the infection to take hold for a time until the defence mechanisms build up sufficiently and overwhelm it. The delay is because the few white cells that are capable of recognizing a particular pathogen for the first time both (a) undergo structural and functional changes and (b) multiply in number. This takes at least a week to occur. Only then can an effective defence be mounted.

The modified white cells formed after contact with a pathogen are termed *memory cells*, and are capable of a very much quicker response if the same infection occurs a second time. You could say that the immune system is a rather slow learner, but once the specific changes to the white cells have occurred as a result of the first encounter with a new pathogen, it never forgets the experience. It is rare for most vertebrates to suffer from the same infectious disease twice in a lifetime. (But you may be wondering 'Then why do I get a cold *every* winter?' The reason is that there are over a hundred different viruses causing 'the common cold'. You can never 'catch' the same one twice, but there are always plenty more in circulation. However, this also explains why colds become fewer as people get older and there are fewer 'new' viruses to encounter.)

Immunological memory can be demonstrated only in vertebrate animals. The response in invertebrates is no faster, no more effective when an infection develops for the second or subsequent time than it was the first time around. However, the lack of a specific immunological memory does not leave invertebrates undefended. They are still capable of detecting and destroying infectious organisms or any other foreign material that enters their bodies.

Invertebrate immune systems are not 'inferior' to those of vertebrates; they simply do not need to maintain long-term surveillance against common pathogens. Because invertebrates live relatively short lives and produce a great many offspring, high mortality from infection can be compensated for by high rates of reproduction. Long-lived organisms such as humans have such long lives that they need an immune system with a 'memory' to defend them against the millions of pathogens they may encounter. In general, their offspring are so few that very high mortality from repeated infections could not be compensated for by increasing the number of offspring produced.

### 5.2.3   Self/non-self recognition

The nervous system has the ability to distinguish between extremely similar objects, patterns, sounds and so on and to recall them years afterwards. The immune system has a similar ability. It has to distinguish accurately between 'me' and 'not me' when it recognizes pathogenic organisms in the body. But the property of self/non-self recognition has far wider applications than its prime task of infection control. The immune system also enables an individual organism to distinguish between its own cells or organelles and those of even its closest relatives. This ability is amply demonstrated by the problem of graft rejection in human recipients of skin or organs, even when the transplant comes from a member of their own family, or from an unrelated individual who by chance has inherited a similar set of tissue genes to those of the patient. The graft is attacked and destroyed by white cells from the transplant recipient. Only the cornea in the eye escapes recognition because white cells cannot penetrate it, so corneal grafts can be made between any donor and recipient without fear of graft rejection. The recognition of small but important differences in the surface chemistry of the membranes of transplanted cells compared with the cells of the recipient requires exquisite accuracy. Moreover, the immunological memory of the chemical 'signature' of a certain graft is very long lasting. If a graft between two individuals has once been rejected, a second graft from the same donor will be rejected by the recipient much more rapidly than on the first occasion, even if a very long time elapses between the two grafts.

Accurate self/non-self recognition between related individuals developed early in evolution. For example, sponges can be passed gently through a sieve, separating the animal into a soup of single cells which migrate towards each other over time and coalesce into a multicelled sponge. If two sponges are sieved together, the cells gradually separate until the two original sponges reform, a process that requires precise recognition between cells of different origin. Moreover, if cells from different individuals are forcibly held together (as in Figure 5.2), then a damaging reaction occurs at the margin between them, which results in widespread cell death. Graft rejection can be demonstrated in enormously diverse animal species: skin grafts between earthworms (*Lumbricus terrestris*) are rejected in much the same manner as grafts between humans; single-celled animals such as *Amoeba* reject organelles from other individuals of their own species which have been gently introduced through the cell membrane via a fine glass pipette. In multicellular invertebrates, graft rejection is mediated by primitive white cells that closely resemble those of vertebrate animals such as ourselves.

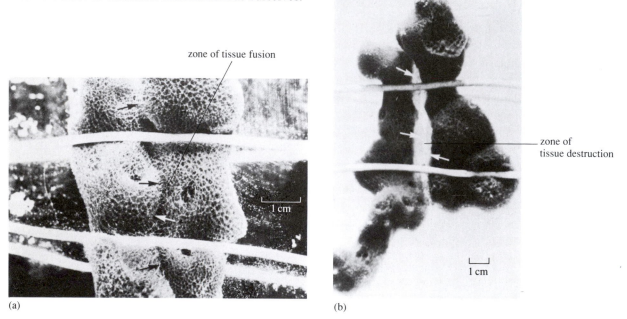

(a)  (b)

**Figure 5.2**  (a) Two branches of a sponge (*Callyspongia diffusa*) from the same individual have been broken off and then held together by plastic-coated wire. They rapidly fuse along the line of contact (shown by arrows) as cells from each branch grow into the other, forming a single mass. (b) When the experiment is repeated with branches taken from different individuals (yet still of the same species), adjacent tissues (shown by the arrows) die as a result of an immune reaction that has much in common with graft rejection in mammals.

☐  At first glance, the ability to reject grafts from other members of the same species appears puzzling. Human tissue transplantation or organ grafting is obviously a contrived situation that cannot happen spontaneously, so why has this extremely subtle level of self/non-self recognition evolved? Can you suggest an explanation? (*Hint:* consider the example of graft rejection in sponges.)

■  In an environment where sedentary animals are crammed together (as on a coral reef) there may be an advantage in being able to 'stake out' one's territory by attacking even close relatives which encroach by overgrowing.

Graft rejection in free-living vertebrates such as ourselves may simply be an evolutionary leftover from ancestral forms.

In conclusion, it can be demonstrated that the immune system operates with a degree of precision and a capacity to learn from experience that is analogous to the properties of the nervous system. But the similarities between the two systems are not simply conceptual 'models' without basis in biological fact. Both systems sample and analyse the internal and external world and react to incoming information in ways that enhance the organism's ability to survive. Both are fundamentally concerned with regulating the internal environment of the body to keep it within strict limits. And most convincing of all, some of the signalling molecules used by neurons and by white cells to communicate information have turned out to be structurally identical. Later in this chapter, the ways in which the immune system interacts with the nervous system and, in particular, common features in their signalling mechanisms will be examined. But first a short detour will be made into the workings of the immune system itself to answer the question: How do white cells recognize pathogens and foreign molecules and destroy them so accurately?

## 5.3   Functions of white cells

The immune system consists of huge numbers of white cells of several different types. In mammals and birds, all of them develop from a single type of cell, termed a *stem cell*, which is found in the bone marrow in the cavities of long bones in the arms and legs, and in the pelvis and breastbone (look back at Figure 5.1). These stem cells are referred to as *multipotent* (or *pluripotent* in some texts) because they give rise by cell division to all the circulating red cells and white cells found in the body, and also to platelets, which have a key role in blood clotting mechanisms (see Figure 5.3, *overleaf*). Red cells carry oxygen to the tissues, and white cells fight infection by various chemical mechanisms.

Between them, white cells have four main methods of eliminating pathogenic cells or molecules, which are summarized in Figure 5.4 (p. 103).

1   **Phagocytosis**. Some white cells can engulf the harmful material, just as *Amoeba* engulfs a particle of food, by drawing it into the cell wrapped in an envelope of cell membrane. Inside the cell are structures known as lysosomes—tiny packets of digestive enzymes and toxic chemicals such as hydrogen peroxide (a bleach), surrounded by a membrane. The lysosome membrane fuses with the envelope of membrane encircling the engulfed pathogen and its chemical contents destroys the pathogen without damaging the rest of the cell.

2   **Cytotoxic contact**. Some white cells can kill infectious organisms such as bacteria and parasites by secreting specialized chemicals onto the surface of the pathogen from close range. These cytotoxic (cell-killing) chemicals include a cylindrical protein which is 'punched' through the opposing cell membrane, opening a channel through which fluids rush in, causing the pathogenic cell to swell and burst.

3   **Inflammation**. Some white cells can release a burst of chemicals around the site of an infection which initiate an intense, short-lived inflammation. The chemicals (which include histamine) cause blood vessels in the area to dilate, so that the skin above the infection site feels hot and appears red. The blood vessels also become leaky so plasma and white cells flood out and distend the area. These reactions dilute the infectious agents and bring large numbers of white cells to attack them. If the reaction goes on too long or is too severe, the inflamed area becomes painful and may 'weep' fluid. Allergy sufferers will recognize these symptoms, which are alleviated to some extent by anti-histamine drugs. (Pain is discussed in detail in Book 3, Chapter 5.)

4   **Humoral factors**. The term *humoral* dates back to the ancient Greek theory that the body contained four kinds of fluid (the humours: namely black bile, yellow bile, phlegm and blood) which had to be in correct balance to maintain health. In modern immunology, humoral factors are molecules that are synthesized by particular white cells after contact with a pathogen and which circulate freely in the body fluids. The most widely-known of these humoral factors are the antibodies (described below), but there are many others. They include interferon, which prevents viruses from replicating by 'interfering' with the translation of their genetic code into new virus particles; anti-bacterial toxins and enzymes that digest bacterial cell walls; chemical attractants that draw white cells towards the source of an infection; and chemicals (opsonins) that stick to pathogens and make them easier for the phagocytic white cells to 'grip' onto and engulf.

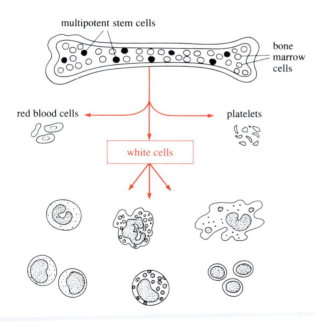

**Figure 5.3**   The development of white cells (leukocytes), red cells and platelets from multipotent stem cells in the bone marrow of mammals and birds.

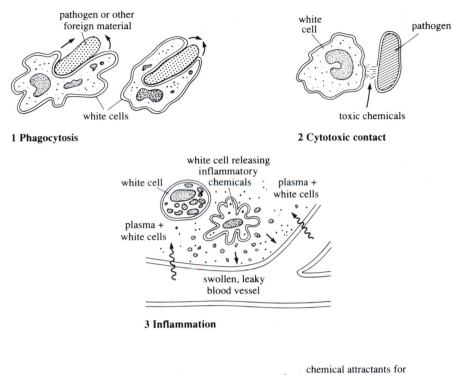

**1 Phagocytosis**

**2 Cytotoxic contact**

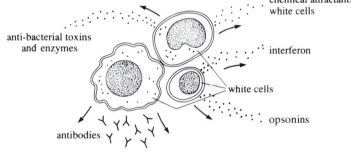

**3 Inflammation**

**4 Humoral factors**

**Figure 5.4**   The four main methods by which the immune system of mammals, birds, amphibians and bony fish destroy pathogenic cells and molecules. For a detailed description, see points 1–4 listed in the text.

**Antibodies** merit a bit more attention because they are mentioned so often in the media. It seems to be common knowledge that after exposure to a pathogen, either as a result of a naturally-occurring infection or when killed pathogens are used to vaccinate children, the body responds by making antibodies. It follows logically that the more antibodies you make, the more effective the immune response is likely to be (or put another way, high levels of antibodies are often taken as evidence of a vigorous immune response). But what are antibodies and how do they help to protect us?

Antibodies are rather simple proteins, with a Y-shaped structure that is relatively constant from one antibody to another, across all the species of animals in which antibodies are found (see Figure 5.5). However, at the tip of each of the

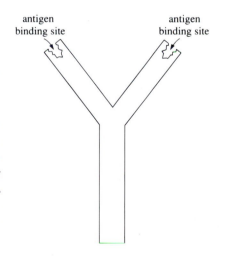

**Figure 5.5**   A stylized sketch of an antibody molecule, showing the location of the two identical antigen binding sites.

outstretched 'arms' of the molecule, there exists a pocket or groove with a highly individual shape and a unique pattern of electrical charges. These pockets are known as the antigen binding sites. You should remember from Section 5.2.1 that the collective noun for any cell or molecule that contains a foreign chemical pattern in its structure is an *antigen*. It follows that antibodies can bind to antigens, but in a highly specific way. The two identical sites on each antibody molecule have such a unique shape and pattern of electrical charges that only a very few 'foreign' chemical structures can fit into these sites. This limits the range of pathogens to which a given antibody molecule can bind. Each antibody molecule can only bind to perhaps one strain of bacteria or virus (or at most a very few closely related strains), or to a particular macromolecule such as a bacterial toxin, because only those pathogens or toxins have the correctly-shaped chemical structure on their surface. This enables a particular pathogen or its products to be 'picked out' by the immune system with great accuracy against a background of millions of other harmless cells and molecules. Elsewhere in this course, you will learn how it has become possible to make antibodies in the laboratory and use them to pick out certain antigens in the test-tube or in slices of tissue on microscope slides.

But the structure of antibody molecules only explains their ability for accurate recognition. How do they protect us once they have bound onto a pathogen? Antibodies are inert proteins—they are not toxic nor do they puncture the pathogens to which they bind—so popular analogies between antibodies and guided missiles are entirely misleading. The function of antibodies is primarily to *label* pathogenic cells and molecules for identification and destruction by white cells that would not otherwise be able to distinguish a legitimate target from the body's own tissues. Many white cells do not have sophisticated receptors that bind only to potentially harmful organisms, so they rely on antibodies to guide them. Any cell or molecule that has antibodies attached to its surface will very rapidly be engulfed by phagocytic white cells or attacked with cytotoxic or inflammatory chemicals. In this way, antibodies greatly enhance the accuracy and hence the safety of the immune response.

Returning to the central theme of this chapter—the interactions between the immune system and the nervous system—one strand in the evidence for the close relationship between these two systems is that they seem to have common origins in the embryo.

# 5.4   Embryological origins of neurons and white cells

The multipotent stem cells, from which all the white cells, red cells and platelets are derived by cell division, are related to embryonic neurons. In the embryo, these stem cells originate in the layer of embryonic cells that also gives rise to the nervous system. The shared embryological (and possibly also the shared evolutionary) origins of white cells, platelets and neurons can readily be demonstrated by examining their surface chemistry and the molecules that they synthesize and secrete. Platelets merit a brief mention before the rest of the chapter focuses on one kind of white cell—the small lymphocyte.

### 5.4.1   Platelets

**Platelets** are fragments of an extremely large cell type which develops from the multipotent stem cells in the bone marrow and then disintegrates, shedding huge numbers of tiny elliptical packets of cell membrane into the bloodstream. The normal concentration of platelets in human blood is between 200 000 and 400 000 per mm$^3$. The common embryological origin of platelets and neurons is revealed by the presence of re-uptake sites on platelet membranes that bind to certain neurotransmitter molecules. You should remember from Section 4.2.3 that some of the neurotransmitter molecules released into synapses bind to so-called re-uptake sites on the neuron and are reabsorbed into the cell. The re-uptake sites for serotonin (Section 4.5.5) on neurons are identical to those found on platelets.

This property of platelets has been known since the 1970s and has been exploited by pharmaceutical companies in tests for the efficacy of anti-depressant drugs. The number of re-uptake sites for serotonin in the brain appears to be lower in severely depressed people than in controls, generating the hypothesis that depression may be caused by oversensitivity to serotonin. (There are flaws in this reasoning which need not concern you here, but Book 6 returns to this topic.) Some anti-depressant drugs are believed to work by affecting these re-uptake sites, so that the neurons recycle serotonin more effectively. It is extremely difficult to test drugs on living neurons, but platelets are a readily available substitute. The ability of putative anti-depressants to affect re-uptake sites for serotonin can be tested on platelets with some confidence that drugs that affect re-uptake sites in platelets will also affect those in the brain.

### 5.4.2   Small lymphocytes

One of the most numerous types of white cell is called the **small lymphocyte**. More than 90% of the white cells in the lymphoid system and about 30% of the white cells in the bloodstream are of this type. The pattern of receptors and re-uptake sites for neurotransmitters on the surface membrane of small lymphocytes is far more complex than that found on platelets and they have also been shown to synthesize and secrete neurotransmitters into the space between closely adjacent white cells. This will be returned to later, but first it is important to sketch the unique functions of small lymphocytes in the immune response. Small lymphocytes are the only type of white cell that can display immunological memory. When an immune response to a particular strain of pathogen is over, some of the small lymphocytes that participated in the attack turn into 'memory cells' which have a very long lifespan. If the same pathogen gets into the body again, these memory cells are activated and proliferate very quickly to form huge numbers of small lymphocytes which bind to the pathogen and usually eliminate it before it has time to cause significant disease (Section 5.3).

Small lymphocytes come in four main kinds (known as four *subsets* by immunologists), each with a distinct function in the immune response (see Figure 5.6, *overleaf*). The B cells (named after the Bone marrow where they mature) synthesize and secrete antibody molecules which, as mentioned earlier, bind to pathogens or to their toxic products and label them as legitimate targets for destruction by other white cells. There are three kinds of T cells, so called because they migrate to the *Thymus* during their maturation (a lymphoid organ close to the heart, which you can see in Figure 5.1, Section 5.2). Cytotoxic T cells are responsible for direct cell-to-cell killing, as their name signifies; they specialize in destroying any of the body's own cells that have become infected with intracellular pathogens such as viruses. The other two types of T cell are known as helper T cells and suppressor T cells; their effects are opposite to each other. The ratio between the two is an important indicator of an immune system in balance: humans normally have about twice as many helper T cells as suppressor T cells.

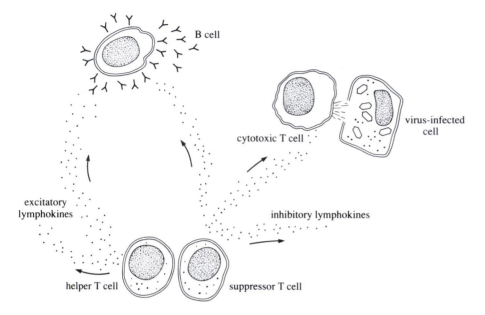

**Figure 5.6**   The four main subsets of small lymphocytes: B cells, which synthesize and secrete antibodies; cytotoxic T cells, which kill pathogenic or infected cells by direct contact with cytotoxic chemicals; and the helper and suppressor T cells, which regulate the immune response.

Helper and suppressor T cells direct the course of an immune response by secreting more than twenty different signalling molecules, known collectively as **lymphokines**, which either promote or inhibit the activity of all the other white cells in the area of an infection. These lymphokines are short-range messenger molecules which have a very short life and which bind to receptors on other white cells in close proximity to the originating cell. When a lymphokine binds to the appropriate receptor, a sequence of chemical events occurs in the responding cell which alters its activity; for example, it may cease producing antibodies, or it may undergo a rapid series of divisions to increase its numbers. Helper and suppressor T cells are active simultaneously during an immune response, fine-tuning the activity of all the other white cells. This is analogous to the activity of excitatory and inhibitory neurons, which fine-tune the output of the nervous system.

# 5.5   Chemical messengers in neurons and small lymphocytes

The lymphokines are an interesting group of chemicals, whose functions are becoming increasingly understood to have a wider range than regulation of the immune response alone. Some of them have turned out to be identical to certain peptide neurotransmitters.

## 5.5.1   White cells secrete endogenous opioids

Helper and suppressor T cells secrete various endogenous opioids (Section 4.5.6) such as the enkephalins and endorphins which, in the brain, seem to be involved in reducing the perception of pain and in counteracting the effects of damage (these will be discussed further in Books 3 and 6). It is not known for sure what their function might be when they are secreted by cells of the immune system. These white cells also have receptors for enkephalins and endorphins on their surface membranes, so they may be communicating with each other by means of some of the same signalling molecules that neurons use. They may even be sending messages to the nervous system about the state of activity during an immune response.

Conversely, the nervous system may use opioid messengers to enhance or inhibit the immune response. When endorphins and enkephalins are administered to experimental animals, there is a curious dose-dependent effect on immunity: high doses of endogenous opioids suppress the immune response and low doses enhance it.

## 5.5.2   White-cell receptors for neuro-active molecules

The possibility of 'cross-talk' between the nervous and immune systems is reinforced by the discovery of other shared signalling mechanisms. Receptors for noradrenalin (Section 4.5.2) are readily detected on small lymphocytes. In addition, these cells secrete a number of peptide hormones, which are also secreted by neurons and which act as neuromodulators in the nervous system (for example, substance P, growth hormone, prolactin and thyroid-stimulating hormone), and they have surface receptors for these peptides and several others. Receptors have also been found for so-called *hormone-releasing* factors which are synthesized in the brain and which stimulate the release of hormones from endocrine glands such as the pituitary and the thyroid. Figure 5.7 (*overleaf*) summarizes the main neurotransmitters, neuromodulators and receptors for such molecules found on the surface of small lymphocytes in mammals (you are not expected to remember the details).

The functions of these varied molecules and their receptors in the operation of an immune response remains a matter for speculation, but the possibility remains that they have a role in regulating the activity of the immune system by carrying messages between participating cells and between neurons and white cells.

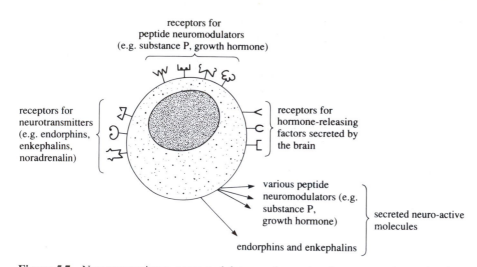

**Figure 5.7** Neurotransmitters, neuromodulators and receptors for neuro-active molecules demonstrated in mammalian small lymphocytes. (The shapes of receptors are purely diagrammatical but in reality they are highly specific for each type of molecule.)

### 5.5.3 Neurons secrete lymphokines

Yet another strand in the chemical evidence of interaction between the nervous and immune systems comes from the discovery that neurons synthesize some of the lymphokines that were formerly thought to be the product solely of white cells. It is theoretically possible, therefore, that the nervous system interferes directly in immune responses by releasing lymphokines which enhance or suppress immunity, 'mimicking' the action of helper and suppressor T cells and using the same signalling molecules. The nervous system might add another level of fine-tuning to the control mechanisms operating from within the immune system itself.

Persuasive though this chemical evidence is, it could be argued that common signalling mechanisms in the nervous and immune systems are simply a vestigial remnant from their common embryological past, without functional significance today. But there is convincing behavioural evidence that the nervous system exerts some regulatory influence over the immune response.

## 5.6 Control of the immune response by the nervous system

Up until the 1970s very little research had been published on the subject of regulation of immunity by the nervous system. A decade later, the trickle of papers had become a steady stream and looked set to turn into a flood. The first International Congress of the newly-created interdisciplinary field of neuroimmunomodulation (sometimes also referred to more simply as neuroimmunology) took place in May 1990 in Florence, Italy, attended by more than 500 scientists from 39 countries. One of its leading researchers and theoreticians, Novera Herbert Spector, described the study of neuro-immunomodulation as 'one of the major areas of biomedical research and perhaps the most rapidly expanding field in all of modern science'.

The first clues that the nervous system might exert an influence on the immune system came from the fluctuations in immune responsiveness that reproducibly occur during the day/night cycle (circadian rhythms) and as seasons change. Later in the course, in Book 5, you will learn more about the precise rhythmic cycles that occur in the levels of various hormones, in body temperature, and so forth, which are mediated by detection of day length and other seasonal changes by the central nervous system. The responsiveness of the immune system is also subject to these periodic fluctuations, giving rise to the hypothesis that the nervous system is able to influence the immune response. There is also good anatomical evidence that the nervous system penetrates deep into the lymphoid organs where many white cells reside, so direct stimulation of white cells may occur.

## 5.6.1  Innervation of lymphoid organs

All the lymphoid organs (look back at Figure 5.1, Section 5.2) are innervated by nerve fibres belonging to a branch of the nervous system called the **autonomic nervous system**, which regulates the activity of the internal organs of the body. The autonomic nervous system regulates the internal environment of the body by (for example) matching heart rate with the body's requirement for oxygen (you will learn more about this in Chapter 8). The lymphoid organs are packed with white cells, some resting and others activated by contact with the pathogen or other foreign matter to which those cells are able to respond. Electron microscope studies of lymphoid organs have shown that axons from the autonomic nervous system branch very widely through all the lymphoid organs and terminate on the surface membranes of small lymphocytes and other white cells.

☐    What evidence would you require, in addition to this anatomical evidence, that the postsynaptic white cells are receiving signals from the neuron axons?

■    The criteria were given in Section 4.4, in the context of communication between adjacent neurons, but the principles apply equally well here. You would have to demonstrate that neurotransmitters were released from the presynaptic neuron endings under normal conditions and that the white cells had specific receptors for those transmitter substances on their surface membranes. Binding of neurotransmitter molecules to the receptors should produce measurable, reproducible alterations in the activity of the postsynaptic white cell. Blocking of the receptors or severing the neuron axons should abolish these changes.

All these criteria have been met in experiments conducted in several different laboratories, primarily on lymphoid organs from rodents. Some of the axons innervating lymphoid organs release noradrenalin, and receptors for noradrenalin have been detected on postsynaptic white cells. These neuron axons can be destroyed in newborn rats by administering a drug that is selectively toxic to noradrenalin-containing axons. When treated animals were exposed to a novel synthetic protein that they could never have encountered in life, their ability to mount an immune response directed against this protein was significantly reduced.

☐  Why should one be cautious about concluding from these experiments that the autonomic nervous system must be 'driving' the normal immune response to foreign substances?

■  The autonomic nervous system has widespread actions in maintaining the internal environment of the body in its optimum state, so its destruction will affect many organ systems and physiological functions, including heart rate, for example. There may be changes in the composition of body fluids, the output of hormones and so forth in treated animals, which could affect the ability of white cells to mount an immune response.

However, other studies have shown comparable effects when the receptors for noradrenalin on rodent or human white cells are chemically blocked. These experiments have shed light on the mechanisms by which the autonomic nervous system could stimulate immunity in the intact animal. For example, T cells whose noradrenergic (noradrenalin-specific) receptors are chemically blocked show a marked reduction in the secretion of lymphokines compared with T cells in untreated animals. Since all white cells are regulated by lymphokine signals, it is possible that the activity of the nervous system enhances certain aspects of immunity by increasing the output of 'helper' lymphokines by helper T cells (Section 5.4.2).

There is also indirect evidence of the involvement of the central nervous system in immune responses. Electrodes implanted in certain areas of the brain have detected an increase in electrical activity in rats that have been immunized by giving them an injection of killed pathogens or foreign proteins. The electrical activity exactly correlates with the appearance, duration and decline of the immune response. It is not possible to say for certain whether this electrical activity is directing any aspect of immunity, or simply responding to it. However, brain activity that correlates with transmitter release from axons in contact with white cells, which in turn correlates with the sequence of the immune response, makes a persuasive story.

## 5.6.2  Classical conditioning of the immune response

Another intriguing clue was discovered in 1924, when students of Pavlov demonstrated that the immune response in laboratory mammals could be modified by classical conditioning (classical conditioning was introduced in Book 1, Section 6.3.2). Various pairs of conditional and unconditional stimuli were investigated, but a closer examination of the process did not occur until the 1980s, when Robert Ader and his colleagues in New York began publishing an influential series of papers on this fascinating phenomenon.

Ader (1985) rediscovered the susceptibility of the immune response to classical conditioning by accident, when he was investigating the conditioning of taste-aversion in rats (discussed in Book 1, Chapter 6). The animals were given a single injection of a toxic drug called cyclophosphamide (the unconditional stimulus or UCS), which made them feel ill and also, serendipitously, suppressed the activity of their immune system. The injection was paired with the arrival of drinking water which had been mixed with saccharin to give it a distinctive flavour (the conditional stimulus or CS). The rats learned to associate the illness (caused by the drug) with the taste of saccharin. Thereafter, the rats expressed a profound aversion to the saccharin-flavoured water, an aversion which declined only very slowly when the solution was offered to them at regular intervals during succeeding weeks without further pairing with the drug. (This is called an *extinction trial*, as you should recall from Book 1, Chapter 6.) But to Ader's surprise, some of the conditioned rats died of infection during the extinction trial and, moreover, the mortality rate varied directly with the amount of saccharin that the rats had consumed at the original conditioning event (i.e. there were more deaths in groups of rats that had been given the most concentrated solutions of saccharin).

☐   Saccharin is harmless to rats in the concentrations used in this experiment, so how might the mortality be explained?

■   Ader concluded that the rats had been conditioned to suppress their own immune responses, leaving them vulnerable to infection. The taste of saccharin became associated with *both* effects of the drug (feeling ill and suppressed immunity), and this association persisted longer if animals were exposed to saccharin during the extinction trial.

Experiments such as this one raise two important questions. What aspects of the immune response are capable of being suppressed by classical conditioning and how is the suppression induced? The first question can be answered but not, as yet, the second. Figure 5.8 shows that the amount of antibodies produced in response to

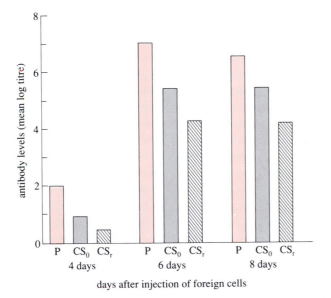

days after injection of foreign cells

**Figure 5.8**   Levels of antibodies (measured as 'mean log titre', a unit which need not concern you here) in the blood of rats at various times after immunization with foreign cells: P refers to the placebo group, (i.e. this group was given a sham injection instead of cyclophosphamide and plain drinking water); $CS_0$ animals were given one dose of the drug paired with saccharin, and drank plain water thereafter; $CS_r$ animals were given one dose of the drug paired with saccharin, but were re-exposed to saccharin-flavoured water daily thereafter.

immunization with foreign cells is greatly reduced in animals with a conditioned suppression of their immune system, when compared with unconditioned controls. Figure 5.9 shows that a significant reduction in the proliferation of white cells in lymph nodes near the site of a tissue graft can be produced by conditioned immunosuppression. This latter finding opens the door to an exciting possibility: could grafted tissue be protected from immune attack by conditioning patients to suppress their own immune response rather than by giving them the immuno-suppressive drugs that are in essential use today?

Another exciting therapeutic prospect is that conditioned suppression of the immune response might provide hope for patients suffering from a group of puzzling diseases in which the immune system attacks normal, healthy body tissues by mistake. These **autoimmune** (anti-self) **diseases** are sometimes treated by immunosuppressive drugs, which greatly reduce the reactivity of the immune system, but have unpleasant side-effects. Robert Ader's research team have been working on an alternative therapy with an inbred strain of laboratory mouse that spontaneously develops an autoimmune inflammation of the kidneys at around 8 weeks of age; all untreated mice die of kidney failure before they are 35 weeks old. However, mice conditioned with paired cyclophosphamide and saccharin, and then repeatedly exposed to saccharin in their drinking water, showed a significant delay in the onset of symptoms of the disease and survived for many weeks longer than untreated mice (see Figure 5.10). Note that there are limitations to this method of treatment; these form the subject of a question at the end of this chapter. Autoimmune diseases are discussed further in Book 6.

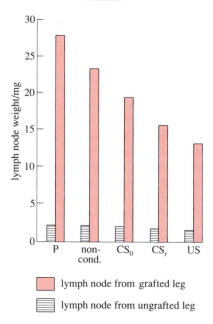

**Figure 5.9** Average weight of the lymph node near the site of a foreign tissue graft in the leg of laboratory rats, compared with the weight of the lymph node from the ungrafted leg. Lymph nodes were weighed five days after the graft was introduced. Group P was the placebo group (i.e. given a sham injection instead of cyclophosphamide); Non-conditioned (non-cond.) animals received one dose of the drug but no saccharin; $CS_0$ animals were given one dose of the drug paired with saccharin, and drank plain water thereafter; $CS_r$ animals were given one dose of the drug paired with saccharin, but were re-exposed to saccharin-flavoured water daily thereafter. US animals were given three small doses of the drug and drank plain water thereafter; this group simply demonstrates the level of immunosuppression that can be achieved with repeated drug use.

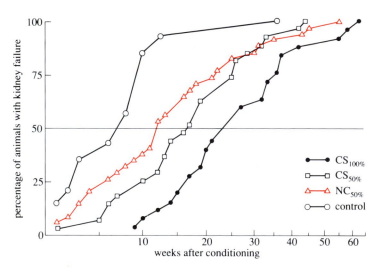

**Figure 5.10** Cumulative rate of kidney failure of mice with a spontaneous autoimmune disease. Controls were untreated; $CS_{100\%}$ animals were given paired cyclophosphamide and saccharin once a week to reveal the extent of symptom control achieved by treatment with an immunosuppressive drug; $CS_{50\%}$ animals were given paired cyclophosphamide and saccharin once every two weeks and re-exposed to saccharin in the intervening weeks to reinforce the association between the drug and the taste of saccharin; $NC_{50\%}$ animals were given the same doses of drug and saccharin as the $CS_{50\%}$ animals, but the stimuli were not paired (they were given a day apart so that the animals never learnt an association between the two stimuli).

It is not yet known precisely how the nervous system produces this remarkable effect, but there are a few clues. Opioids such as the enkephalins and endorphins have been shown to be involved in classical conditioning of immune responses, and conditioning can be blocked by drugs that block receptors for these neurotransmitters.

# Summary of Chapter 5

Regulation of the internal environment and control of the impact of external forces on the body are functions which the nervous system and the immune system have in common. This chapter has looked at how the defence of the internal environment and the maintenance of its physical integrity against pathogens involve both the immune and the nervous systems. The nervous and immune systems may have evolved from common ancestral cells far back in evolution, which subsequently diverged and specialized to sense and respond to different kinds of stimuli. Neurons and white cells share a common origin in the embryo and some of their signalling molecules are identical. It may prove to be simply an historical accident that the two systems have been studied in isolation for so long, and they are now increasingly seen as part of a single interactive network. Books 5 and 6 will return to the subject of the immune system to ask: What happens to the immune response when an organism is under stress? And how does the immune response contribute to degeneration, damage and disease?

# Objectives for Chapter 5

When you have completed this chapter you should be able to:

5.1     Define and use, or recognize definitions and applications of each of the terms printed in bold in the text.

5.2     State the grounds for describing the immune system as a sort of 'mobile brain' and explain the limitations of this analogy. (*Question 5.1*)

5.3     Summarize the evidence that the nervous system and the immune system interact in the course of a normal immune response, and suggest what function such interactions might serve. (*Question 5.2*)

5.4     Evaluate the evidence that interactions between the nervous system and the immune system might be exploited to improve the health of certain groups of patients. (*Question 5.3*)

# Questions for Chapter 5

**Question 5.1** (*Objective 5.2*)
Is it legitimate to describe an animal as having a memory of previous encounters with infectious organisms? Explain your answer.

**Question 5.2** (*Objective 5.3*)

The concentration of receptors for noradrenalin on the surface of mammalian T cells has been shown to be significantly greater on suppressor T cells than on helper T cells. Does this undermine the evidence given in Section 5.5 that the action of noradrenalin released by autonomic nerve axons in contact with white cells is predominantly to *enhance* the immune response? Explain your answer.

**Question 5.3** (*Objective 5.4*)

Weigh up the evidence shown in Figure 5.10 (Section 5.6.2) that conditioned immunosuppression may be a possible therapy for autoimmune diseases.

# References

Ader, R. (1985) Behaviourally conditioned modulation of immunity, in Guillemin, R., Cohn, M. and Melnechuck, T. (eds), *The Neural Modulation of Immunity*, Raven Press, New York, pp. 55–69.

# Further reading

Blalock, J. E. and Smith, E. M. (1985) The immune system: our mobile brain? *Immunology Today*, **6**, pp. 155–117.

Davey, B. (1989) *Immunology: A Foundation Text*, Open University Press, Milton Keynes.

# CHAPTER 6
# NERVOUS SYSTEMS IN INVERTEBRATES

## 6.1   Introduction

The preceding chapters introduced you to neurons and how they communicate with one another using electrical and chemical signals. In Chapter 2 the structure and function of sensory receptors and motor effectors was described, but animal behaviour depends upon the integrative properties of the nervous system as a whole. Now that the basic element of the nervous system, the neuron, has been introduced, the ways in which neurons are connected to form complete systems in animals can be investigated, along with the ways in which those systems function.

It might seem to be too daunting a task to explain how a whole nervous system might function, given the complexity of even a single neuron, which can have a multitude of excitatory and inhibitory inputs and a highly branched axon with many outputs. However, the anatomy of the nervous system, where neurons which receive sensory information and which innervate muscles are connected to each other, can reveal a lot about how the system operates. Detailed knowledge of neuroanatomy is a very necessary part of understanding animal and human behaviour. Inevitably such descriptions will contain new terms; particular structures in the nervous system have particular names. Many animals have common structures and common structures often function in similar ways, so that knowledge of a function derived from one group of animals can often be applied to another.

There is a striking diversity of animal life. The relative abundance of some of the groups of living animals is shown in Figure 6.1 (*overleaf*). Those multicellular animals that do not have a backbone (animals such as worms, insects and snails) form a group called the **invertebrates**. In fact, most multicellular animals belong to this group. As you can see from Figure 6.1, they greatly outnumber those animals with backbones such as fishes, amphibians, birds, reptiles and mammals—the **vertebrates**.

There are two reasons why it is useful to begin a description of nervous system organization with the invertebrates. One is their numbers and importance in the world; the other is that many of them have nervous systems that contain relatively few neurons, some of which are relatively very large in size. Many fundamental discoveries about how nervous systems work have been made by studying invertebrates.

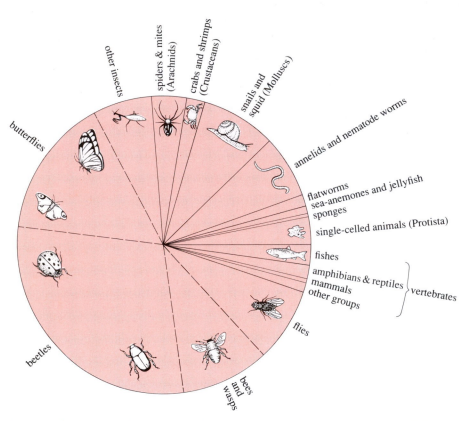

**Figure 6.1** Diagram showing the relative abundance of the known species of living animals. Notice the tiny proportion taken up by the vertebrates. Scale is 1 degree equals 3 715 species.

## 6.2 Nerve nets

If you look into a rock pool at the beach, the chances are that you will find a sea-anemone (Figure 6.2). This animal is a living example of what the first multicellular animals may have been like.

The nervous system in sea-anemones and jellyfish consists of a 'net' of electrically excitable cells: the **nerve net**.

When the tide is in, the anemone looks more like a plant with its long and often highly coloured tentacles. But this is not a plant; it is an animal that needs to catch prey in order to survive. A small shrimp passes close by and becomes stuck to a tentacle; soon other tentacles close over it, the prey is moved to the mouth and ingested. When the tide goes out the sea-anemone changes its shape, retracts the delicate tentacles and turns into a rather boring slimy lump. Now it can withstand exposure to the air until the return of the next tide.

The structure of the sea-anemone is shown in Figure 6.2a. The main body is composed of two layers of cells separated by a non-cellular layer; an outer tough protective cell layer and an inner one of cells that are specialized to digest food. Both the outer and inner cells have extensions that contain contractile filaments rather like muscles. Contraction of the outer cells causes the animal to elongate, while contraction of the inner cells causes the animal to shorten. Localized contractions cause the animal to bend. The tentacles can also move and are equipped with specialized stinging cells that are responsible for catching and paralysing prey. From this description it can be seen that the sea-anemone is composed of several different types of cell that perform different tasks. The activity of these cells is controlled by the nerve net.

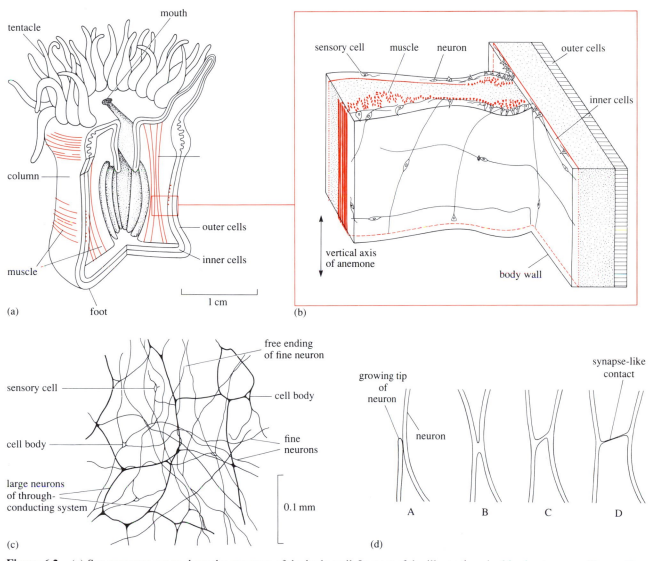

**Figure 6.2**   (a) Sea-anemone cut to show the structure of the body wall. In most of the illustrations in this chapter you will see a line called a calibration bar. Its size tells you how much the object has been enlarged—in this case the calibration bar represents 1 cm. (b) Enlarged view of a section of the body wall to show the internal structure and the nerve net. (c) A portion of a nerve net seen with a high-power microscope. (d) Development of synaptic contact between two neurons. Arrows indicate direction of growth.

The nerve net also receives information from specialized cells that are sensitive to touch and chemicals (e.g. released by those tasty shrimp morsels!). The nerve net is responsible for coordinating the behaviour of the sea-anemone, from responding to the first contact by food on the tentacles to controlling the movements that transfer the food to the mouth and ingest it.

If a tasty morsel such as a small shrimp touches a tentacle it will become attached to it by the action of the stinging cells. Other nearby tentacles then move over to enclose the shrimp and convey it to the mouth. If you were to touch a tentacle gently, the sea-anemone would retract it—the withdrawal response. The difference in the two responses to touch depends upon the activation of different types of sensory receptors in the tentacles.

As described in Book 1, Chapter 2, responses to stimuli are not necessarily always the same. If the anemone is touched gently a number of times, the withdrawal response will decrease until the animal fails to retract at all.

☐ What is the name given to such a waning of response to repeated stimuli?

■ Such a decrease in response to non-harmful stimuli is called habituation (Book 1, Chapter 6).

This habituation to non-harmful stimuli has obvious survival value, since it allows the anemone to continue feeding when there is no danger. It illustrates a very important property of all nervous systems: their ability to change their activity to suit changes in conditions. In this sense, habituation is a kind of learning (Book 1).

## 6.2.1 Structure of the nerve net

The cells in this nerve net look rather different from the neurons you are familiar with from earlier chapters (Figure 6.2), but they function in the same way and will be referred to as neurons.

Although all the neurons in Figure 6.2c appear to be joined together, each of the *fine* neurons is actually separate. As a neuron grows (Figure 6.2d) it may pass close to another neuron. A connection is formed at the point of closest contact and is called a synapse. It is similar in function to synapses in other nervous systems, but the precise details of its function are not known at present.

The large neurons form a closed system in which there is continuity between neighbouring neurons. This forms a *through-conducting* nerve net, so-called because there are no synapses between these large neurons. You will learn more about nerve nets in Chapter 7.

It is possible to stain the complete nerve net in *Hydra*, a smaller relative of the sea-anemone, and then view the whole animal with a light microscope (Chapter 2). The nerve net shows up clearly (Figure 6.3), and it covers the whole of the animal. Around the mouth there are slightly more neurons, presumably because feeding requires a greater amount of sensory feedback and control.

Excitation spreads in all directions over the nerve net from the point at which an action potential is stimulated. Conduction along the neurons can be in either direction and so can conduction across the synapses. This contrasts with the

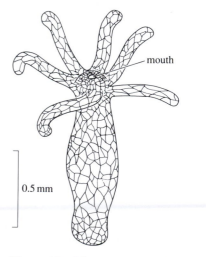

**Figure 6.3** Diagram showing the nerve net in *Hydra*, a small freshwater relative of the sea-anemone.

situation in most nervous systems where neurons normally conduct in one direction only and chemical synapses are not able to transmit action potentials in both directions.

## 6.2.2   The nerve net and behaviour in the jellyfish

Jellyfish belong to the same group of animals as anemones; they also have two layers of cells and they have nerve nets (Figure 6.4). Jellyfish are active swimmers, however, collecting food by first swimming upwards then slowly sinking down, trapping small organisms under the bell and then ingesting these with the mobile mouth. Their nerve nets show some interesting adaptations related to their more active way of life.

### Receptors

At the depths inhabited by the small animals and plants on which jellyfish feed, light penetrates the water from the surface. Jellyfish have light receptors which communicate with the nerve net. There are also receptors that signal the animal's orientation and movement. These are cells equipped with fine hair-like processes that extend into a fluid-filled cavity. Movement of the fluid (caused by movement of the animal) excites these cells which transmit the information to the nerve net. There is a remarkable similarity between the structure of these light and orientation receptors across a wide range of animal species, including ourselves.

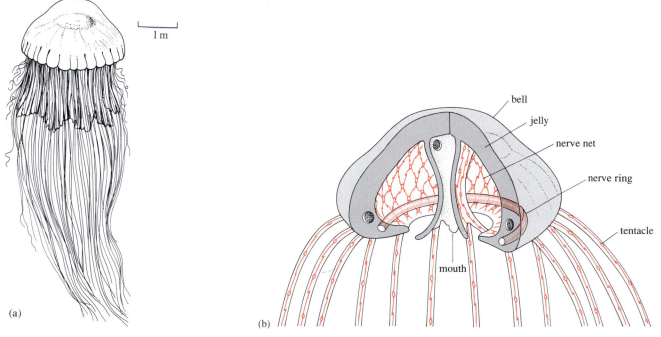

**Figure 6.4**   (a) A giant jellyfish (*Cyanea*). (b) A diagram showing the internal structure. Note the dense nerve net forming a kind of ring around the base of the bell.

**Effectors**

Jellyfish swim by making regular pulsing contractions of the bell which forces water out of the bell, propelling the animal upwards. These regular pulsations are generated by a specialized part of the nerve net which forms a ring that innervates the contractile cells round the base of the bell.

The ability to generate rhythmic activity is another important general feature of networks of neurons. Many animals generate regular contraction of muscles innervated by groups of neurons acting as rhythm generators—from insect flight (Chapter 7) to our own regular breathing and walking movements. In order to be effective in producing movements suitable for the occasion, such motor systems must be closely controlled by sensory information, allowing the animal to move appropriately.

### 6.2.3 What can be learned from examining such simple nervous systems?

This brief look at these rather simple animals tells us some of the basic rules of how nervous systems function and are organized. The animal receives relevant information from the external world. The sensory receptors are specialized excitable cells that respond to particular stimuli. This sensory information is transmitted to the nervous system which is responsible for coordinating the response of the animal to these external stimuli. The nervous system is a highly structured network of excitable neurons; it receives sensory information, interprets it, and generates the appropriate responses by activation of effector organs such as muscles.

Two of the more important properties of nerve networks are (1) their capacity to change their response to a given stimulus under certain circumstances, and (2) their ability to generate rhythmic activity. Both of these properties depend on the way neurons communicate with one another using electrical and chemical signals. The nervous system of more complex animals can also perform these functions. However, their nervous systems are constructed along very different lines, which allows them to perform additional functions, as will be described in the following sections.

# 6.3 Central and peripheral nervous systems

In a two-layered aquatic animal like the sea-anemone (Figure 6.2a), sufficient oxygen can be obtained by simple diffusion from the surrounding water. Similarly, waste products diffuse from the cells into the surrounding water. More complex mechanisms for getting oxygen to the tissues and for removing waste products have evolved in larger organisms since diffusion over a distance greater than a few cells cannot take place quickly enough. The specialized tissues that perform these functions are usually collected together in organs which lie in a cavity within the body. Inside the body cavity of animals such as an earthworm, a lobster, a snail or a human are organs concerned with providing oxygen and nutrients to the cells of the body, removing waste products, and digesting food. Often several organs work together to perform a function, acting as a 'system', e.g. the respiratory system, circulatory system, digestive system, and nervous system.

Although the sea-anemone has quite a large behavioural repertoire, it is very limited compared to most of the invertebrates. In contrast to the anemone nerve net, the nervous systems of most invertebrates consist of distinct groups of neurons rather than the more uniformly distributed nerve net. The coordination and control of more complex behaviour requires more complex neural networks than can be provided by a simple nerve net (although nerve nets are still retained to control some organs such as the gut). In these animals the neurons are grouped together allowing a far greater interchange of information, and many are functionally specialized to perform particular tasks (e.g. the interpretation of information from the sense organs, the control of movement).

The nervous systems in all vertebrates and invertebrates (other than sea-anemones and their relatives) can be divided into two parts—the central nervous system and the peripheral nervous system. An example of this was given in Chapter 1. The central nervous system (CNS) largely contains whole neurons as well as the cell bodies of neurons whose processes are outside the CNS. The peripheral nervous system (PNS) contains the sensory receptors and their axons together with the axons which connect the CNS with peripheral effectors such as muscles and glands. The axons in the PNS are often collected together in discrete bundles of nerve fibres.

As will be discussed in a later chapter, the CNS in all vertebrates and many invertebrates consists of the brain and a nerve cord. In vertebrates the nerve cord is encased by the vertebral column and is called the spinal cord; the PNS consists of those neurons and axons outside the brain and spinal cord. However, there are some fundamental differences in the position and structure of the CNS in invertebrates and vertebrates. One obvious difference is that the invertebrate CNS is a structure situated towards the animal's belly rather than its back. This location is termed **ventral**. The vertebrate CNS is a structure running down the animal's back. This location is termed **dorsal** (Figures 6.5a and b).

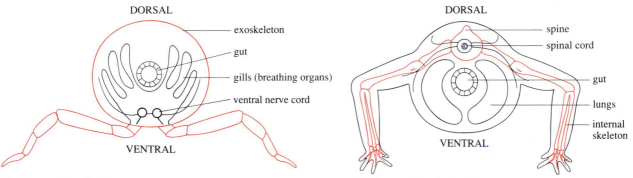

(a)  Cross-section of a lobster

(b)  Cross-section of a lizard

**Figure 6.5**   The position of the nerve cord in an invertebrate (the lobster described in Section 6.6.2) and the spinal cord in a vertebrate (lizard). Notice also that the skeleton in this invertebrate is an external structure (for this reason it is called an exoskeleton, 'exo' meaning 'outside'), while it is an internal structure in vertebrates.

121

The distinction between central and peripheral nervous systems is not always obvious. Thus in many animals there are collections of neurons found outside the CNS which regulate the function of local organs such as the gut. In general, however, the CNS contains the bulk of those neurons that act as the integration centre for the behaviour of the animal.

The extracellular environment surrounding all neurons is closely regulated, and this permits the sensitive electrically excitable cells to function correctly. Often there are special mechanisms to ensure a reliable supply of oxygen and nutrients.

☐   Which cells are responsible for regulating the local environment of the neurons?

■   The glial cells.

In Chapters 2 and 3 the specialized glial cells that surround many of the axons in the vertebrate nervous system were described. Some of these glial cells form a coating around the axons called myelin.

☐   What effect does the presence of myelin around an axon have on the function of that axon?

■   You should recall from Section 3.8 that the presence of myelin greatly increases the speed of action potential conduction along the nerve.

The speed of conduction of axons is dependent on both the diameter and whether or not myelin is present. Some motor neurons have a conduction velocity of $100 \, \text{m s}^{-1}$. A typical figure for the fast axons in the sciatic nerve of the frog is $30 \, \text{m s}^{-1}$. As a contrast, an unmyelinated axon of around $1 \, \mu\text{m}$ in diameter will have a velocity of less than $2 \, \text{m s}^{-1}$.

Myelin is only found in vertebrates: no invertebrate species has this kind of glia, although their neurons and axons are surrounded by glial cells. This means that, on the whole, speed of communication between neurons in invertebrates is slower than that in vertebrates. In those situations where speed is necessary, producing fast contractions for escape responses when danger threatens, for example, the speed of conduction is increased by increasing the diameter of the axon.

☐   Can you recall from Chapter 3 an example of such a large diameter axon that has provided important information concerning the mechanism of action potential conduction?

■   Hodgkin and Huxley used the giant axon of the squid to investigate the mechanism of action potential conduction.

Most animals are 'built' in a modular fashion (see Figure 6.6) in that they consist of a series of repeated units or segments—their bodies show **segmentation**. They are also bilaterally symmetrical, meaning that they can be divided into two 'mirror-image' left and right halves by a line ( the mid-line) running from head to tail. **Bilateral symmetry** is one of the basic organizational features of most animals and is related to the way they develop. The bilaterally symmetrical segmental body plan is clearly visible in invertebrates such as the earthworm, leech or lobster. It is also shown in many vertebrates as the segments of the spine—each individual bone, or vertebra, that makes up the spine is a segment—and in fish as a repeated pattern of the muscles of the body.

This bilaterally symmetrical segmental arrangement is also seen in the structure of the nervous system in both invertebrates and vertebrates.

### 6.3.1   The organization of the invertebrate CNS

There are obvious differences between the nervous systems of the invertebrates illustrated in Figure 6.6 (the earthworm, leech and lobster), but their nervous systems have the same basic organization of repeated units. Among the invertebrates the organization is clearest in the earthworm and the leech. The nerve cord is actually double, with the two halves running alongside each other. In each body segment the nerve cord is expanded to form a pair of ganglia (single: **ganglion**), each of which contains collections of the cell bodies of neurons (Figure 6.6a). Figure 6.7 (*overleaf*) shows the anatomy of a ganglion in the leech. The neuron bodies are situated around the outside, and are protected by a thick fibrous sheath. The inner part of the ganglion, the **neuropile**, contains the axons of the cells as well as their dendrites; it is here that the synaptic contacts between the neurons are made. The ganglia are joined to those in neighbouring segments by bundles of axons called longitudinal **connectives**. The two ganglia in each segment are connected to each other across the mid-line by axons forming the **commissures**. Nerves connect each pair of ganglia with peripheral sensory receptors and motor effectors (muscles and glands) within each segment.

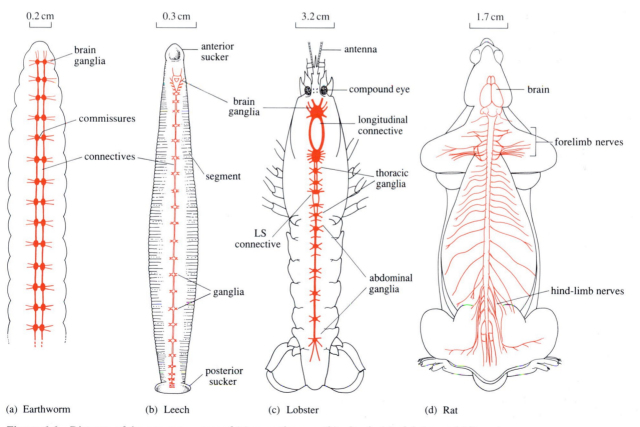

**Figure 6.6**   Diagram of the nervous system of (a) an earthworm, (b) a leech, (c) a lobster, and (d) a rat.

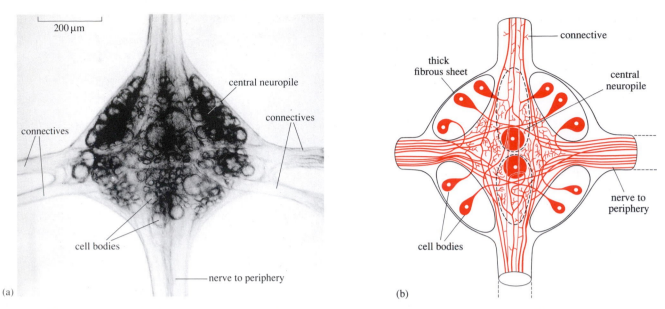

**Figure 6.7** (a) A photograph of a ganglion in a leech. The ganglia have been dissected out of the animal and, if bathed in a suitable fluid, the cells will stay alive so that their activity can be investigated. Although they have not been stained the cells inside are clearly visible through the protective outer layer. It is possible to identify neurons which occupy the same position in each ganglion in different individuals of the same species. (b) A drawing of the arrangement of cells and their processes within the ganglion.

☐ Suggest a functional reason why all the ganglia in the lobster in Figure 6.6c are not the same size?

■ The ganglia are not the same because the segments in which they lie have different roles to play in behaviour. For example, the ganglia controlling the leg-bearing segments are larger than those in the abdomen. The enlargement reflects the greater functional requirement of the ganglia in controlling activity of the legs.

In addition to variations in the sizes of ganglia, the organization and connections of neurons within particular ganglia will vary according to the function of the segment in which they lie. The kinds of sensory inputs and motor outputs of different segments will obviously vary. For example, inputs from sensory receptors to the ganglia controlling legs will be quite different from those to the ganglia operating the mouthparts.

Most animals have a head end and a tail end. The CNS in nearly all animals also has a noticeable enlargement of the ganglia at the head end; this is called **cephalization**.

☐ Why should there be this enlargement of ganglia at the head end?

■ It is obviously important for an animal to be aware of what it is approaching. Therefore the head or leading end is usually equipped with special sense organs together with the neurons required to interpret the sensory information and to direct appropriate motor actions.

Usually, the head also contains the largest number of neurons. This concentration of neurons plays an important role in coordinating the behaviour of the whole animal. In most invertebrates this concentration takes the form of a pair of enlarged ganglia at the head end which can be regarded as the brain, although, strictly speaking the word brain refers to that part of the CNS enclosed within the skull in vertebrates.

Within the invertebrate brain are groups of neurons which collectively perform various tasks such as interpreting information from the sense organs on the head. They have extensive connections with the other ganglia which are linked by the longitudinal connectives. These connectives, on the basis of the direction of travel of action potentials, make both *ascending* (towards the brain) and *descending* (away from the brain) connections.

To complete this list of basic descriptive terms about information flow in nervous systems, in general the axons that carry information *to* a particular group of neurons are called **afferent** axons, and those carrying information *away* from a group of neurons are called **efferent** axons.

The shape of many invertebrate neurons is rather different from the basic shape described in Chapter 2. The axon of an invertebrate neuron often arises from the dendritic tree rather than the cell body. Figure 6.8 illustrates this using the examples of a motor neuron in a locust ganglion and some neurons from the brain of a fly. It is often difficult to tell which is an axon and which a dendrite. With a microscope it can be seen that many of these processes contain both pre-synaptic and post-synaptic structures; they both release transmitter and contain membrane receptors. Despite these differences, the way in which these neurons receive and integrate synaptic inputs from many sources and influence other neurons is fundamentally the same as described for vertebrate neurons in Chapters 2, 3 and 4.

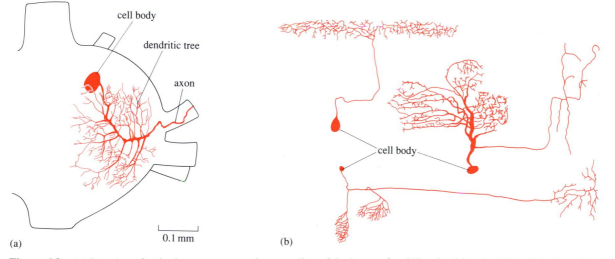

**Figure 6.8**   (a) Drawing of a single motor neuron in a ganglion of the locust after filling it with a dye. Not all the branches have been completely filled so some appear with breaks in them. (b) A variety of neurons from the CNS of a fly stained using the Golgi technique (Box 2.3, Section 2.3.1).

Within certain segmental ganglia there are neurons that generate rhythms, for example to produce rhythmic locomotory patterns. However, the output from the ganglion depends upon three factors: (a) the input from receptors, (b) the input from the brain, and (c) intrinsic rhythmic activity. Inputs to the ganglia originate from sensory receptors within that segment (detecting muscle stretch or contact with the ground, for example) as well as from descending connections from the brain, which coordinates the activities of the different ganglia. In this way the motor output is controlled both by local sensory information and also from the brain.

The role of local versus 'higher' (i.e. brain) control of movement can be demonstrated in segmented marine worms that swim by undulating waves passing down their bodies. If a cut is made through the nerve cord just behind the head in such a segmented worm, the segments below the cut will still make swimming movements but such movements will be more violent and uncoordinated. The influence from the brain on the other ganglia tends to be one of inhibition as well as organization. The movements made by each segment are coordinated with those of its neighbours. The longitudinal connectives are important in this coordination: if the nerve cord is cut midway down such a segmented worm, the segments below the cut will still make swimming movements but they will not be synchronized with those in the front half of the worm.

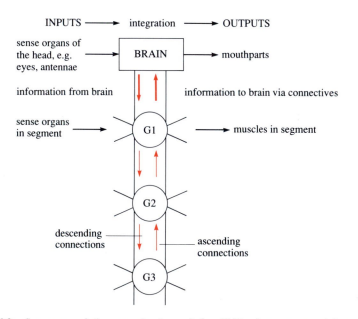

**Figure 6.9** Summary of the organization of the CNS of a segmented invertebrate illustrating the flow of information between various parts. G1–G3 are the ganglia of the first three segments below the head.

The detailed arrangement of the cells in a given segmental ganglion is often very repeatable from one individual to the next within a species, and also between ganglia with similar functions. This makes them ideal for studying the structure and function of neural cells (see Chapter 7) since individual cells can be identified using relatively low-power microscopy. In addition, invertebrate neurons can tolerate changes in their environment much better than the cells of vertebrates so that study of isolated ganglia, or even isolated cells, is feasible. A summary of the organization of the CNS of a segmented invertebrate is shown in Figure 6.9. Only three segmental ganglia are shown, but this illustrates the flow of information between various parts of the nervous system.

## 6.3.2   Molluscs

The molluscs are the second most numerous group of invertebrates (the largest being the arthropods, discussed in Section 6.3.3). Snails, oysters and the octopus are familiar members of this group. They are built on a segmental plan (which is often not obvious) and have a bilaterally symmetrical nervous system which is found close to the gut.

### Aplysia

You have already come across the sea slug *Aplysia*, sometimes also known as the sea hare on account of its large sensory tentacles that look like ears (Book 1, Chapter 6). It is the mollusc famous for its use as a subject in the study of learning. This marine herbivore is related to slugs and snails. Figure 6.10 shows the location of the major features of the nervous system in *Aplysia* plus an enlarged view of the abdominal ganglion.

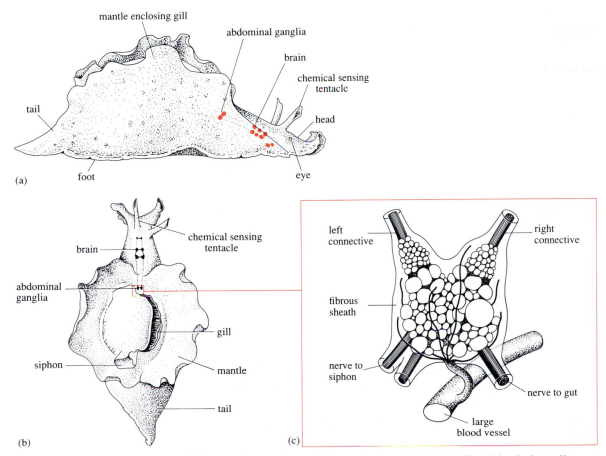

**Figure 6.10**   (a) Side and (b) top views of *Aplysia* showing the CNS. (c) The abdominal ganglion.

The *Aplysia* brain receives information from chemoreceptors located on a pair of tentacles. The eyes have a rather simple design. They are nothing like as sophisticated as human eyes, consisting of photoreceptors and associated neurons which respond to general variations in light intensity rather than patterns of light and dark in the visual image. This animal, like its relatives the slugs and snails, moves by regular waves of contraction passing from head to tail along its muscular foot. The two ganglia in each segment are very close together so that the commissure is not visible. The longitudinal connectives are bilaterally symmetrical, but the nerves that innervate the siphon (part of the respiratory system) and the huge gill are not symmetrical, being found only on one side.

## Cephalopods

The squid, cuttlefish and octopus are all cephalopods. Cephalopods are highly evolved, predatory marine molluscs whose nervous system reflects their active lifestyle. The most obvious difference in the nervous system of these molluscs is the huge size of the brain, especially the region receiving input from the well developed eyes (Figure 6.11). Notice that their eyes look remarkably like human eyes; in fact they work on the same principle as the vertebrate eye with a lens to focus light rays onto the light receptors at the back of the eye (in the same way as the lens in a camera focuses the image onto the film). They can also interpret highly patterned visual information. The cephalopods communicate with one another using very elaborate visual displays. The elaborate visual systems and the large size of the brains of both squid and octopus mean that they can be trained to learn complex visual discrimination tasks.

The arrangement of the axons connecting the eye to the brain is precisely ordered so that neighbouring photoreceptors send their axons to neighbouring neurons in the brain. This kind of projection is called a **topographic** projection. Since neighbouring photoreceptors are stimulated by light coming from neighbouring parts of the visual scene, such a topographic projection provides the nervous system with information concerning the location of visual stimuli in space. In effect, the animal has an internal representation of the patterns of light and dark falling on the retina which bears a direct relationship with the spatial localization of objects in its environment. Such a precise ordering of sensory inputs to the CNS is a very common feature in both invertebrates and vertebrates.

Unlike the slow moving slugs and snails, squid and octopus can quickly escape from danger by forcing a jet of water out through the siphon (Figure 6.11a). This jet drives the animal backwards. To get maximum force the muscles must contract synchronously and quickly.

☐ How is a high speed of conduction of signals to these muscles achieved?

■ The axons that innervate these muscles have a very large diameter which provides a high speed of conduction of action potentials. Recall that large diameter axons have a higher conduction speed than small diameter ones (see Section 6.3).

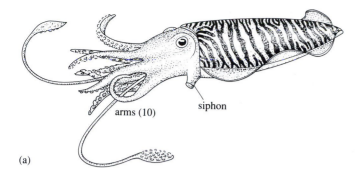

(a)

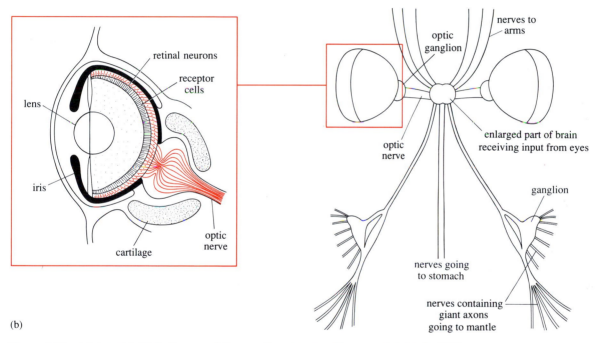

(b)

**Figure 6.11** (a) A squid. (b) A diagram of the eye of an octopus with connections to the CNS.

### 6.3.3 Arthropods

Arthropods make up the largest and most diverse group of invertebrates. They include the crustaceans (e.g. lobsters, crabs and shrimps), the insects, and the arachnids (spiders and mites). All arthropods have a hard external skeleton called the exoskeleton which supports and protects the inner organs, muscles and nervous system. They are all clearly segmented (Figure 6.12, *overleaf*); their ancestors were segmented worms similar to earthworms. The arthropods are an extremely successful group of animals occupying almost every available habitat on earth. They come in a range of sizes and shapes, and this variation is also reflected in the structure of their nervous systems, as illustrated in Figure 6.13 (*overleaf*).

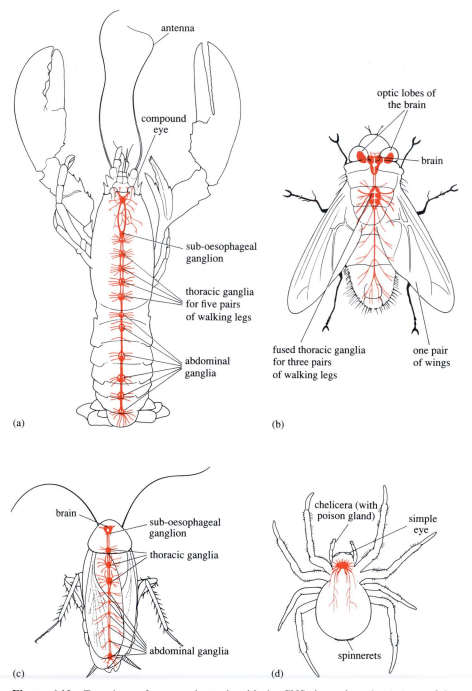

antenna

compound
eye

sub-oesophageal
ganglion

thoracic ganglia
for five pairs
of walking legs

abdominal
ganglia

(a)

optic lobes of
the brain

brain

fused thoracic ganglia
for three pairs
of walking legs

one pair
of wings

(b)

brain

sub-oesophageal
ganglion

thoracic ganglia

abdominal ganglia

(c)

chelicera (with
poison gland)

simple
eye

spinnerets

(d)

**Figure 6.12** Top views of some arthropods with the CNS shown in red. (a) A crayfish
(crustacean), (b) a fly (insect), (c) a cockroach (insect), and (d) a spider (arachnid).

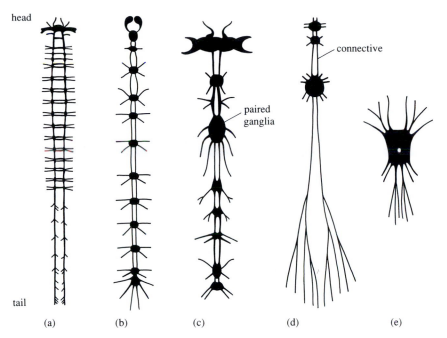

**Figure 6.13**   Diagrams showing the variability in the arrangement of the ganglia in different arthropods. (a) Woodlouse (terrestrial crustacean), (b) caterpillar (insect), (c) honey-bee (insect), (d) water-bug (insect), (e) mite (arachnid). In the mite the ganglia are all fused together.

The bodies of arthropods can be divided up into three regions, the head containing the brain, the thorax which bears the legs and wings (if present), and the abdomen which contains the digestive, excretory and reproductive organs. (Notice that these regions are a bit different from those with the same names in vertebrates.) As you can see from Figures 6.12 and 6.13, in some arthropods these three regions have become fused together.

The head contains a pair of enlarged ganglia, the front one lying above the gut and the back one lying below it. Sense organs on the head include the usually prominent antennae (there may be several pairs) and the eyes. The antennae are long jointed structures equipped with fine hair-like mechanoreceptors sensitive to touch and air movements. They also contain chemoreceptors; some moths have especially elaborate antennae which are acutely sensitive to the signalling molecules released by prospective mates.

Arthropod eyes are of various types, with some being very simple like those described in *Aplysia*. Spiders often have several pairs of eyes, each specialized for a particular task. The crustaceans and insects also have much more complex eyes which bear no resemblance to either the simple eyes of molluscs or the 'camera-like' eyes of cephalopods and vertebrates. This type of eye is called a **compound eye** because it is made up of an array of separate units each having its own lens and photoreceptors. The compound eye forms an image made up of lots of separate dots rather like a newspaper photograph, each separate unit looking at a separate region of space. Figure 6.14b (*overleaf*) is a photograph of the compound eye of a fly. As was discussed for the cephalopods, the neuronal connections between the eye and the CNS are topographically ordered. Many insects are active during the day and rely on vision. This is reflected in the structure of their brains, which have enlarged regions that receive input from the eyes. The beautifully ordered arrangement of the cells and axons in this region of the brain in a fly is illustrated in Figure 6.14c.

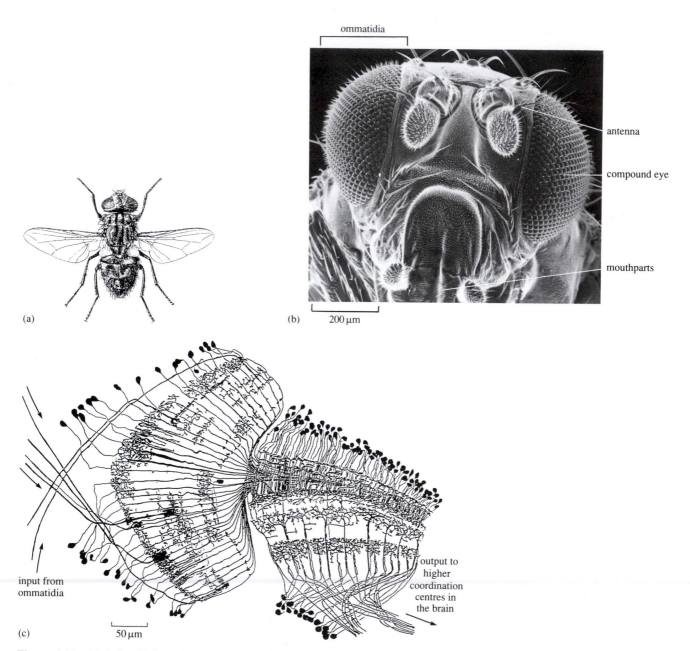

(a)

(b)  200 μm

ommatidia

antenna

compound eye

mouthparts

input from ommatidia

output to higher coordination centres in the brain

(c)  50 μm

**Figure 6.14**  (a) A fly. (b) Scanning electron micrograph of the head of a fly showing the compound eye. The facets of each separate unit are clearly visible. (c) Drawing showing the intricate orderly pattern of connections in the part of the brain receiving input from the compound eye in the fly. The preparation was stained using a modification of the Golgi technique.

The thoracic segments behind the head bear the walking legs (five segments in crustaceans, four in spiders and three in insects, of which two may also bear the wings). Behind the thoracic segments are the abdominal segments that contain the bulk of the digestive, excretory and reproductive organs.

The neurons in each thoracic ganglion control the movement of the limb and wing (if present) on its side of the body. Each ganglion receives sensory information from local receptors providing information about contact with the ground, the angle of the various parts of the jointed limb and tension in the muscles. Coordinated walking movements are generated by interaction between the thoracic ganglia on the two sides via the commissures and the longitudinal connectives (which also carry information to and from the brain). The small number of neurons in the ganglia together with their relative simplicity provides a good opportunity to study the structure and function of neuronal circuits controlling, for example, flight in locusts, as will be discussed in Chapter 7.

In addition to the sense organs on the head, many insects have special sense organs on other parts of their bodies. For example, one of the thoracic segments in some moths and locusts contains a region where the exoskeleton is very thin, providing the animal with a kind of ear drum to detect sounds. Such 'thoracic ears' provide nocturnal moths with a very sensitive bat-detection system—see Book 1.

Mechanoreceptive hairs sensitive to air movements are not only found on the antennae. The two special structures protruding from the back of the abdomen of a cockroach (Figure 6.12) contain mechanoreceptors that pick up air movements. Excitation of these receptors produces a very quick escape response which makes them almost impossible to swat!

The abdominal ganglia are invariably smaller than the thoracic ganglia, with the size of the ganglia giving some indication of the number of neurons contained within them. Most crustaceans move by walking, but shrimps and lobsters have evolved a method of rapidly propelling themselves out of danger. You may have noticed how shrimps and lobsters can shoot off backwards using a rapid flick of the tail (which is very muscular). The motor neurons in the abdominal ganglia that innervate the tail muscles are activated by large diameter axons in the longitudinal connectives that come from neurons in the brain.

☐   Why might the axons of these neurons be large in diameter?

■   Like the giant axons in the cephalopods, in these large diameter axons the speed of conduction of action potentials is increased and the escape response is activated quickly.

Many insects show remarkable feats of learning. Bees learn to visit particular flowers at those particular times of day when the nectar is available. Furthermore, they can communicate their knowledge to other members of the hive. However, there are only a relatively small number of neurons in the insect nervous system. This means that there is a limit to the range of neural interactions possible. Insects are less able to vary their behavioural repertoire greatly when external circumstances may require it. The success of insects at colonizing a wide range of habitats lies in their reproductive fecundity and evolutionary adaptation to changes in the environment rather than the ability to change their behaviour quickly as a result of learning, in order to survive such changes.

# Summary of Chapter 6

This chapter has looked at the nervous systems of some invertebrates and has drawn some comparisons and contrasts both (a) between different invertebrates, and (b) between invertebrates as a group and vertebrates. The chapter started by looking at the most simple kind of nervous system: nerve nets in the sea-anemone and *Hydra*. The nerve net consists of a collection of electrically excitable cells taking the shape of a net and located in the body wall of the animal. Though relatively simple, the nerve net contributes to behaviour that is appropriate to the circumstances. That is to say, it allows for specific responses to stimuli to be performed (e.g. capture of prey in anemones and swimming in jellyfish). Habituation of the withdrawal response can be observed in sea-anemones: the response to a harmless and non-food stimulus decreases in magnitude with repeated stimulation.

Other invertebrates (such as arthropods and molluscs) have more complex nervous systems than those involving simply a nerve net. Their bodies show segmentation. In their case, a CNS (consisting in large part of whole neurons and the cell bodies of neurons) and a PNS (consisting in large part of the axons of neurons) can be discerned. The brain and nerve cord make up the CNS in such invertebrates. The nerve cord may consist of paired longitudinal connectives with paired ganglia in each segment. Unlike the vertebrates, the nerve cord is not surrounded by bone and is therefore not described as a spinal cord.

Collections of nerve cell bodies are termed ganglia and are found at regular locations in the invertebrate CNS, associated with particular body segments. Within certain ganglia of the invertebrate nervous system there are neurons that can generate rhythms. The output from such a ganglion (to control, for example, motor action) would depend upon (a) the output of rhythm generating neurons, (b) input from sensory receptors, and (c) input from the brain.

Invertebrate axons lack the myelin sheaths that provide high conduction speed in vertebrates. In invertebrates, high speed can only be achieved by their axons having relatively large diameters (for example, the giant axon of the squid).

# Objectives for Chapter 6

When you have completed this chapter you should be able to:

6.1 Define and use or recognise the definitions and applications of each of the terms printed in **bold** in the text. (*Question 6.1*)

6.2 Describe the structure and function of the nerve net in sea-anemones and jellyfish, and relate these to their respective lifestyles. (*Questions 6.2 and 6.3*)

6.3 Explain the significance of habituation in a response to repeated presentation of the same non-harmful stimulus. (*Question 6.4*)

6.4 Describe the basic organization of the nervous system in invertebrates. (*Question 6.4*)

6.5     Explain the importance of myelination when considering the difference between the nervous systems of vertebrates and invertebrates. (*Question 6.5*)

6.6     Explain why invertebrates are often chosen by neurophysiologists to investigate neural function. (*Question 6.6*)

6.7     Compare the structure of the nervous system and the function it serves in some relatively simple invertebrates such as sea-anemones and some more complex invertebrate animals such as insects or molluscs. In particular, relate the structure and function to their lifestyles and behaviour. (*Questions 6.5 and 6.6*)

# Questions for Chapter 6

**Question 6.1** (*Objective 6.1*)
How are sensory inputs to the CNS arranged to give the animal spatial information about the external world?

**Question 6.2** (*Objective 6.2*)
What are the general properties of nervous systems that the nerve net illustrates?

**Question 6.3** (*Objective 6.2*)
In what way does the lifestyle of the sea-anemone differ from that of the jellyfish? How is this related to differences in the tasks that their nervous systems perform?

**Question 6.4** (*Objectives 6.3 and 6.4*)
What is the importance of habituation and rhythm generation in nervous systems? What basic structures are involved?

**Question 6.5** (*Objectives 6.5 and 6.7*)
How is the speed of conduction of action potentials enhanced in (a) vertebrates, and (b) invertebrates?

**Question 6.6** (*Objectives 6.6 and 6.7*)
What is the function of the giant fibre system in the squid and what feature makes it useful for investigations about the nature of the action potential?

# CHAPTER 7
# NERVOUS SYSTEMS AND CONTROL OF BEHAVIOUR

## 7.1    Introduction

This chapter explores the way in which the separate elements of the nervous system combine with muscles to produce recognizable behaviour patterns. This will mean drawing on your knowledge of behaviour from Book 1 and of neurophysiology from Chapter 3 of this book, but you will also make use of simple control systems theory as a useful analytical tool. As you now know from Book 1, the description and analysis of behaviour patterns is not easy. The description of the underlying biological mechanisms is also difficult but the conservation of structure that has occurred during evolution means that there are similarities in function in all nervous systems and in muscles. Furthermore, since evolution has been, generally, a process of increasing complexity with time, the function of 'simple' nervous systems in evolutionarily ancient groups of animals can be investigated, and the principles used to describe the more complicated behaviour patterns and neural systems of, for example, mammals.

This distinction between 'simple' and 'complex' nervous systems is often used, but it is a highly arbitrary one. The contraction of a single muscle in a horse may involve hundreds of neurons and their interconnections, but a single muscle contraction in an insect might involve only three or four neurons. Thus, from the point of view of an investigator, the nervous system of an insect is simple by comparison with the horse. The unravelling of the relation between the nervous system and behaviour is, initially, a more practical proposition in the insect. The principles of operation of the nervous system will not be simpler, but there is at least some prospect of discovering them.

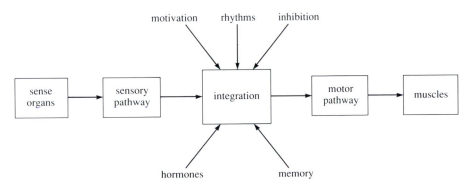

**Figure 7.1**    Block diagram of a generalized behavioural pathway.

Animal behaviour is the result of the coordinated action of effectors, usually muscles, with the coordination being provided by the nervous system. The stimulus for a particular behaviour pattern may come from within the animal or from external sources. A particular behaviour pattern can be generalized as a block diagram of the type shown in Figure 7.1, with the stimulus being provided by a sense organ.

This diagram shows a flow of information through the animal from sensory system to motor system. It leaves out a number of key pathways, as you will see, e.g. information about the state of muscles also flows in the reverse direction. However, it provides a good starting point. You have already come across hormones, memory and motivation in Book 1. In this chapter you will learn about the sensory and motor pathways, inhibition and rhythms. Not all the features shown in Figure 7.1 are found in all animals, but the figure provides a context for analysis of the 'simple' neural pathways underlying behaviour in sea-anemones and, later on in the chapter, the rather more complicated pathways in the locust.

# 7.2 Shell climbing behaviour in sea-anemones

Sea-anemones are very good models for the study of important general phenomena, for example, electrical conduction in living tissues and sensory reception. Their behaviour can be described using terminology derived from studies of vertebrates and it is possible to provide a partial explanation of the neural mechanisms underlying the behaviour. You were introduced to the sea-anemone and nerve nets in Section 6.2.

A typical sea-anemone is illustrated in Figure 7.2. You can find this anemone on most rocky shores in Britain, attached to a rock by the foot (the pedal disc). When the tide is out and the animal is exposed it looks just like a shapeless blob of red jelly. When covered by water, the body and the tentacles expand (Figure 7.2b).

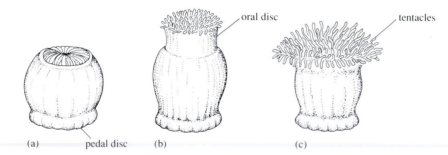

**Figure 7.2** The sea-anemone *Actinia* (a) in the contracted state, (b) starting to expand, and (c) in the expanded state.

In this section you will learn how behaviour patterns can be broken down into discrete components, each associated with a particular group of muscle contractions and with particular events in the nerve net. After reading it you should be able to appreciate the links between nerve net, muscles and behaviour but you will not need to memorize the names of all the muscles or all the components of behaviour in the sea-anemone.

## 7.2.1   Muscles and movement

Although anemones appear to be firmly and permanently attached to rocks, they are able to move around, albeit slowly, and some anemones climb onto and attach themselves to mollusc shells. Shell climbing behaviour in the large anemone *Calliactis* can be more easily understood if it is subdivided into easily recognizable stages (Figure 7.3, *overleaf*). There are a number of discrete behavioural building blocks, each of which can be linked with specific muscle contractions. Figure 7.4 (*overleaf*) shows the behavioural building blocks that have been recognized by research workers. The muscles responsible for each of these blocks are shown in Table 7.1. Shell climbing behaviour involves a sequence of movements and a corresponding sequence of muscle contractions. The actual sequence of behavioural building blocks (using the standard numbers shown in Figure 7.4) is

$$3 \rightarrow 4a \rightarrow 8 \rightarrow 6 \rightarrow 2 \rightarrow 5 \rightarrow 9 \rightarrow 5 \rightarrow 1 \rightarrow 7$$

The individual stages may overlap and, of course, there will be variation between individuals but this is the basic sequence. How is the sequential contraction of muscles brought about? The next section looks first at the properties of the electrical conducting systems and then relates these to shell climbing behaviour.

**Table 7.1**   A description of the muscles which may be involved in producing the shape changes shown in Figure 7.4. You are not expected to remember the details in this table.

| Movement | Muscles involved | Symmetrical (S) or local contraction (L) | Excitation (E) or inhibition (I) |
|---|---|---|---|
| 1.  Column shortening | Parietals | S | E |
| 2.  Column extension | Column circulars | S | E |
| 3.  Local contractions of tentacles and oral disc | Tentacle longitudinals and oral disc radials | L | E |
| 4.  Closure (a) partial, (b) complete | Sphincter and retractors | S | E |
| 5.  Column bending | Parietals | L | E |
| 6.  Column wall contraction | Column circulars | L | E |
| 7.  Oral disc expansion | Oral disc radials | S | I |
| 8.  Pedal disc detachment | None | – | – |
| 9.  Pedal disc expansion | Pedal disc circulars and basilars? | S? | I |

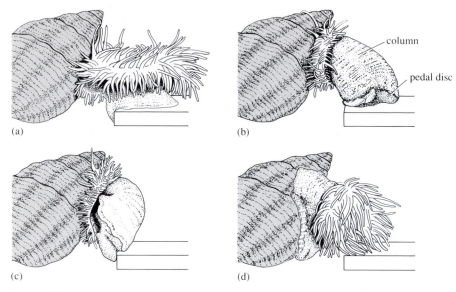

**Figure 7.3** Shell climbing behaviour in the anemone *Calliactis*. (a) Initial contact with the shell is made by the tentacles. (b) After 6 minutes the pedal disc is partly detached. (c) After 8 minutes the column is bending, bringing the pedal disc close to the shell. (d) After 28 minutes the anemone is firmly attached to the shell by the pedal disc.

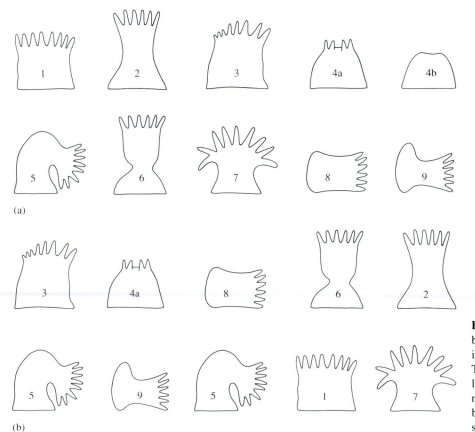

**Figure 7.4** (a) Behavioural building blocks in *Calliactis* (only the more important changes in shape are shown). The numbers refer to Table 7.1, which lists the muscles responsible for the movements. (b) The sequence of behavioural building blocks that make up shell climbing behaviour (see text).

## 7.2.2   Electrical conducting systems

The neurons in sea-anemones are dispersed in thin layers, apparently at random. They form a network known as a nerve net (recall Figure 6.2 and the description of nerve nets in Section 6.2.1). Nerve nets are the simplest, and probably the 'oldest' (in evolutionary terms) form of nervous system, and yet they provide the basis for the quite complicated behaviour patterns seen in anemones. Nerve nets are not restricted to anemones, but occur in the peripheral nervous system (PNS) of other invertebrates and in the gut of vertebrates, including humans. The neurons in sea-anemones have long, very fine processes that criss-cross to form a very diffuse network (see Figure 6.2). Where the processes cross over one another they make synaptic contact. There is generally no preferred direction of conduction of action potentials, so a stimulus at any one point tends to be conducted radially away through the nerve net. The small size of the neurons makes it difficult to insert recording electrodes and so little is known about synaptic conduction in nerve nets.

Experimental work on anemones like *Calliactis* suggests that there may not be just a single nerve net (Figure 7.5). There is certainly evidence of more than one system capable of conducting electrical signals. If a recording electrode is attached to the tentacle of *Calliactis* to record extracellular potentials and the column is stimulated by a short electrical pulse about 4 cm away from the recording electrode, three separate events can be detected (Figure 7.6a). These same events can also be recorded from the other tentacles (Figure 7.6b). Such events will be referred to here as 'action' potentials although, as you will see later, they show some differences from action potentials recorded in other nervous systems.

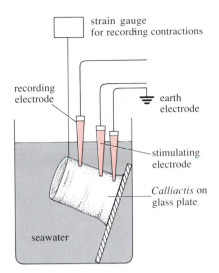

**Figure 7.5**   Recording electrical activity from the nerve net of an anemone.

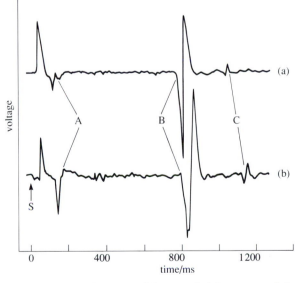

**Figure 7.6**   Action potentials recorded from two of the tentacles of *Calliactis*. The stimulus was a single shock to the column 4 cm away from the recording electrode in trace (a), given at point S (time = zero). Trace (b) shows the same electrical events recorded by an electrode on a neighbouring tentacle.

☐ Look at the upper trace in Figure 7.6. For each action potential, measure the time delay after the stimulation.

■ Action potential A starts about 40 ms (milliseconds, see Box 7.1) after the stimulus, B about 800 ms after, and C about 1 020 ms after.

☐ From these delays you could get an estimate of conduction velocities. How do your estimates for A and B compare with other conduction velocities that you have come across in Chapter 6?

■ The conduction velocity for action potential A is 100 cm s$^{-1}$ (see Box 7.1 on scientific notation). This conduction velocity is calculated as follows. It takes 40 ms for the action potential produced by the stimulus to travel the 4 cm to the recording electrode. So in 1 ms the action potential travels 4 cm divided by 40, which is 0.1 cm (0.1 cm in 1 ms equals 100 cm in 1 s). The conduction velocity for B is 5 cm s$^{-1}$. This is very much slower than the figure of 30 m s$^{-1}$ which is typical for frog axons and 100 m s$^{-1}$ for mammalian myelinated axons.

These three pulses have such different conduction times that they are thought to represent conduction in three different parts of a single nerve net, or just possibly three different nerve nets. Each part will be considered in turn. The first is the main nerve net, called the through-conducting nerve net. The other two systems are termed conducting systems since their relationship to the main nerve net is unclear.

---

## Box 7.1　Scientific notation

In everyday language you may well refer to speed as 'miles per hour' or 'feet per second'. Science uses internationally agreed units based on the decimal system—hence metres and kilograms—and standard abbreviations, for example 's' for seconds and 'm' for metres. So, miles per hour becomes kilometres per hour, but it is written as km h$^{-1}$. The '$^{-1}$' is equivalent to 'per'.

---

## The through-conducting nerve net or TCNN

Action potential A is a single action potential from the through-conducting nerve net (TCNN). There is a clear similarity between the function of the TCNN and the function of nervous systems in other animals. Both mechanical and electrical stimulation applied to the outside of the animal will produce responses from the animal. Activity in the TCNN evokes action potentials, and subsequently contraction, in muscles. The muscles can contract slowly or rapidly. Both fast and slow contractions are initiated by activity in the TCNN. Each muscle contracts optimally at a particular frequency of stimulation. Different muscles have different optimal frequencies so the frequency of action potentials occurring in the TCNN at any instance will influence the pattern of muscle contraction.

There is also some spontaneous activity. Bursts of action potentials at 10–15 minute intervals have been recorded. Each burst contains a number of action potentials at 3–4 s intervals. The timing of this activity suggests that there are **pacemakers** scattered through the nerve net that provide signals at regular intervals, rather like a clock ticking. Unfortunately the function of spontaneous activity is unknown, although it may play a part in the respiratory (breathing) rhythm.

## The slow systems (SS1 and SS2)

Action potential B is from the conducting system known as slow system 1 (SS1) because of the much lower conduction velocity of 5–12 cm s$^{-1}$ (compared with 100 cm s$^{-1}$ for the TCNN). If the column of the anemone is stimulated repetitively, repetitive potentials can be recorded from the SS1 system. For each stimulus one action potential is produced, but there is only a one-to-one relationship between stimulus and response if the interval between stimuli exceeds 100 ms (Figure 7.7a). These action potentials are unusual and do not behave in the same way as those found in other nervous systems. If the interval is less than 100 ms only some of the stimuli produce action potentials. Even at intervals as large as 10 s the response potentials decrease in size (Figure 7.7b). This suggests that the rate at which action potentials can be conducted is limited by the properties of the system. The period following an action potential during which the system cannot conduct another one is called the absolute refractory period (Section 3.8). It appears that the SS1 system has an absolute refractory period of 100 ms when no action potential can be generated and a long **relative refractory period**, the period after a potential when the system is recovering and when action potentials are smaller than normal.

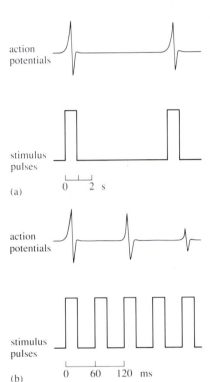

☐ How do the action potentials in the anemone nerve net differ from those described in Section 2.3.2?

■ They do not obey the all-or-nothing principle, i.e. action potentials in the anemone are not always of the same size.

Action potential C in Figure 7.6 is a potential from a second slow conducting system, SS2. It is even slower than SS1 and it has a long refractory period. Both its known actions are inhibitory. Activity in the SS2 inhibits certain body wall muscles, but more interestingly SS2 activity slows the TCNN pacemakers. Recall from the previous discussion of the TCNN that a muscle contracts optimally at a particular frequency of stimulation by action potentials. Different muscles have different optimal frequencies. It is probable that the frequency of action potentials in the TCNN is linked to the rate at which the pacemakers produce signals. So, if the SS2 system can alter the rate of the pacemakers then it may consequently alter the pattern of muscle contraction. This is a complicated control mechanism since it involves three separate elements, the slow system SS2 modifying the pacemakers in the TCNN which in turn modifies the contraction of groups of muscles.

Here, then, is an important part of the control mechanism that underlies behaviour, so the next section now returns to shell climbing behaviour to see how far it is possible to go in linking the behavioural building blocks to activity in the nerve net and slow systems.

**Figure 7.7** (a), (b) Responses recorded in the SS1 system (upper trace) to electrical stimulation of the column of an anemone by short pulses (lower trace). (a) As the interval between stimulus pulses is very large there is a one-to-one relationship between stimulus and response. However, in (b) the interval between pulses (60 ms) is less than the absolute refractory period (100 ms) so there is not a one-to-one relationship between stimulus and response. The second and third pulses are reduced in size because it takes the SS1 system nearly 10 s to recover before it can transmit another full size potential..

### 7.2.3 Coordination of behaviour, and shell climbing

Touch a sea-anemone and it will contract. The harder you poke it, the greater will be the contraction. This illustrates a basic building block in the nervous system— the reflex response (Book 1, Sections 2.2 and 6.3.3). The response is fast, indicating that the connection between the point of stimulus and the muscles that contract must be the TCNN, rather than the slow systems. The nature of the receptors is still unknown but their presence can be deduced. The rapidity of this response is atypical of behaviour in the anemone, but speed is a property of many reflexes found in animals. A reflex provides a fast, stereotyped response to a stimulus and can be the basis for escape or avoidance behaviour.

Most behavioural activity of anemones, however, is probably based on slow muscle contraction. There is a complex cycle of slow contractions that constitutes a respiratory rhythm. This rhythm is thought to result from a respiratory pace-maker in the SS2 system. The SS2 system is inhibitory, so the pace-maker is likely to produce action potentials that rhythmically alter activity in the TCNN, producing rhythmical changes in the contractions of muscles.

☐ What is the probable action of the SS2 system on the TCNN?

■ It probably acts directly on the TCNN pacemakers and, because it has an inhibitory effect, it slows them down.

So, the contractions of the muscles during the respiratory rhythm are produced by a decrease in activity in the SS2 system which removes the inhibitory effect on the TCNN pacemakers. This system is summarized in Figure 7.8.

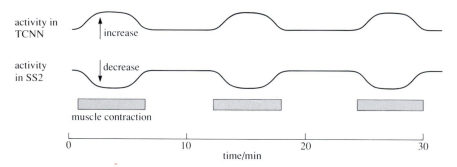

**Figure 7.8** Summary of the control of the respiratory rhythm in *Calliactis*.

Shell climbing behaviour was illustrated in Figure 7.3 and the behavioural building blocks that contribute to the behaviour were illustrated in Figure 7.4. The behaviour pattern is coordinated by the SS1 and SS2 systems and it can be divided, broadly, into five stages:

1   tentacles attach to the shell,

2   pedal disc detaches,

3   detached pedal disc moves onto the shell,

4   pedal disc fixes onto shell, and

5   tentacles release and anemone returns to its normal posture.

When the tentacles make contact with the shell, the resulting stimulus produces action potentials in both the SS1 and SS2 systems. The SS1 action potentials cause the pedal disc to detach from the rock. The SS2 potentials, as you might now be able to predict, inhibit the TCNN pacemakers. This means that the normal rhythmic contraction of muscles is abolished and the only contractions that occur are responses to stimuli. The contractions of the muscles that move the anemone onto the shell are produced by pulses in the SS1 system. The way in which the sequence of contractions is controlled is not known. However, there appear to be receptors in the column that respond to stretching as the anemone tilts towards the shell. The activity of the stretch receptors causes low frequency action potentials in the TCNN and these initiate swelling of the pedal disc during attachment.

Notice how far this description is from being a complete explanation of the nervous control of behaviour, even in a comparatively simple animal with a 'simple' nervous system! However, it is possible to see the properties of the nerves and muscles that provide the elements of the control system:

1    different muscles contract optimally at different frequencies of stimulation,

2    pacemakers maintain rhythms,

3    inhibitory neurons alter pacemaker activity,

4    inhibitory neurons alter muscle contraction, and

5    reflex responses can be fast.

Shell climbing behaviour is only one of the recognizable behaviour patterns in sea-anemones, but it is the one which can provide the most complete explanation. In Book 1 you read how some behaviour patterns are common to a wide range of species, and one such behaviour pattern is recognizable in anemones.

## 7.2.4   Aggression

Aggression in the anemone involves a complicated behaviour pattern, like shell climbing, and the neural mechanisms underlying the behaviour are not completely worked out yet. Describing the behaviour of an anemone as aggression may not seem appropriate, but some anemones are able to attack, maim and sometimes destroy other anemones of the same species. Similar behaviour in other species would be called aggressive. It is an impressive behavioural sequence, particularly because anemones give the appearance of being such sedentary animals. The sequence lasts 2–10 minutes and has been studied in another species of sea-anemone, *Actinia*. Three stages in the behavioural sequence are illustrated in Figure 7.9 (*overleaf*). The response is initiated when an anemone contacts some part of another anemone with its tentacles. The stimulus provided by tentacle contact must differ in some way from contact with a hard surface, contact with another of the animal's own tentacles, or with food. It can be deduced that there are either different groups of receptors, or receptors that respond differently to different stimuli. Also, the anemone must have a means of distinguishing between itself and another anemone (Chapter 5).

The anemone responds to the stimulus of tentacle contact initially by withdrawing the tentacles, but then it extends them again. If contact with the other anemone is resumed there is an asymmetric contraction of the column muscles that pushes batteries of stinging organs against the other anemone (Figure 7.9b). The effect of the stinging cells on the 'victim' is contraction of column muscles followed by loosening of the pedal disc. Thus the victim withdraws from the 'aggressor' by detaching from the rock surface. The waves in the sea may then carry it away, leaving the aggressor in possession.

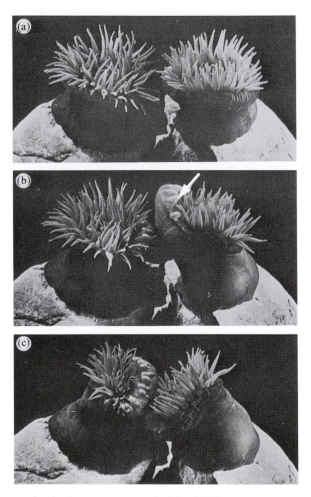

**Figure 7.9** Aggression in the sea-anemone *Actinia*. (a) The two anemones make contact with their tentacles. (b) The right-hand anemone responds. The column on the side facing the other anemone expands bringing the stinging cells (arrowed) forward. (c) The stinging cells are pushed into the side of the left-hand anemone inflicting a wound.

The response of the victim contains some of the behavioural building blocks that were recognized in shell climbing behaviour, and similar events would be expected to occur in the nervous system. To analyse the neural control of aggression or of shell climbing it would be necessary to record electrical activity during behaviour, which is technically very difficult. However, by choosing an appropriate animal it is possible to make recordings from the nervous system while behaviour is in progress and Section 7.3 examines such a model. Many of the properties of the nervous system of the anemone also appear in this model, but some additional features are present.

## Summary of Section 7.2

In sea-anemones the nervous system is divided into a number of discrete, but interconnected, cells that form nerve nets. Nerve nets are found in most animals, including humans, and studying anemones increases our understanding of some important general phenomena, for example:

1    conduction and coordination in nerve nets,

2    simple reflexes,

3    interactions of nerves and muscles and control of behaviour,

4    pacemakers in the nervous system.

Although simply organized, anemones have a relatively wide range of behaviour patterns some of which, such as aggression, are very complex. Aggression in anemones is equivalent, in behavioural terms, to aggression in other animals.

# 7.3    Introduction to control mechanisms in insect flight

The remaining sections of this chapter are concerned with the control mechanism involved in insect flight. As you study these sections you will be introduced to the process of muscle contraction, the mechanism by which rhythms are generated, and the principles of sensory feedback.

Imagine that you are trying to catch a grasshopper. You creep up upon it cautiously. Despite your careful movements the grasshopper jumps. That jump is a response to a stimulus. It is a response that gets the animal out of danger.

☐    What stimuli might elicit that response?

■    A movement within the animal's visual field is the most obvious one, but it is probably the vibration produced by your movements that is detected by the animal.

☐    What elements of the nervous system might be involved in the jump?

■    One or more sense organs are involved. Axons from the sensory organs will carry action potentials to the CNS where they will affect central neurons via synapses. Neurons in the CNS will make contact with motor neurons that send action potentials to the leg muscles, producing a jump.

This sequence of events is summarized in Figure 7.10. The animal may well start to fly after it has jumped, the jump having been converted into a take-off. Once the 'decision' to take off has been made the forewings and hindwings maintain a flight rhythm. What are the neural elements underlying this behaviour pattern?

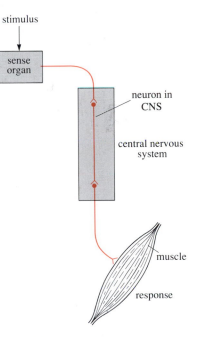

**Figure 7.10**    Block diagram of a generalized behavioural pathway.

# 7.4  Locust flight

## 7.4.1  Locusts in tethered flight

The movement of the wings of a locust can be 'frozen' during flight by illuminating the animal with flashes of light using a stroboscope (see Box 7.2). If the time between flashes is the same as the wing-beat frequency then the wings will appear to be stationary.

The locust has two pairs of wings. They move out of phase with each other in a cycle that lasts 50 ms. (If each cycle lasts 50 ms, then dividing 1 000 (the number of milliseconds in a second) by 50 gives a frequency of 20 cycles per second.) The hindwings always lead the forewings by 7 ms (the *phase difference* is 7 ms), which means that the wings do not collide. In addition to moving up and down, the wings also rotate around their long axis during each cycle, which improves their aerodynamic performance.

There are two main questions that can be asked: how is this pattern of wing movement produced by the nervous system, and how is it maintained in flight? Firstly, however, the initiation and termination of flight will be looked at.

---

**Box 7.2  The stroboscope**

A stroboscope contains a timing device and a very bright light. The light source provides very brief flashes of light at regular intervals determined by the timer. In addition to its entertainment value in discos, it is used wherever rapidly occurring and repetitive events need to be observed. For example, a rotating fan can be made to appear stationary if illuminated with a flash of light at the same point in each rotation. When the fan appears to be stationary, the time between each flash equals the time taken for the fan to rotate once. By adjusting the rate of flashing until the fan appears to be stationary, the speed of rotation of the fan can be measured.

A stroboscope thus provides a means of making a fast repetitive movement visible but it also provides a precise way of measuring the rate at which the movement is occurring.

---

## 7.4.2  Sensory control of locust flight

The tethered locust provides a simple way of investigating the stimuli for flight. Blowing on the locust with a hair-drier will usually make it fly, but the stimulus is most effective if the air stream is directed onto the front of the head. This suggests that the receptors that detect wind are sited there. A coat of nail varnish over the front of the head abolishes flight. Peeling off the layer of varnish restores flight.

When a locust is on the ground it does not fly, predictably. If a tethered locust is flying in an air current, touching the tip of a leg will stop it flying, showing that contact with the ground, a bush or a tree inhibits or terminates flight.

# 7.5   Locust flight muscles and wing movement

Each wing is acted on by two sets of muscles, one set which raises the wing (the elevator muscles) and one set that lowers it (the depressor muscles). Because the muscles produce opposite effects they are said to be **antagonistic** to each other. Muscles that work together are **synergistic**. Muscles contract when stimulated electrically but they are unable to expand actively. Some other force is thus required to stretch them after a contraction so that they are able to contract again. This restoring force is generally provided by antagonistic muscles.

The main flight muscles are shown in Figure 7.11 (*overleaf*). They are inside a skeletal box called the thorax. The skeletal plates that make up the thorax are flexible and this flexibility contributes to muscle contraction. The muscles that raise the wing are grey in the figure; they are the elevator muscles. The depressor muscles are shown coloured red in the figure. The main depressor muscles can be divided into two groups. Two are attached *directly* to the wing and their mode of action is obvious. When they contract they pull the wing down. However, one is attached to the skeletal plate of the thorax and acts *indirectly*. When it contracts it distorts the thorax, drawing in the ends and pushing up the top plate. This contributes to the downward movement of the wing. The elevator muscles are attached to the top plate of the thorax and when they contract they pull the plate down, raising the wing.

Since the locust has so many muscles, they are numbered by biologists according to a standard system, for easy reference. Rather than invent a new system for this course, the standard reference numbers have been retained, seen on later figures. A similar standard numbering system is applied to neurons—the size of the numbers gives an indication of just how much work has already been done on identifying individual muscles and neurons in the locust!

The muscles are quite large and it is possible to insert fine copper wires into them (Figure 7.12a, *overleaf*) to record the electrical activity during contraction. This electrical activity is shown in Figure 7.12b (*overleaf*). When combined with a graph of the wing movement the relation between movement and muscle activity can be seen. Each muscle is activated at a particular point in the flight cycle. At the top of the upstroke (point A) the depressor muscles are activated (indicated by red rectangles on Figure 7.12b). At the bottom of the downstroke the elevators are activated. Look at the contraction of the direct depressors (muscles 128 and 98) for the hindwing and the forewing.

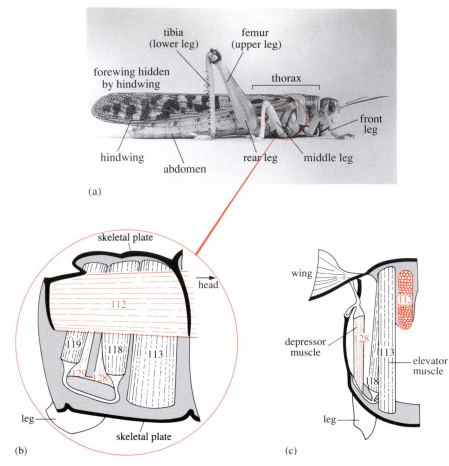

**Figure 7.11** (a) An adult locust. (b) The major flight muscles of the locust. A side view of a section through the thorax of to show the large flight muscles. (c) A cross-section through the thorax.

☐ What is the time delay between the electrical activity in the forewing and the hindwing direct depressor muscles?

■ About 7 ms.

☐ How does this correlate with the wing movements observed with a stroboscope?

■ It matches the phase difference of 7 ms between the forewings and the hindwings.

These observations have assumed, quite correctly, a link between electrical activity in muscle and muscle contraction. What is the nature of that link? In the next section the structure of muscle, the electrical activity associated with contraction and the mechanical properties of muscle, are all looked at.

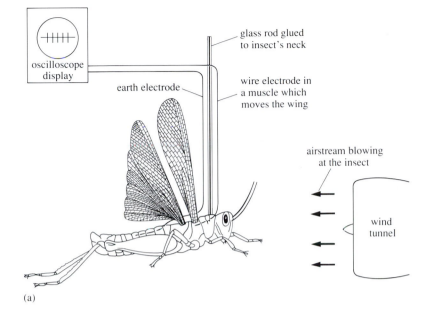

(a)

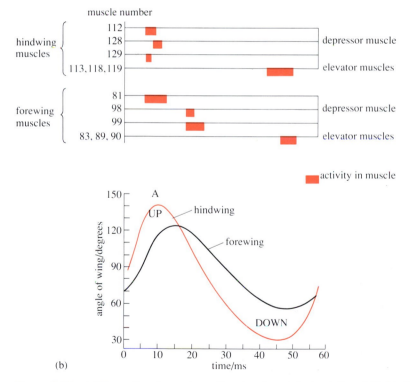

(b)

**Figure 7.12**   (a) Recording the motor pattern in a locust during tethered flight. (b) Pattern of electrical activity in major flight muscles and the wing position during one complete cycle of the wing beat.

# 7.6 Muscles as mechanical systems

This section covers the structure and function of muscles and describes the way in which an action potential in a motor neuron arriving at the muscle causes a contraction. You should be able to describe the characteristics of a muscle contraction and describe the main events leading up to it. You do not have to be able to reproduce the detailed diagrams of the microscopic structure of muscle, but you should be aware of the principal features of the mechanism of muscle contraction.

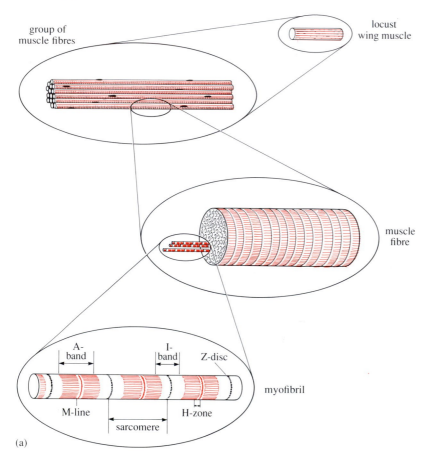

(a)

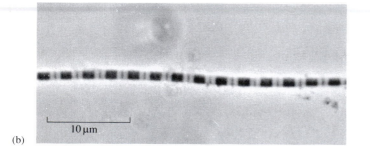

(b)

**Figure 7.13** (a) A striated muscle consists of a large number of long muscle fibres. Within each fibre there are several thousand myofibrils. (b) The characteristic banding pattern on a single myofibril shows up with the light microscope. The repeating units are the sarcomeres, each of which is broken down into lettered bands and zones (10 μm is 1/100 mm).

## 7.6.1   Microscopic structure of muscle

Basic muscle structure and function is similar over a wide range of animals, and insect flight muscle is organized in the same basic way as vertebrate muscle. The muscle cells are long fibres, each surrounded by a membrane. They are unusual cells in that they have several nuclei. Muscle cells are more usually known as *muscle fibres*. Each fibre contains a large number of cylindrical sub-units called myofibrils (Figure 7.13a). When myofibrils are examined microscopically using polarized light they can be seen to be divided into light and dark transverse bands (Figure 7.13b). The striated appearance of the myofibrils led to this type of muscle being called **striated muscle**. The other main type of muscle is non-striated or **smooth muscle**. In striated muscle there is a repeating pattern of striations along the length of each myofibril and the repeating units are called sarcomeres (Figure 7.13a). A single sarcomere is shown in the electron micrograph in Figure 7.14. The photograph shows that the banding pattern is produced by overlapping filaments in the myofibril. Two filamentous proteins, *actin* and *myosin*, form these filaments (Figure 7.14). The interaction between the filaments provides the basic contractile mechanism of muscle.

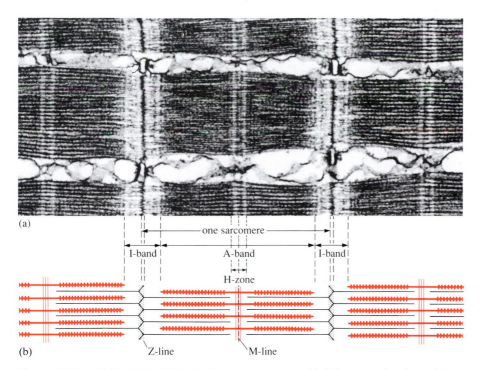

**Figure 7.14**   (a) Electron micrograph of a sarcomere. (b) Schematic drawing of the sarcomere to show the interleaving of the filaments.

If you divide a new pack of cards into two equal piles, place the piles side by side, shuffle them, and then push the piles together, the cards slide over each other and interleave (Figure 7.15a, *overleaf*). The filaments in muscle behave in a similar way when a muscle shortens. The individual filaments remain a constant length but the actin filaments slide into the array of myosin filaments shortening the overall sarcomere length and hence the length of the muscle. In the card analogy, force is necessary to get the cards to interleave (i.e. the piles have to be pushed together). By contrast, in the muscle force is *generated* by the interleaving process that shortens the muscle. The force is the result of projections on the myosin filaments, called cross-bridges, 'stepping' along the actin filaments and pulling them into the myosin arrays (Figure 7.15b).

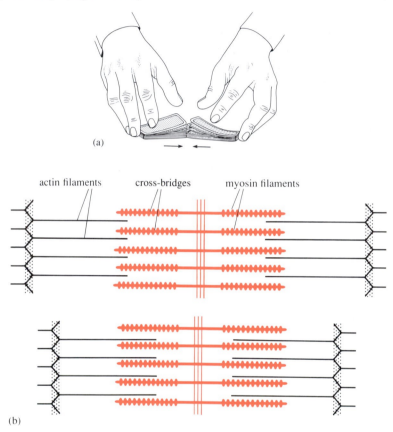

(a)

actin filaments          cross-bridges          myosin filaments

(b)

**Figure 7.15**  (a) Two piles of playing cards being interleaved. (b) Movement of the actin and myosin filaments of an individual sarcomere during muscle contraction.

The process of muscle contraction is initiated by action potentials in the motor neurons that innervate the muscle. The electrical events in muscle during contraction will now be discussed, together with the link between these events and the movement of the actin and myosin filaments.

## 7.6.2  The muscle action potential

A motor neuron usually innervates a large number of muscle fibres, forming a **motor unit**. Normally a large number of motor units make up one muscle. However, in insects there are only a small number of motor neurons innervating each muscle and in the flight muscles the number is further reduced, so that a motor unit may be a whole flight muscle. Where there is more than one motor unit in a muscle the units may have different characteristics, e.g. their thresholds of response may differ. The action potential from the motor neuron causes release of transmitter at the synapse (the neuromuscular junction) with each muscle fibre. The transmitter causes a depolarization of the muscle fibre membrane which triggers a muscle action potential that spreads over the surface of the fibre. These action potentials are the signals that were recorded by the thin copper wire electrodes used in the experiment illustrated in Figure 7.12. Muscle action potentials generally last longer than nerve action potentials, e.g. the potentials recorded in the experiment shown in Figure 7.12a last up to 10 ms.

The muscle action potential spreads over the surface of the muscle fibre but it is also conducted into the fibre along a series of fluid-filled tubes. These conduct the action potential into each individual sarcomere (Figure 7.16). The tubes run at right angles to the sarcomere and they are called, therefore, the transverse tubule system or the T-system. The sarcoplasmic reticulum contains calcium ions in a high concentration. When a muscle action potential is conducted along the T-system, calcium ions are released from the lining of the tubing into the space around the muscle filaments. The effect of the calcium ions is to initiate the myosin stepping along the actin which results in muscle shortening or contraction. When the action potential is over, calcium ions pass back into the T-system and the bonds between actin and myosin are broken.

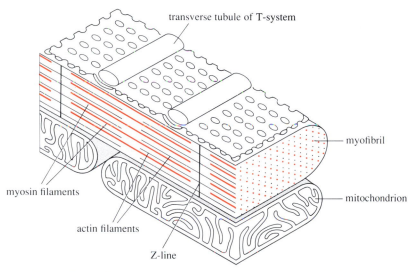

**Figure 7.16**   The T-system for a single sarcomere of locust flight muscle.

☐   How do the filaments separate so that a further contraction can occur?

■   In Section 7.5.2 you read how muscles can only contract, and cannot actively lengthen. The restoring force is usually provided by the action of an antagonistic muscle which pulls the actin and myosin filaments apart again.

### 7.6.3   The muscle twitch

When a single action potential activates a muscle the resulting muscle contraction is called a muscle twitch. Muscle contraction can be recorded from an isolated muscle by fixing one end and connecting the other to a strain gauge, an instrument that converts the pull exerted by the muscle when it contracts into an electrical signal that can be displayed on an oscilloscope. The muscle can be stimulated to contract by applying a short pulse of electricity to the motor nerve. Figure 7.17 shows the experiment and the type of record obtained. If low level stimulus pulses are used the muscle does not twitch, but as the intensity of stimulation is increased a point is reached where the twitch appears. This point is the threshold and the response reflects the fact that the muscle action potential is an all-or-nothing event.

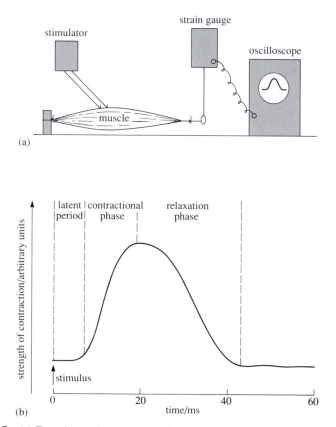

**Figure 7.17** (a) Experimental arrangement for recording the strength of contraction of an isolated muscle when stimulated directly. (b) A single muscle twitch from a locust muscle.

☐ How does the time course of the muscle twitch compare with the time course of an action potential?

■ The twitch lasts longer. An action potential in a neuron lasts about 1 ms (Section 3.4). In a locust flight muscle the muscle action potential can last up to 10 ms. The muscle twitch from a leg muscle shown in Figure 7.17 lasts about 40 ms. In some vertebrate muscles a single twitch may last 400 ms.

If a train of pulses is applied to the motor nerve, the muscle produces a series of twitches. The stiffness of the strain gauge is such that the muscle does not shorten appreciably during contraction and the force generated by the muscle is transferred to the gauge. This muscle twitch is, therefore, an *isometric* twitch, one in which the length of the muscle does not change. Although not relevant to this experiment, it is also possible to keep the load on the muscle constant and thus measure length changes during contraction. This is called an *isotonic* twitch.

☐   What predictions can you make about the record that would be produced by stimulating the motor nerve with a train of pulses at a rate of 40 per second?

■   You might have suggested that muscle has a refractory period like nerves, so that increasing the frequency of stimulation would not increase the number of twitches. However, in practice you get a record of the type shown in Figure 7.18b. The individual twitches merge and summate as there is insufficient time for the muscle to be stretched before the next stimulus.

Summation of responses demonstrates that as the rate (frequency) of stimulation increases, the degree of contraction of the muscle increases. However, note that the single twitches are still all-or-nothing responses.

A further increase in the stimulation frequency would produce a sustained contraction (Figure 7.18c) called **tetanus**. In locust flight muscle this is not a normal occurrence since the frequency of stimulation needed to induce tetanus is higher than would ever occur naturally.

The single twitch produced in the experiment was described earlier as an all-or-nothing response. However, muscles can show a graded response where each level of response has a different threshold. If a flight muscle from a locust is stimulated with single shocks that gradually increase in intensity the size of the twitch increases in steps (Figure 7.19).

☐   Can you offer an explanation for the three steps shown in Figure 7.19?

■   In Section 7.6.2 you learnt how muscles may be made up of one or more motor units. The explanation of the three steps in Figure 7.19 is that there are three motor units in the muscle, each with a different threshold.

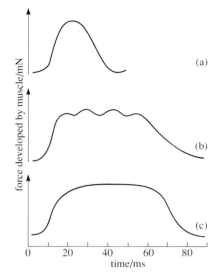

**Figure 7.18**   Responses of locust muscle to stimulation. (a) A single muscle twitch. (b) Summated response to stimulation at 40 stimulus pulses per second. (c) Tetanic response. Force is measured in Newtons (N). A milliNewton (mN) is one thousandth of a Newton.

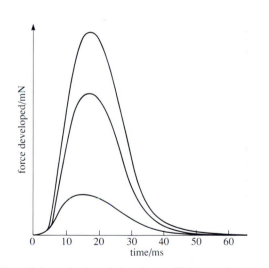

**Figure 7.19**   Recording of three single twitches from a flight muscle, superimposed on the same axes. The stimuli were of increasing intensity and produced responses of greater magnitude.

157

## 7.6.4   Muscle contraction and power output

You now know of two factors that influence the degree of contraction developed by the locust flight muscle:

1   the number of motor units that are active,

2   the frequency and pattern of action potentials in each motor neuron, which affects the degree of summation and the duration of the summated response.

If the muscle is to produce maximum power, then the pattern of action potentials in the motor nerves must be optimal. It is possible to determine the optimum conditions for maximum power output, but the techniques are complicated and outside the scope of this book. However, it is possible to draw some general conclusions from the experimental results. Recall from Section 7.4.1 that the wing beat frequency of locusts is 20 Hz. This means that the flight muscles contract in a cyclical pattern of lengthening and shortening. You will also recall that there is a latent period between the stimulus reaching the muscle and the twitch starting. There is also a delay between the start of the twitch and the development of maximum power output. The relationship between stimulus, force of contraction and muscle length is shown in Figure 7.20 for an experimental situation. When the time relationships between muscle contraction and maximum power output derived from experiments were compared with those obtained from the muscles during flight (Figure 7.12), it was clear to the experimenters that there was a good agreement between the figures. Thus, in the flying locust, the timing of muscle contraction is such that the muscles produce the maximum power that they are capable of producing.

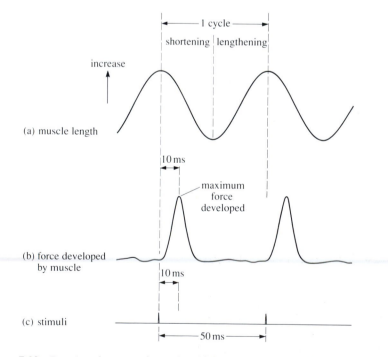

**Figure 7.20**   Results of an experiment in which a muscle was artificially lengthened and shortened (a). The maximum force developed by the muscle (b) occurs when the stimulus (c) for the twitch comes at the onset of the shortening phase of the cycle.

A further point that has been established in experiments is that multiple stimuli to the muscle give an increase in power output of about 20%. The optimum is three stimuli, each 4 ms apart. In recordings from tethered locusts in flight, a similar frequency of action potentials in the motor neurons has been observed.

Therefore there is good agreement between experimental observations on isolated muscles and the information obtained from the whole animal. The system depends upon accurate timing of the action potentials in the motor nerves. How is this accuracy produced? Section 7.7 looks at pattern generation in the nervous system, again using locust flight as the example.

## Summary of Section 7.6

Insect flight muscle is organized in the same basic way as vertebrate muscle. Muscle fibres contain cylindrical myofibrils which are divided up into light and dark bands when viewed using polarized light—hence the term striated muscle. Muscle fibres are innervated by motor neurons; in insects only a small number of motor neurons innervate each muscle. The muscle action potential initiates contraction. Within the muscle fibre, interleaved filaments of actin and myosin interact, with the actin filaments sliding further into the array of myosin filaments, producing contraction.

A single action potential produces a short contraction known as a twitch. Successive action potentials, if close together, produce a summated response which may develop into a sustained or tetanic response if the frequency of action potentials is high enough. In insect flight muscle the pattern of action potentials in the motor neurons is such that the contraction produces the maximum power output.

# 7.7 · The locust central pattern generator

Pattern generation in the nervous system probably underlies most rhythmic behaviour such as walking, swimming or flying. Locomotory rhythms are useful in the study of the link between neurons and behaviour because they are composed of a series of short, identical sequences repeated a very large number of times. Some animals will perform these activities in the laboratory almost as they would in their natural habitat so it is perhaps not surprising that locust flight was one of the first rhythmic patterns for which a pattern generator was sought, and found.

## 7.7.1   Evidence for existence of the central pattern generator

In Section 7.4.2 the role of wind in maintaining flight was described. In experiments involving tethered locusts the wind has to be directed onto the head to maintain flight. There are wind-sensitive hairs on the head which, when they are distorted, produce signals in sensory neurons that pass information to the brain. However, if the connections between the brain and the rest of the nervous system are severed, the locust is still able to fly when tethered. So, although the brain is involved in flight, the basic flight rhythms must be generated outside the brain.

The basic arrangement of the locust nervous system is shown in Figure 7.21. The points at which cuts are made to isolate the brain from the rest of the nervous system are marked with arrows. By looking at the figure you can see that the organization of the nervous system in locusts is very different from that found in sea-anemones. There is no diffuse nerve net; instead there is aggregation of neurons into larger units—nerves and ganglia (Chapter 6). The nerve cord running down the animal, beneath the gut, is expanded at intervals to form ganglia. This nerve cord constitutes, with the brain, the CNS (Chapter 6). Most neuronal cell bodies are located in the ganglia and neural control pathways are routed through them. Motor neurons branch out from the nerve cord to the effectors, and sensory information is brought into the nerve cord from the periphery by sensory neurons. Interneurons, which are found only in the CNS, make interconnections within the cord and greatly enhance integration. Within each ganglion are identifiable regions with different functions (Figure 7.21b). The neuropile is of interest in the locust flight story since this is the region where synaptic contacts between neurons are made.

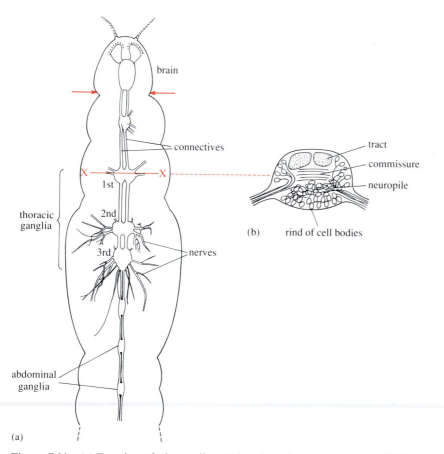

**Figure 7.21** (a) Top view of a locust dissected to show the nervous system. (b) Transverse section through a ganglion.

Flight is possible without the sensory input from hairs on the head, and it is possible to remove other sources of sensory input without destroying the basic rhythm. A variety of receptors provide information about the position of the wings and this information is conveyed along sensory neurons to the thoracic ganglia. It is possible to cut the axons of these neurons, eliminating the input of sensory information from the wings. Flight still occurs but the rhythm is not so steady and, interestingly, is only half the normal speed. The pattern of action potentials during flight can be recorded from the motor nerves leading from the thoracic ganglia to the wings, and can still be recorded if the wings and the flight muscles are removed. The locust CNS has by now been simplified to the point where it is only an isolated thoracic nervous system.

Young locusts do not have wings, and yet it is still possible to record the flight pattern in the motor nerves. These experiments show that the basic flight pattern is generated in the nervous system independent of sensory information.

So, the evidence for a central pattern generator independent of sensory input is clear enough but is it possible to get further information about its neural basis?

## 7.7.2 Microelectrode recordings from the CNS

Identifying neural elements of the central pattern generator has been possible using microelectrodes that can penetrate individual neurons within the thoracic ganglia. The practical problem facing the experimenter is to ease a very fine glass electrode through the tough outer sheath of the ganglion without breaking it and then penetrate the membrane of a neuron that is part of the flight system. Once inside the ganglion the tip of the electrode cannot be seen. A technique that has often been used to locate the recording site is to leave a mark at the electrode tip after all the recordings have been made. Later microscopic examination of the ganglion then shows the recording site.

At one time, burning was used as a marker—a burst of high frequency radio waves was sent down the microelectrode and the resulting high energy at the tip produced a small burn mark. However, dyes (introduced through the microelectrode) are now used extensively because some of them have the interesting property of spreading through the whole neuron and thus displaying all its connections. A typical picture obtained by this method is shown in Figure 7.22. If nothing else, this picture reveals how, once again, a 'simple' system turns out to be enormously complicated when examined closely. Let us see how these two techniques of intracellular recording and staining can be applied to identifying elements in the central pattern generator.

A locust is dissected to reveal the thoracic ganglia and nerves and most of the thoracic nerves are cut to eliminate all the sensory input but retain some motor neurons intact. Three recording electrodes are used in this case, one fine wire in a wing muscle to record flight activity, and two microelectrodes in neurons in the neuropile. The sensory neurons from the wind receptors on the head are left intact so that when the experimenter blows on the locust's head, 'flight' is initiated and the electrodes record flight activity. Typical records are shown in Figure 7.23 (*overleaf*). You will notice that the action potentials look very different from the idealized potentials illustrated in Chapter 3. These records are tracings taken directly from the display on an oscilloscope screen.

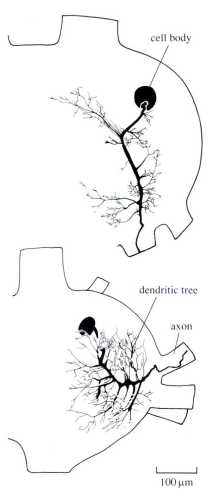

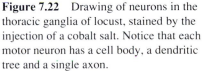

**Figure 7.22** Drawing of neurons in the thoracic ganglia of locust, stained by the injection of a cobalt salt. Notice that each motor neuron has a cell body, a dendritic tree and a single axon.

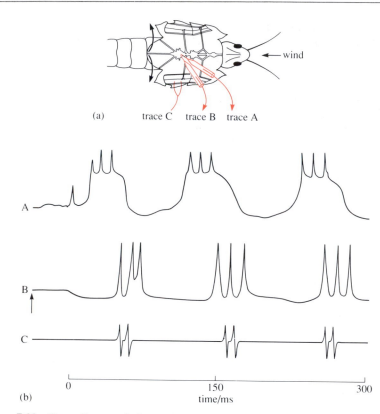

**Figure 7.23** Recordings made from a locust during flight activity. (a) The experimental arrangement. (b) The records from the three electrodes. A is the record from a motor neuron that stimulates an elevator muscle to raise a wing, B is the record from a depressor motor neuron, and C is the record of muscle action potentials from a depressor muscle.

☐ What is the frequency of the flight rhythm in Figure 7.23? How does this compare with the natural rhythm (Section 7.4.1)? How do you explain any difference?

■ First measure the time between bursts of action potentials in the flight muscle: 100 ms. Dividing 1 000 (the number of ms in a second) by 100 gives the number of cycles per second: 10 Hz. This is half the normal flight frequency of 20 Hz, the explanation being that in this experiment all the sensory inputs from the wings have been eliminated.

The records from the microelectrodes show that after the wind stimulus (arrow on Figure 7.23) the motor neuron to the elevator muscle first produces a burst of action potentials (trace A) while the motor neuron to the depressor muscle is inactive (trace B). This ties in well with behavioural observations. When a locust starts to fly the wings are first raised.

☐ How does the pattern of action potentials in the elevator and depressor motor neurons match the wing movements in flight?

■ The pattern of action potentials is entirely consistent with wing movement. The alternation of elevator and depressor activity is what you would expect from the flapping of the wings.

You can satisfy yourselves that the activity in the motor neurons is directly related to flight by looking at the muscle action potentials in the depressor muscle (trace C in Figure 7.23). As predicted, they follow the action potentials in the depressor motor nerve (trace B).

It would be possible to devise a theoretical model in which flight, once started, was maintained by direct interactions between motor neurons. However, evidence from experiments with this system have demonstrated that the flight pattern is not generated within the flight motor neurons themselves.

☐   What structural feature would you expect to find on motor neurons if they were to interact directly?

■   You would expect to find synaptic connections between elevator and depressor motor neurons.

In fact, such synapses have not been located by dye staining. Also, electrical signals in one motor neuron do not appear in others, as would be expected if there were synapses connecting them. Thus it is necessary to look inside the ganglia of the CNS for the pattern generator and to examine interneurons.

### 7.7.3   Interneurons

Interneurons can be studied in much the same way as motor neurons. It is possible to insert microelectrodes, record electrical activity and inject dye. However, there are many interneurons in the thoracic ganglia and mapping them is a long and complex process. Fortunately it appears that the number involved in the central pattern generator for flight is relatively small and some have already been identified, for example interneurons 301 and 501.

The structure of interneuron 301 is shown in Figure 7.24. The branching structure is characteristic of interneurons. The axon spreads through two thoracic ganglia (the second ganglion and the third ganglion), with a single link via the connective. Each blind-ending axonal branch probably represents a synaptic connection to another neuron. The cell body of the interneuron lies in the second ganglion (indicated by an arrow in Figure 7.24) and its axon runs down the connective to the third ganglion.

Interneuron 301 is rhythmically active at the flight frequency. This does not necessarily mean that it is generating the rhythm itself—it could be that it is following the rhythm produced by another neuron. One of the tests that can be applied to resolve this point is to insert a stimulating microelectrode into the interneuron and force a change in the rhythm by providing an external signal. If this change produces a change in the flight rhythm, and if the rhythm resets itself as soon as the stimulus ends, the interneuron *is* part of the pattern generator. Interneuron 301 meets these criteria.

A second interneuron, 501, has its cell body in the third thoracic ganglion with its axon passing through the connective into the second thoracic ganglion. The axonal branches thus overlap with the dendrites of 301. Intracellular recording from 501 shows that it too is rhythmically active, the rhythm coinciding with that of depressor muscles.

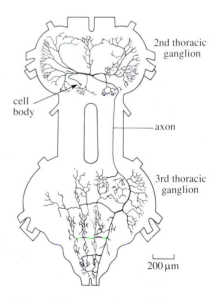

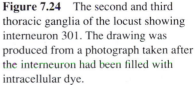

**Figure 7.24**   The second and third thoracic ganglia of the locust showing interneuron 301. The drawing was produced from a photograph taken after the interneuron had been filled with intracellular dye.

It is possible to record from 301 and 501 simultaneously and the records that are obtained show a close linkage between the two interneurons. When a flight sequence is stimulated 301 produces rhythmical bursts of action potentials. Following each action potential an excitatory potential appears in 501 after a delay of 6 ms (Figure 7.25a). Three milliseconds after the action potential in 501 there is a change in 301 (Figure 7.25b). This change in voltage in the interneuron prevents it producing action potentials; it is inhibited by 501. When the inhibition ends 301 is able to produce action potentials again and the cycle is repeated. This cycle of excitation and inhibition is at the heart of the central pattern generator. The timings give some further information. It takes a measurable amount of time for a signal to cross a synapse from one neuron to another (synaptic delay, Section 4.2.1). So, by measuring the time delay between an action potential in one neuron and the action potential appearing in a neighbouring neuron it is possible to estimate how many synapses the action potential has crossed.

The delay of 3 ms between the action potential in 501 and that in 301 (Figure 7.25b) is very short, which suggests that the connection between the two is *monosynaptic*, i.e. that there is only one synapse between them. Thus it can be deduced that 501 is directly connected *to* 301. However, the link back *from* 301 to 501 is not necessarily monosynaptic as there is a delay of 6 ms. This suggests that there are two synapses, with another interneuron providing a delay.

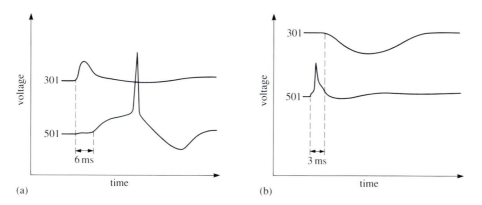

**Figure 7.25** (a) The response of interneuron 501 to an action potential in interneuron 301. The response of 501 is shown on an expanded vertical scale compared with 301 to show the details of the shape more clearly. (b) The inhibition of interneuron 301 by an action potential in 501.

This third interneuron, 511, links 301 with 501 (Figure 7.26). Bursts of activity in 301 inhibit 511 and while it is inhibited activity occurs in 501. So, 501 is normally inhibited by 511 and only produces action potentials when 511 is itself inhibited by 301. In turn the potentials in 501 inhibit 301. This looping of inhibition is the basic mechanism by which the flight pattern is generated once the system has been started by, for example, wind on the head. The next section turns to the sensory input that influences the interneurons of the central pattern generator.

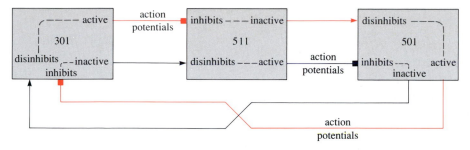

**Figure 7.26**   The links between three key interneurons in the central pattern generator. The diagram shows what happens when the interneuron 501 is either active (red path) or inactive (black path).

## Summary of Section 7.7

There is good evidence that the flight pattern in the locust is generated in the CNS by a central pattern generator. The flight pattern can be recorded from motor neurons leading to the flight muscles, even if the muscles themselves and the wings are absent.

The neural elements of the central pattern generator and their connections have been identified using microelectrode staining. Direct synaptic connections between the motor neurons for the elevator and depressor muscles have not been found, indicating that the flight pattern is not generated within the motor neurons. A small number of interneurons have been identified in forming the central pattern generator, with three of them linked together to form a loop. The delays produced by synapses, together with inhibitory connections in the feedback part of the loop, generate the repetitive flight pattern.

# 7.8   The sensory input in locust flight

There are a number of receptors that influence flight. You have already read about wind receptors on the head and sensors that detect vibration. The eyes and ears will also provide information that could trigger flight as an escape response. However, of particular interest here are receptors that feed information into the CNS and influence the central pattern generator.

☐   Where might such receptors be found?

■   Recall from Section 7.7.1 that if sensory axons from the wings are cut, the flight rhythm changes. This suggests that there are sensory receptors in the wings that influence central pattern generation.

## 7.8.1   Stretch receptors

The sense organs that detect wing position are called **stretch receptors**. Each stretch receptor consists of a single sensory neuron attached to an elastic strand that stretches between the two sides of the wing hinge. There is one stretch receptor for each wing. The axon from the stretch receptor runs into the thoracic ganglion and has branches in both the second and the third ganglia. The axon makes synaptic connections to flight motor neurons and interneurons, but only those associated with depressor muscles.

Although the sensory nerve containing the stretch receptor neuron is very small it is possible to hook a tiny wire around it and seal it in place so that the output from the stretch receptor can be monitored during tethered flight. A fine copper wire inserted into a flight muscle records the muscle action potentials. In addition, wing position can be monitored by an electronic position detector. A typical result from such an experiment is shown in Figure 7.27. The stretch receptor fires when the wing is close to the top of its beat.

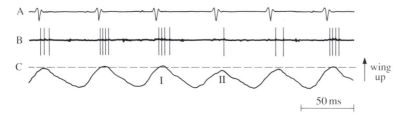

**Figure 7.27** Wing stretch receptor activity during flight in a tethered locust. Trace A represents depressor muscle activity, B stretch receptor activity, and C wing movement. The dotted line on the trace represents a standard wing level, to highlight changes in the wing movement between cycles.

☐ The number of action potentials produced by the stretch receptor varies with time. From the record can you suggest a reason?

■ The number of action potentials is directly related to the movement of the wing. The further up it moves the greater the number of action potentials.

☐ What reasons can you suggest for the variation in wing movement between cycles?

■ The wing is not moving in a uniform air flow. In the natural state there may be turbulence resulting from wind, the 'wash' from other insects or the insect changing its flight path. Also, of course, there may be slight changes in the flight rhythm that would produce larger or smaller wing movements. For example, if the depressor muscle contracts late, the wing will have moved further up before starting its downward movement.

In fact, there are continual changes in the flight pattern produced by the central pattern generator as a result of the activity in the stretch receptors. Look at Figure 7.27 and compare the three traces. The time relationship between the muscle action potentials, the stretch receptor potentials and the wing movements varies. If the wing movement is large (I), the action potentials in the stretch receptor start just before the wing reaches the top of its cycle. They start *during* the muscle action potential. However, if the wing movement is small (II) the single action potential from the stretch receptor occurs just after the wing has reached the top of its cycle, after the end of the muscle action potential. These changes in relative timing are called phase changes.

Detailed analysis of these phase changes is too complex for inclusion here, but it is possible to draw general conclusions about them. In the question above it was pointed out that the timing of the contraction of the depressor muscle would in part determine the amount of upward movement of the wing. The number of action potentials in the stretch receptor is, therefore, related to the timing of the depressor action potential. If the depressor muscle action potential is late, then the wing will have moved higher and the stretch receptor will produce more action potentials. The action potentials from the stretch receptor influence the depressor motor neuron. If it is very late in producing a potential the stretch receptor kicks it into action, thus forcing it back into the correct timing in the next cycle. So, the stretch receptors are an integral, and important, part of the central pattern generation.

### 7.8.2    Inputs from the outside world

The most important receptors in flight are those that monitor internal states, but those that provide information about the outside world also have inputs into flight control. The sensory hairs on the head initiate and maintain flight. Each hair has a sensory axon and the axons from the hairs pass to the brain and then down through the connectives to the thoracic ganglia. You might expect to find them in the same area of the ganglion as the pattern generating neurons, but in fact they occupy a different part of the neuropile. This means that any connection that they have to the pattern generating neurons cannot be monosynaptic but would have to be via other interneurons. The sensory axons make connections with interneurons whose cell bodies lie in the brain. These neurons are called descending interneurons because their cell bodies lie in the brain but their axons pass down the connectives. The next section examines the role of the brain.

### Summary of Section 7.8

There are a number of sensory inputs that influence flight in locusts. The eyes, ears and wind receptors feed information to the CNS. In addition, stretch receptors in the wings influence central pattern generation. The phase relationship between muscle action potentials, wing movements and stretch receptor potentials provides a mechanism for re-setting the flight rhythm if it starts to drift.

Flight is initiated and maintained by the brain integrating sensory inputs from hairs on the head. The sensory axons make connections with the pattern generating neurons via descending interneurons whose cell bodies lie in the brain.

# 7.9    Integration in locust flight

With the exception of the wind receptors, all the neural elements of flight generation considered so far have been sited outside the brain and perhaps the impression has been created that the brain has no role to play in flight. However, this is far from being the case. Although a tethered locust *will* fly if the brain connectives to the thoracic ganglia have been severed, this does not mean that it could fly free in the air under all conditions. The central pattern generator provides a basic rhythm, but this is modulated (regulated) by a range of sensory inputs processed by the brain.

### 7.9.1  Inputs to the brain

In Section 7.8.2 you read that wind movement and visual information reaches the thoracic ganglia via descending interneurons from the brain. The axons of these interneurons are large and so they have attracted the attention of experimenters. Four neurons have been studied extensively and all receive information from receptors that respond to light. The locust has two large compound eyes which are prominent on the head, but there are also three much smaller 'eyes' called ocelli. Three of the four interneurons receive input from ocelli. The fourth receives input from the eyes.

### 7.9.2  Multimodal neurons

Single neurons may receive inputs from more than one receptor type. This provides an integrative function. The four interneurons that receive information about light also receive information from other receptors, particularly the wind receptors on the head. They are, therefore, called *multimodal neurons*. The three interneurons that receive inputs from the ocelli have a role in maintaining the locust on its flight path and are known as 'deviation-detecting' neurons for that reason. The deviation-detecting neurons and the central pattern generator both have inputs to a pre-motor interneuron whose output is an integration of the two inputs.

The pre-motor interneuron acts like a gate, only allowing activity from the deviation-detecting neurons through at particular parts of the cycle of the central pattern generator. The action potentials from the pre-motor interneuron are passed to the flight motor neurons and modify their activity. So, if a deviation is detected, activity in the detecting neurons increases but is integrated with the central pattern generator so that it only influences the motor neurons at the correct part of the cycle.

### 7.9.3  Role of sensory feedback

The receptors on the head that detect wind can also detect the wing movement since the wings generate air movement. The pattern of air movement generated by the wings will, of course, be cyclic like the wing movements themselves. The fourth of the descending interneurons, the one carrying information from the compound eyes, is rhythmically excited and inhibited by the wind receptors at the flight frequency. This information about the wing beat frequency is fed back to flight interneurons, resetting the flight rhythm.

### 7.9.4  Constructing a flow diagram for the control of flight in the locust

It is now possible to produce a flow diagram that summarizes the control of flight in the locust. A good picture has emerged of the major elements of the nervous system that are involved, but equally it should be clear to you that it has not been possible to present a complete description of how locusts fly. For example, there must be a whole network within the brain that produces a 'decision' about whether or not to take off so, although all the basic elements of the flight control system are in the nerve cord, the brain must initiate take-off and hence flight.

All the elements of the flight system that you have examined, together with the links between them, are shown in Figure 7.28.

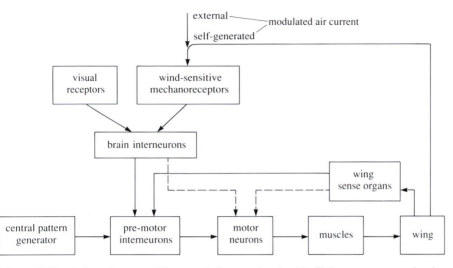

**Figure 7.28**   A flow diagram of the neural elements involved in flight pattern generation in the locust.

Before finishing this discussion of rhythm generation for flight it is worth mentioning that rhythmic behaviour can be generated in muscles themselves. The flight muscle of some insects, for example flies, wasps and bees, generates its own rhythm. The nervous system still has a role to play in providing motor action potentials to stimulate the muscle but the timing of the flight cycle is generated from within the muscle rather than from within the nervous system.

## Summary of Section 7.9

Behaviour patterns in locusts, like those in sea-anemones, are the combination of patterns of contraction of muscles, the effectors. Information from sensors can produce responses directly from effectors, but for complex behaviour patterns some processing is necessary. Rhythmic behaviour may be produced as a result of an internal rhythm generated in the nervous system, and in fact this is probably the normal situation. However, rhythmic behaviour can be generated in muscles themselves.

The central pattern generator in the locust provides a framework of signals for the generation of the wing movement cycle, but the fine tuning of the pattern and the matching of it to prevailing conditions is carried out through the integration that goes on in interneurons, particularly multimodal neurons. A particular feature of the flight system is that information about performance is monitored and fed back to the CNS continually, almost on a cycle to cycle basis. This information is processed in such a way that it modifies the flight pattern and keeps it centred on a specific frequency, the optimum frequency.

# Summary of Chapter 7

Looking at simple behavioural patterns in the nervous systems of insects and other animals can give us an insight into the changes in neural function that underlie changes in behaviour. The structure and function of the components of the nervous system are similar over a wide range of animal species, and so conceptual models derived from these animals can provide a framework for exploring the neural mechanisms responsible for controlling behaviour in other, more complex organisms.

# Objectives for Chapter 7

When you have completed this chapter you should be able to:

7.1    Define and use, or recognize definitions and applications of each of the terms printed in **bold** in the text.

7.2    Give a brief description of the three major neural systems found in sea-anemones, and their role in producing 'behavioural building blocks'.

7.3    Give a description of locust flight behaviour and the stimuli that initiate and terminate it. *(Question 7.6)*

7.4    Describe the characteristics of a single muscle twitch and the circumstances under which it is produced. *(Questions 7.1, 7.2 and 7.3)*

7.5    Describe how twitches summate and eventually produce tetanus. *(Questions 7.1 and 7.3)*

7.6    Explain why rhythmic behaviour is easier to analyse in neurophysiological terms than most other types of behaviour. *(Question 7.4)*

7.7    Describe some basic techniques available for identifying neural elements in a system.

7.8    Describe how the properties of the neurons in the central pattern generator, and the links between them, produce a repetitive pattern. *(Question 7.5)*

7.9    List the types of sensory input that modulate the output of the central pattern generator in locusts. *(Question 7.6)*

7.10   Describe the role of the brain in the control of flight in locusts. *(Question 7.6)*

# Questions for Chapter 7

**Question 7.1** *(Objectives 7.4 and 7.5)*
Which of the following statements about the muscle action potential is false?

(a) The muscle action potential spreads over the surface of the muscle fibre.

(b) The muscle action potential is conducted into the muscle fibre by the fluid-filled T-system.

(c) Calcium has a crucial role to play in linking the muscle action potential and contraction.

(d) The duration of the muscle action potential is very short by comparison with the nerve action potential.

(e) Muscle action potentials that are close together in time produce a summated response.

## Question 7.2 *(Objective 7.4)*

Which of the following statements about a single locust muscle twitch are true?

(a) It has a latent period.

(b) At the end of the contraction phase the muscle actively relaxes.

(c) A muscle twitch develops the maximum force that the muscle is capable of.

(d) The relaxation phase lasts longer than the contraction phase.

(e) Active contraction lasts longer than the action potential that stimulated it.

(f) All fibres in the muscle always contract when the muscle produces a single twitch.

(g) Successive single twitches in a muscle will always generate the same force.

## Question 7.3 *(Objectives 7.4 and 7.5)*

Which of the following is the correct definition of tetanus in a muscle?

(a) In tetanus successive muscle contractions do not fuse.

(b) Tetanus is a smooth contraction in which individual twitches cannot be distinguished.

(c) Tetanus is when the muscle is working to its maximum capacity.

(d) Tetanus is a contraction produced by simultaneous excitation of many motor neurons.

(e) Tetanus is an unusually strong contraction of a muscle.

## Question 7.4 *(Objective 7.6)*

What are the practical advantages of investigating a behaviour pattern composed of a series of short cycles, repeated many times?

## Question 7.5 *(Objective 7.8)*

What criteria are used to determine whether a neuron involved in flight in insects is rhythmically active?

## Question 7.6 *(Objectives 7.3, 7.9 and 7.10)*

A number of sensory inputs that influence flight have been described. Mark these on the outline diagram of the flying locust (Figure 7.29, *overleaf*). Underline those that influence pattern generation only, rather than initiation or termination of flight.

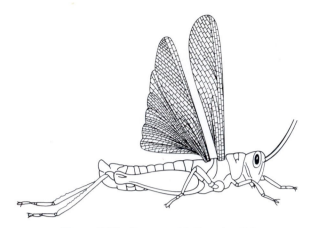

**Figure 7.29**   For use with Question 7.6.

# CHAPTER 8
# THE VERTEBRATE NERVOUS SYSTEM

## 8.1 Introduction

This chapter describes the organization of the nervous system in the group of multicellular animals to which humans belong. The vertebrates, like the invertebrates, have an internal body cavity in which the various organs of the body are found. The structures in any vertebrate body can be recognized easily because they are fundamentally similar to those in our own bodies. Thus you could label the brain, heart, kidneys and liver in a fish, frog, lizard, bird or mammal.

You learnt in Chapter 6 some of the differences between the nervous systems of invertebrates and vertebrates. While the central nervous system (CNS) in invertebrates lies ventrally beneath the gut, the vertebrate CNS is a dorsal hollow structure consisting of the brain enclosed within the skull and the spinal cord enclosed within the vertebral column or backbone. Like the invertebrate CNS, it is bilaterally symmetrical and segmented. The segmental arrangement is very obvious in the vertebral column, which is divided into separate segments by each vertebra, although the spinal cord is a continuous tube rather than a chain of separate ganglia, as in the invertebrates.

As discussed in Chapter 6, one of the important differences between vertebrates and invertebrates is simply size. With vertebrates the CNS is enclosed within an internal rather than an external skeleton. With an internal skeleton there is less restriction on size as long as the animal can be well supplied with oxygen and nutrients. Thus most vertebrates have a larger body size than invertebrates. The control of movement in larger animals involves monitoring activity in more muscle fibres and controlling the activity of their associated motor neurons, and the increased surface area of the body brings with it an increase in the number of sensory organs. All these changes demand more neurons in the CNS, and especially in the brain. In the more recently evolved vertebrates such as mammals and birds the development of huge arrays of interconnected neurons in the brain can be seen. Many of the connections in these arrays are specified through use and experience during early life, as will be discussed in Book 4. This mechanism for specifying neuronal connections provides mammals and birds with a greatly improved ability to adapt to changing external circumstances during an individual's own lifetime. The strategy for survival of vertebrates is thus rather different from that of the invertebrates such as the insects. There are far fewer species of vertebrates, they are usually large in size and have much longer lives, often with a very protracted and vulnerable developmental period. These differences are linked to the complexity and size of their nervous systems.

In addition to the CNS, vertebrates have a second nervous system called the autonomic nervous system (ANS, Chapter 5) which is specifically concerned with regulating the activity of the various systems (e.g. the circulatory, excretory and digestive systems) that are responsible for maintaining normal body functions and a stable environment for the cells of the body. The basic difference between the CNS and the ANS is in the kind of effector cells. Whereas the CNS motor neurons innervate skeletal muscles that move various parts of the body, the output neurons of the ANS innervate muscles of the internal organs (e.g. the heart and the gut), blood vessels, and also various glands (e.g. sweat glands, salivary glands). Details of the organization of the ANS are given in Section 8.5. The CNS and ANS are closely connected to each other and also influence the immune system which protects the animal from infection (Chapter 5).

Both the CNS and the ANS contain interconnected neurons which are usually grouped together to perform various functions. Such a group is often referred to as a **nucleus** (not to be confused with the nucleus of a cell—see Chapter 2). Groups of neurons lying outside the CNS are usually called ganglia. In common with the invertebrate nervous system, the peripheral nervous system (PNS) contains the axons that connect the CNS and the ANS with sensory receptors and motor effectors in the periphery.

Although a lot is known about the nervous system in vertebrates, and especially humans, exactly how the nervous system works to produce behaviour is far from understood. The vertebrates as a group share many more characteristics than do the invertebrates, and so their nervous systems also share many common themes. This chapter is intended to provide you with a basic understanding of the way that the vertebrate nervous system is assembled.

The chapter begins by explaining how the brain is orientated so that its anatomy can be described, i.e. 'getting your bearings'. This is followed by a description of the internal structure of the spinal cord. The vertebrate brain is a complex structure but, once you understand that all vertebrate brains are built on the same plan, you will find it much easier to learn what the various parts of the brain do and what they are called.

The description of the brain begins by considering the brain of a mammal, the human brain, which will give you some idea of basic anatomy. A brief comparison of brains from different vertebrate groups is then made to illustrate how their structure can be related to the animal's lifestyle and also how the structure of the brain has evolved. You have been provided with two aids to learning and understanding the anatomy of the human brain: a plastic model together with an audiotape entitled *Exploring the Brain*, and a videocassette entitled *The Human Brain*. These two teaching aids should be used as you read through this chapter. Finer details of structure and function of particular parts of the mammalian nervous system will be presented in later chapters.

## 8.1.1 Getting your bearings: the naming of parts

In order to describe the anatomy of the body (or the brain) it is necessary to know how to look at it. Description must be more precise than just saying 'in front of' or 'behind', etc. To make things simpler, neuroanatomists refer to a set of coordinates that are clearly defined and can be transferred from one brain to the next. All vertebrates are bilaterally symmetrical; the plane of symmetry is the *midline* (Figure 8.1a).

Looking at a fish (or a cat or a whale) head on, dorsal is up and ventral is down. Within each half of the fish, towards the midline is **medial**, away from it is **lateral**. Looking at the fish from above, **rostral** is towards the nose, **caudal** towards the tail, and medial and lateral as before (Figure 8.1). Structures on the same side of the midline are described as being **ipsilateral** to each other, while those on the opposite side are said to be **contralateral** to each other.

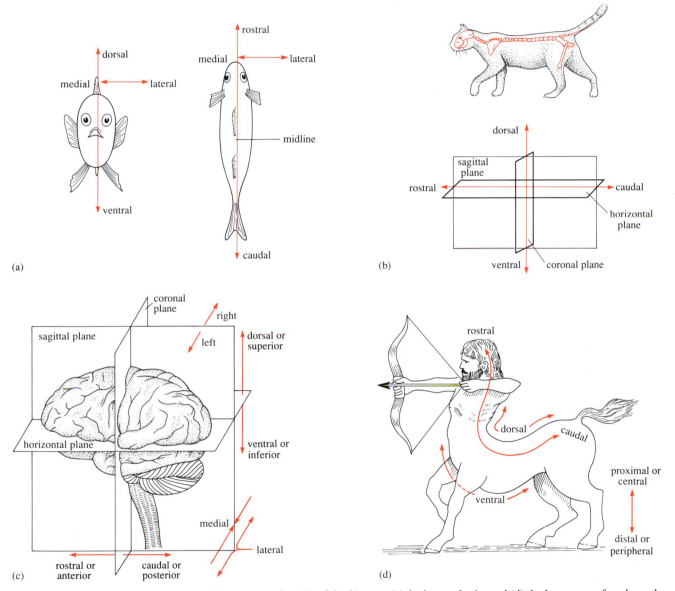

**Figure 8.1**   The planes of symmetry and the anatomy for: (a) a fish, (b) a cat, (c) the human brain, and (d) the human as a four-legged animal.

When the brain or body is sliced to show its internal structures, one of three standard cutting planes is used. The *sagittal* plane is parallel to the plane passing down the midline that divides the animal into right and left halves, the *coronal* (when referring to the head or brain) or *transverse* (when referring to the body or spinal cord) plane slices the brain or body across its long axis into rostral and caudal halves at right angles to the sagittal plane, and the *horizontal* plane divides the structure into dorsal and ventral halves. These planes of section are illustrated in Figure 8.1b. You can see from Figures 8.1c and d that these definitions are a bit different in the case of upright humans, and because of the 'bending upwards' of the human brain, the terms rostral and caudal are less applicable. Instead, the terms **anterior** (towards the front) and **posterior** (towards the back) are used. Additionally, **superior** and **inferior** are often used instead of dorsal and ventral. In this chapter all descriptions of horizontal vertebrates will use the more general terms defined above. When describing structures in the body the terms *proximal* (nearest or most central) and *distal* (farthest or most peripheral) are often used to indicate the part of the structure being described. This is most easily understood in limbs, such as the leg in Figure 8.1d, where proximal refers to the part of the leg closest to the centre and distal refers to the hoof end closest to the periphery.

## 8.2 The structure of the spinal cord

The structure of the spinal cord is fundamentally similar in all vertebrates. A transverse section (a slice made across its length) of the vertebrate spinal cord shows two different regions clearly visible to the naked eye (Figure 8.2). In preserved specimens there is a pale, greyish, butterfly-shaped region (the **grey matter**) which is surrounded by noticeably whiter areas (the **white matter**). The dorsal half of the grey matter consists of the two dorsal horns, and the ventral half consists of the two ventral horns. The central canal is the hollow centre of the tube from which the brain and spinal cord are formed.

In fresh tissue the grey and white areas have a definitely pinkish tinge since they are well supplied by blood vessels. The grey matter contains mainly the cell bodies of neurons and their dendrites.

☐ Can you remember where the cell bodies in the invertebrate CNS ganglia are located?

■ In invertebrate ganglia the cell bodies are arranged around the outside of the neuropile which contains the dendrites and axons (Section 6.3.1).

In each segment of the spinal cord (i.e. the section of spinal cord contained within a single vertebra) there are two bundles of axons on each side forming the bilateral spinal nerves (Figure 8.3). The bundles entering the dorsal side of the spinal cord are called the dorsal roots and contain the axons of sensory neurons. The bundles on the ventral surface, the ventral roots, contain the axons of the motor neurons.

☐ What connections do motor neurons make?

■ Motor neurons innervate muscles in the periphery (Sections 1.2 and 2.4.2).

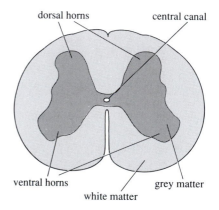

**Figure 8.2**   Transverse section of the spinal cord.

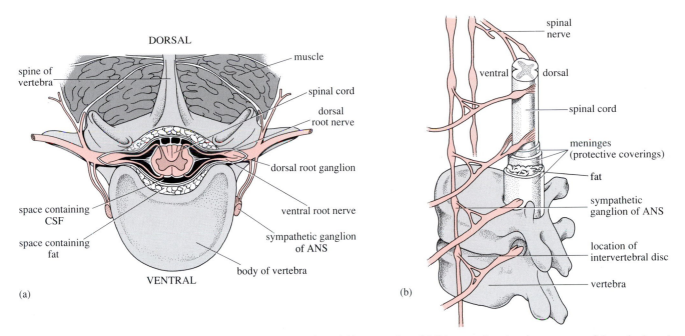

**Figure 8.3**   (a) Transverse section through the spinal cord lying within a vertebra. (b) Diagram showing the structure of the spinal cord and its associated spinal nerves, in a section of the vertebral column.

The motor neurons are the output neurons of the nervous system. Many are very large, with large cell bodies and huge and complex dendritic trees extending over a large part of the grey matter of the spinal cord (Figure 8.4).

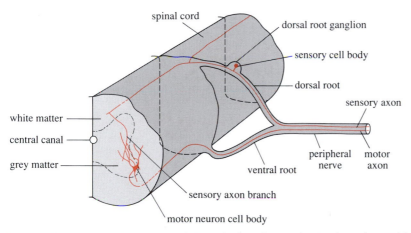
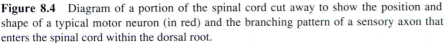

**Figure 8.4**   Diagram of a portion of the spinal cord cut away to show the position and shape of a typical motor neuron (in red) and the branching pattern of a sensory axon that enters the spinal cord within the dorsal root.

The cell bodies of motor neurons are located within the grey matter, but the cell bodies of the sensory neurons are found outside the spinal cord in enlargements of the dorsal roots called the dorsal root ganglia (see Figures 8.3 and 8.4).

The central grey matter in the spinal cord also contains many neurons other than sensory and motor neurons. Some of these have short axons that make local connections with other neurons. These are usually referred to as interneurons (Section 7.7.3). Others relay information—or *project*—to other parts of the nervous system and the brain. These are called **projection neurons**. You will find this distinction between local interneurons and longer distance projection neurons occurring frequently in descriptions of other regions of the CNS. As was described in Section 6.3.1, axons from projection neurons carrying information *to* a particular part of the CNS are described as afferent axons, while those carrying information *away from* the region are described as efferent axons. You will find that many neuroanatomical texts describe axon pathways as if the axons themselves were moving. For example, nerves 'run', 'enter' 'branch' or 'exit'. As you are now well aware, axons (at least in adult animals—see Book 4) do not move much, but the information they conduct does. The dynamic nature of the nervous system is emphasized by these kinds of descriptions.

The white matter consists mainly of large numbers of myelinated axons—the myelin is responsible for the glistening white appearance of white matter. Many of these axons are arranged in large longitudinal bundles, or tracts, that lead to or from the brain. As in the description of the invertebrate CNS, these connections are described as descending (from the brain) or ascending (to the brain), depending upon the direction of information flow (Section 6.3.1). Other axons in the white matter connect neighbouring segments of the spinal cord together.

☐   What is myelin?

■   You should remember from Section 2.4.4 that myelin is the insulating sheath around axons formed by glial cells. This insulation, made up of layers of cell membrane, surrounds many vertebrate axons and increases the speed of conduction of action potentials.

The dorsal root ganglion cells convey information from sensory receptors in the periphery to the spinal cord. They therefore have rather an unusual structure: they have no dendrites and one axon which branches very close to the cell body. One branch extends out to the periphery where it contacts sensory receptors (or has its own special sensitive ending like the mechanoreceptor in Figure 2.13). The other branch enters the spinal cord. The peripheral axon branch may branch many times, innervating sensory receptors over a wide area. Action potentials travel from the periphery all the way to the spinal cord without, in general, involving the cell body of the dorsal root ganglion cell.

The dorsal root axons again branch many times within the spinal cord. Some branches synapse locally in the dorsal horn, while others make synapses in neighbouring segments. Often there is one main branch that ascends towards the brain along one of the dorsal fibre tracts of the white matter.

# 8.3    Segmental organization in the spinal cord

Each segment of the spinal cord (enclosed in its vertebra) is concerned with controlling a particular part of the body. It receives sensory information from that part and coordinates the activity of its muscles and other effectors. Although the spinal cord looks like a continuous structure, its segmental organization betrays its evolutionary history. However, in vertebrates the function of individual segments is far more closely integrated with the rest of the CNS than in the invertebrates. The large ascending and descending tracts connecting the brain to the spinal cord reflect this increase in the brain's control over the function of individual segments.

In fishes the segments of the spinal cord are all very similar. They each innervate a block of muscular tissue. In animals with limbs there is an obvious increase in the number of neurons in the spinal cord segments serving the limbs, leading to an increase in the thickness of the spinal cord in that area. The different segments in these animals are described according to the areas they innervate. The **cervical** segments include those in the neck and those supplying the forelimbs; the **thoracic** segments innervate the thorax (chest); the **lumbar** segments innervate the hind limbs and the abdomen (lower body); and the sacral segments innervate the tail.

# 8.4    Introduction to the brain

This section introduces you to the basic plan of the vertebrate brain and its cellular structure. The main landmarks of the mammalian brain are then introduced. One of the more externally obvious and easily identified landmarks is the cerebral cortex, which is, as you will see later, of particular interest when comparing different species. The videocassette *The Human Brain* and the model brain together provide a guide to the structure of the human brain and introduce you to basic brain anatomy. You will need to study the model brain and the audiotape *Exploring the Brain* after reading Section 8.4.2. You will find that the drawings that you label during your study of the model will be of use to you when you read later sections of this chapter.

## 8.4.1    The basic plan of the vertebrate brain

The CNS of all vertebrates develops from a hollow tube of cells. The brain is an enlargement of the rostral end of this tube and it can be divided into three regions. To a large extent, each region receives and analyses sensory information from a particular type of sensory receptor. Therefore one way of looking at the organization of the vertebrate brain is that shown in Figure 8.5 (*overleaf*). The **forebrain** receives chemical information from the nose via the olfactory nerves. The **midbrain** receives visual information from the eyes via the optic nerve. The **hindbrain** receives vibration and orientation information from the ears and balance organs via the auditory and vestibular nerves, respectively. This simple three-lobed structure is seen during the early development of all vertebrates. The central core of the midbrain and the hindbrain is called the **brain stem**. Each of these regions contains groups of neuronal cell bodies which are collected together to serve a particular function. This central core has a structure similar to that of the spinal cord, with the neuronal cell bodies in the grey matter surrounded by white matter.

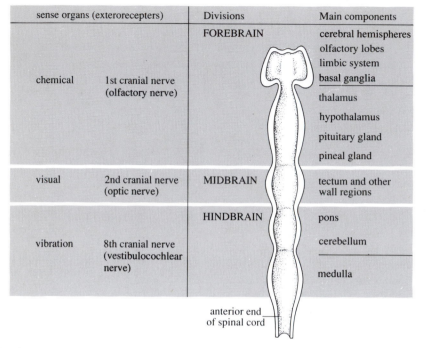

| sense organs (exterorecepters) | | Divisions | Main components |
|---|---|---|---|
| | | FOREBRAIN | cerebral hemispheres<br>olfactory lobes<br>limbic system<br>basal ganglia |
| chemical | 1st cranial nerve<br>(olfactory nerve) | | thalamus<br>hypothalamus<br>pituitary gland<br>pineal gland |
| visual | 2nd cranial nerve<br>(optic nerve) | MIDBRAIN | tectum and other<br>wall regions |
| | | HINDBRAIN | pons |
| vibration | 8th cranial nerve<br>(vestibulocochlear<br>nerve) | | cerebellum<br><br>medulla |

anterior end of spinal cord

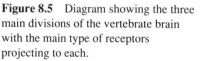

**Figure 8.5** Diagram showing the three main divisions of the vertebrate brain with the main type of receptors projecting to each.

The interconnected cavities within each enlargement are called ventricles; these are the remnants of the tube from which the brain developed and are continuous with the central canal in the spinal cord. The brain ventricles and central canal are filled with a special fluid called the cerebrospinal fluid which also surrounds the brain, cushioning it from knocks. The cerebrospinal fluid does not contain red blood cells and its composition is rather different from the composition of the fluid part of the blood (plasma). This difference is the result of the activity of special cells which form what is known as the blood–brain barrier (Section 2.4.4). The existence of the blood–brain barrier protects the neurons in the CNS from harmful substances; it also affects how easily drugs can enter the extracellular environment of the CNS.

There are ten or twelve nerves (depending on the species) that innervate various regions of the head. These are known as the cranial nerves. The position and function of a particular cranial nerve is the same in all vertebrates. Anatomists usually refer to each by a number (sometimes written in Roman numerals) or a name. Table 8.1 is a list of the cranial nerves, their site of exit from the brain and their function in humans. The nerves are all visible from the ventral side of the brain (Figure 8.6) and you will see the key ones that you need to remember on the model brain.

The function of the cranial nerves in other vertebrates differs only in detail (e.g. the presence of gills and no larynx in fish). You do not need to learn the whole list, although it would be useful to learn those in italic type in Table 8.1 since you will keep coming across them later in the course. Remember that these names, numbers and functions apply to all vertebrates. This means that the location of, say, the optic nerve can be identified fairly easily in a fish, a snake or a human.

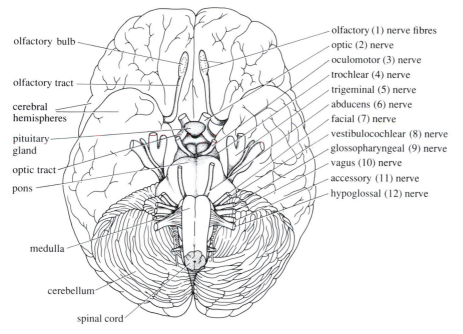

olfactory bulb

olfactory tract

cerebral
hemispheres

pituitary
gland

optic tract

pons

medulla

cerebellum

spinal cord

olfactory (1) nerve fibres
optic (2) nerve
oculomotor (3) nerve
trochlear (4) nerve
trigeminal (5) nerve
abducens (6) nerve
facial (7) nerve
vestibulocochlear (8) nerve
glossopharyngeal (9) nerve
vagus (10) nerve
accessory (11) nerve
hypoglossal (12) nerve

**Figure 8.6**   The ventral surface of the human brain showing the twelve cranial nerves.

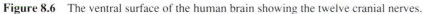

**Table 8.1**   Summary of the cranial nerves (in humans).

| No. | Name | Exit from brain | Function |
|-----|------|-----------------|----------|
| 1 | *Olfactory* | forebrain | sense of smell |
| 2 | *Optic* | diencephalon | vision |
| 3 | Oculomotor | midbrain | control of eye muscles, pupil muscles |
| 4 | Trochlear | midbrain | control of eye muscles |
| 5 | Trigeminal | hindbrain | sensory input from head<br>control of jaw muscles |
| 6 | Abducens | hindbrain | control of eye muscles |
| 7 | Facial | hindbrain | control of muscles of facial expression<br>and sensory input from tongue |
| 8 | *Vestibulocochlear*<br>(vestibular + auditory<br>nerves) | hindbrain | sense of balance (vestibular nerve) and<br>hearing (auditory nerve) |
| 9 | Glossopharyngeal | hindbrain | sensory input from tongue<br>control of throat muscles |
| 10 | *Vagus* | hindbrain | sensory input from external ear, tongue<br>and internal organs<br>control of muscles in throat and larynx<br>parasympathetic axons to heart and<br>internal organs |
| 11 | Accessory | hindbrain | control of muscles in the ear |
| 12 | Hypoglossal | hindbrain | control of tongue muscles |

### 8.4.2   The human brain

The dominant feature of the human brain is the highly folded cerebral hemispheres, as you saw in Chapter 1. These enfold, and partly obscure, many of the other structural details. From the outside, three distinct structures stand out: the cerebral hemispheres, the brain stem and the cerebellum. These are illustrated in Figure 8.7.

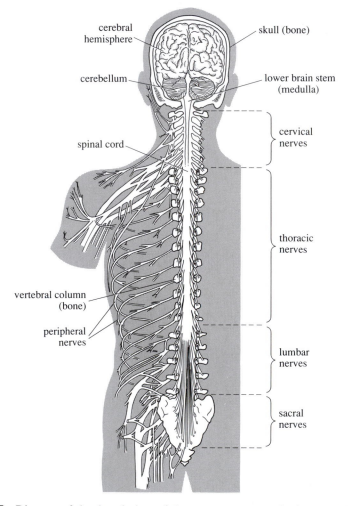

**Figure 8.7**   Diagram of the dorsal view of the nervous system of a human. The spinal nerves are shown on the left side only, though they do of course occur on both sides.

The distinction between forebrain, midbrain and hindbrain that was made in Section 8.4.1 for the vertebrate brain can be applied to the human brain, although the divisions are less clear. The cerebral hemispheres and the diencephalon (Figure 8.8) make up the forebrain. The midbrain is the upper part of the brain stem. The pons, medulla and cerebellum together make up the hindbrain. Each of these regions will be considered in turn.

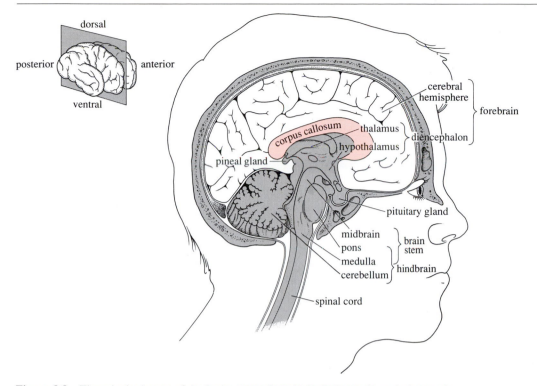

**Figure 8.8**   The principal parts of the brain, seen when the brain is cut down its long axis, a sagittal section. This is the same cut as that made in the model brain. The cut corpus callosum is shaded in red; other structures that have been cut are shaded in grey.

### 8.4.3   The forebrain

The forebrain consists of the two large cerebral hemispheres and the diencephalon. The cerebral hemispheres are largely separated by a longitudinal division (Figure 8.8). They are connected by bundles of myelinated axons, the largest group of which is the corpus callosum, shown shaded red on Figure 8.8.

The outer layer of the cerebral hemispheres is called the cerebral cortex, a layer of cells that is about 3 mm thick. Notice that the structure of the cortex is rather different from that of the spinal cord—here the cells are on the outside of the white matter. You will learn later how the addition of this large extra layer of neurons is an important feature both in the evolution of the mammals and the increase in the complexity of their behaviour. The cerebral cortex is responsible for analysing sensory information, especially vision, touch and hearing, and coordinating motor responses. The ventral part of the cerebral hemispheres is concerned with olfaction. In many mammals (especially nocturnal small mammals such as rats and shrews) this region is relatively larger in size than in humans, where vision rather than olfaction is the dominant sense. The axons running to and from the neurons in the cerebral cortex are in the white matter beneath it.

In humans the cerebral cortex is highly folded and has a very large surface area.

☐   What are the valleys called? (recall Chapter 1).

■ The valleys are called the sulci.

The patterns of these deep folds make very useful landmarks dividing the cortex into areas, as shown in Figure 8.9.

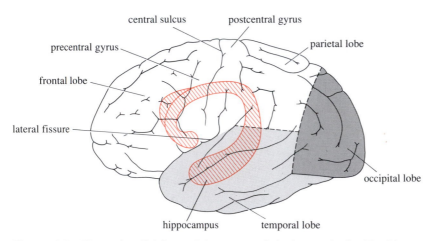

**Figure 8.9** The major divisions of the cortex of the human brain. The hippocampus connects the cortex with the rest of the forebrain.

The importance of the cerebral cortex in controlling behaviour is reflected in its size and also in the organization of its inputs and outputs. The major functional divisions of the cortex are shown in Figure 8.10a. Each half of the cerebral cortex receives visual, tactile and auditory inputs from the opposite side of the body. Each sensory input is mapped topographically onto particular areas of the cortex called the **primary sensory cortex**. The term 'topography' originates from a Greek word describing the practice of providing an accurate scaled representation of a city, town or tract of land. At its most basic, a topographic map provides a representation in which the relative positions of the parts of the original structure(s) are preserved. The tactile and visual maps are topographically arranged; they provide information about the location of a stimulus relative to the body. The size and area devoted to particular senses and regions of the body reflects their importance in life. The auditory map is arranged rather differently in order to provide information about the frequency (pitch) of the sound (see Book 3). There is also a **primary motor cortex**: a (topographically) well-ordered output that connects, through motor neurons, with specific groups of muscles in the opposite side of the body. The size of the area of cortex devoted to specific motor functions is related to the intricacy of the movements. In Figure 8.10b notice the size of the areas devoted to the control of the thumb and the tongue.

Lying outside the primary sensory and primary motor areas are the areas of **association cortex**. In these, information from memory is compared with the primary sensory information to give the input context and fuller meaning. The association areas are areas of higher processing; they do not receive a *direct* sensory input and nor do they have a *direct* output to motor neurons.

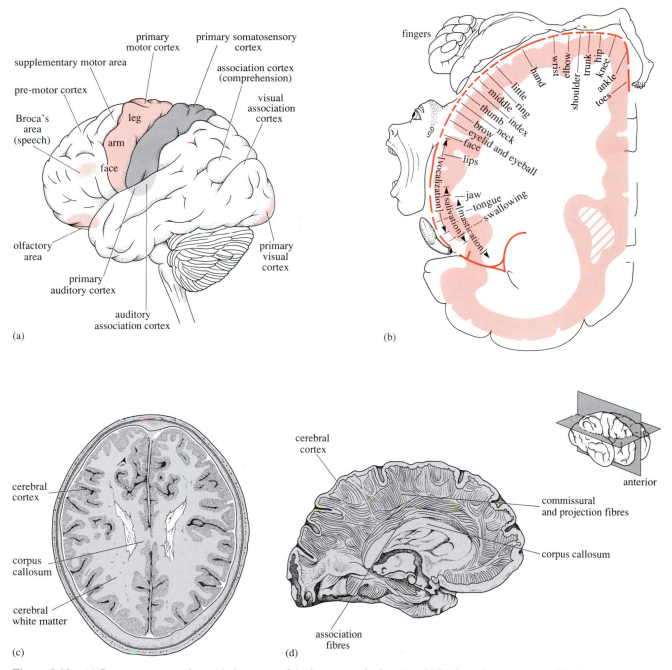

**Figure 8.10**   (a) Sensory, motor and association areas of the human cerebral cortex. (b) Body regions represented in the motor cortex of humans. The diagram shows a cross-section through the right cerebral hemisphere of a person standing facing you. The size of each body part in the illustration roughly relates to the size of the cortical region that controls that part. (You do not need to memorize the detail of this figure.) (c) A horizontal section through the cerebral hemispheres. (d) A sagittal section through the left cerebral hemisphere to show the fibre groups of the white matter.

The cerebral cortex is closely connected with most other brain areas; the tracts of fibres entering (ascending tracts) and leaving (descending tracts) it are therefore very large. The white matter that underlies the cortex consists of myelinated axons running in three principal directions (Figures 8.10c and d). These axons are the *association* fibres that connect different gyri of the same cerebral hemisphere, the *commissural* fibres that connect equivalent gyri in opposite hemispheres, and the *projection* fibres that transmit action potentials from the cerebral cortex to other parts of the brain and spinal cord.

In the ventral part of the mammalian forebrain are found a number of interconnected nuclei called the basal ganglia. These play an important role in supporting the control of movement by the cortex. Details of how the basal ganglia help to regulate movements will be given in Chapter 9.

The hippocampus is a special structure which connects the cerebral cortex with the rest of the forebrain. This highly ordered structure (Figure 8.9) plays an important role in controlling how the animal responds to stimuli. It seems to play a role in putting sensory experiences into the context of past experiences. It has important links with regions of the brain that are involved in motivation and emotional responses. Collectively these structures are called the limbic system. While the cerebral cortex is involved in the analysis of sensory stimuli and the direction of motor commands, the limbic system provides the emotional responses, the link with deeper feelings and past experience. The limbic system is closely connected with both the olfactory sense (which may account for the emotional effects produced by many odours) and the hypothalamus. Stimulation of limbic structures produces changes in blood pressure and respiration, and also causes movement such as chewing and other feeding related activities.

The diencephalon is the caudal half of the forebrain; it contains the thalamus and the hypothalamus (Figure 8.8). With the evolution of the cerebral cortex the thalamus became very important as the relay centre between the cerebral cortex and the rest of the brain. The thalamus contains many small groups of cells which relay different kinds of information to and from the cortex: tight groups of neurons that together perform a particular function. A particular group of these, the **specific thalamic nuclei**, relay visual, touch and auditory information to the primary sensory areas, and are topographically arranged. There are many other nuclei which are involved in relaying less specific sensory information (the non-specific nuclei). The only sensory input not received by the thalamus is olfactory input from the nose.

There are some thalamic nuclei that relay motor output from the cortex and yet others that are involved in integrating cortical activity with the activity in the rest of the brain. The evolution of the cerebral cortex in mammals has resulted in a great increase in the complexity of the thalamus which might be regarded as one of the important 'gateways' to and from the cerebral cortex.

Below the thalamus is an area called the hypothalamus ('hypo' means below) that plays an important role in controlling hormonal systems and the ANS. It is therefore very much concerned with emotional and motivational states of the animal and has strong links with the limbic system.

### 8.4.4   The midbrain

The midbrain has a specialized role controlling orientation to sensory information, especially visual and auditory. The midbrain is the upper part of the brain stem (Figure 8.8), and is made up of the tecta, one in each half of the brain, which are tucked under the posterior part of the cerebral hemispheres. Each tectum is divided into two regions, with the more anterior part forming a pair of small bumps called the superior colliculi (singular, colliculus) which receive visual, auditory and tactile inputs and are concerned with eye movements and orientation to external stimuli. As in other vertebrates, these projections come from the contralateral side of the body and are topographically arranged so that neighbouring points in visual or auditory space project to neighbouring points in the tectum. The superior colliculi have extensive connections to and from the cerebral cortex (via the thalamus) and the cerebellum. In the posterior part of the tectum there is another pair of bumps called the inferior colliculi. These are devoted to the analysis of acoustic information, which is then relayed to the primary auditory cortex, also via nuclei in the thalamus.

### 8.4.5   The hindbrain

The hindbrain is continuous with the spinal cord and contains three major divisions (Figure 8.8). The most prominent one is a large cauliflower-like structure, called the cerebellum. Although the cerebellum is also a paired symmetrical structure, the two halves are so closely joined together that it is usually referred to in the singular.

The cerebellum in most mammals is well developed. Its structure and physiology have both been analysed in detail, but how it controls movements and posture is still unclear. Like the cerebral cortex, the cells of the cerebellum form a cortex surrounding the white matter. This complex structure is concerned with coordinating body movements rather than initiating them, and ensures that intended movements can be executed. It therefore receives commands from the optic tecta, and information from movement sensors or proprioceptors via the spinal cord and vestibular apparatus. These sensory projections are ordered, but the order is rather different from the simple topographic arrangement in the tecta. The role of the cerebral cortex in the initiation of movements means that it is very closely connected to the cerebellum, the link being through the second major area of the hindbrain, the pons. The pons is the relay point for information from the cerebral cortex to the cerebellum in addition to providing the principal output from the cerebellar cortex to the spinal cord motor neurons. The pons also contains fibres that link (form a bridge between) the two halves of the cerebellum.

The third major area of the hindbrain is the medulla. The medulla and pons together form the most posterior part of the brain stem which connects with the spinal cord. This part of the brain stem performs many vital roles such as controlling breathing and circulation of the blood. Loss of blood supply or damage to this region of the brain always results in death. Many of the cranial nerves enter or exit the brain here, including the tenth, the vagus, which controls the heart and gut and is an important part of the ANS.

How is the function of these separate parts of the brain coordinated to direct the behaviour of the whole animal? First, there are extensive connections between the various brain regions and between the two halves of the brain. Second, there is a complex network of cells in the brain stem extending from the midbrain to the medulla, called the reticular formation, which has extensive connections with all other brain regions. The reticular formation coordinates and controls the activity in the various brain areas, as well as controlling information passing between the brain and the spinal cord. The cells in the reticular formation receive inputs from many different types of sensory receptors. These inputs are not topographically arranged, and often a single reticular cell is contacted by axons carrying widely different types of sensory information from different parts of the body. The complex organization and function of the reticular formation makes it difficult to unravel how it works, although its function has been described as 'activating' or 'priming' other parts of the brain and spinal cord in a very general way.

## Summary of Section 8.4

The most important change in the structure of the mammalian brain during evolution was the increase in size and importance of the dorsal part of the cerebral hemispheres in the control of behaviour. The increase in the number of interconnected neurons in the cerebral cortex provides for a substantial increase in the complexity and adaptability of behaviour. The dominance of the cerebral cortex is reflected in the topographically arranged sensory inputs to the primary sensory cortices. These inputs arrive via the thalamus which has an important role filtering the incoming information. Each kind of sensory information (touch, hearing, vision) has its own special nucleus in the thalamus whose input is also topographically organized. The cerebral cortex is responsible for analysing incoming sensory information and initiating appropriate responses. The hippocampus seems to be concerned with ensuring the appropriateness of the responses in the light of past experience.

The increased role played by the cerebral cortex has important consequences for the function of the midbrain. The superior colliculi are involved in orientation to stimuli while the inferior colliculi are involved in analysing sounds.

Before examining the structure of the mammalian brain in more detail (Section 8.8), it is important to describe the ANS, which plays such an important role in the maintenance of the internal environment of the body.

# 8.5   The mammalian ANS

The ANS in all vertebrates regulates the internal organs responsible for maintaining optimal living conditions for the cells of the body. Signals involved in this control come from receptors responding to internal stimuli such as the amount of oxygen in the blood, blood pressure, concentration of salts in the blood, or temperature (Chapter 5). Obviously such control systems become very important in vertebrates such as mammals and birds in which body temperature is maintained at a high level through physiological rather more than by behavioural means. The name 'autonomic' derives from the idea that such a system would operate autonomously, independently of the CNS. It is now known that the ANS is closely controlled by the CNS, but the old name has remained. As discussed in the introduction to this chapter, the ANS can be thought of as the motor system controlling the muscles of the internal organs and blood vessels rather than the muscles that move the limbs. The ANS has the same basic pattern in all terrestrial vertebrates. Figure 8.11 compares the arrangement of sensory afferents and motor efferents in the CNS and the ANS. Sensory inputs reach the ANS via the dorsal roots of the spinal cord. This account describes the ANS in mammals, although its organization is similar in most vertebrates.

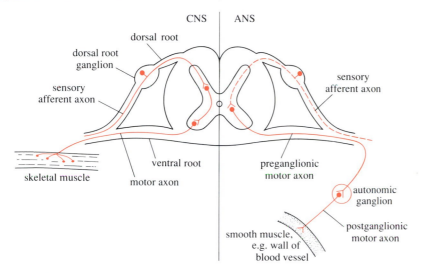

**Figure 8.11**   The afferent and efferent pathways in the ANS (to the right) and the CNS (to the left). Sensory information to both arrives via the dorsal root ganglia. The CNS motor neurons innervate the skeletal muscles directly but the output from the ANS makes a synapse within the autonomic ganglion before innervating muscles in, for example, the heart, gut or blood vessels. The connections within the spinal cord of both systems may involve additional interneurons.

The outputs of the ANS can be divided into two divisions called the **sympathetic division** and the **parasympathetic division**, which have rather different arrangements of ganglia and by and large have opposing actions. The sympathetic division has pairs of ganglia on each side of each of the thoracic segments of the spinal cord just outside the vertebral column (Figure 8.12). The ganglia of the parasympathetic division are situated in the periphery within the effector organs themselves. The preganglionic axons of the parasympathetic division arise from the brain (exiting along some of the cranial nerves) and the sacral segments of the spinal cord. You can see from Figure 8.12 that no region of the brain or spinal cord innervates both sympathetic and parasympathetic divisions of the ANS. You will also notice that most of the organs are innervated by both systems. You are not, of course, expected to remember all the details on this figure!

☐   What do the cervical and lumbar segments of the spinal cord innervate?

■   These segments contain the many motor neurons that innervate the limb muscles, which may account for the absence of an autonomic output in these segments.

The inner part of the adrenal gland (the adrenal medulla) lying above each kidney is an important output of the sympathetic nervous system. Electrical stimulation of the sympathetic axons innervating the adrenal glands causes the release of the hormones adrenalin and noradrenalin (also known as epinephrine and norepinephrine, respectively) into the blood. Adrenalin has widespread action in the body, speeding up the heart beat, dilating the air passages in the lungs, decreasing movement of the stomach wall, and mobilizing glucose in the liver. This activity prepares the body for 'fight or flight' by increasing the blood-flow to skeletal muscles, making glucose (an energy source) readily available, and increasing heart rate while shutting down unnecessary activities in the gut (Book 1, Section 2.9).

☐ Why, acting in this context, is adrenalin considered to be a hormone rather than a neurotransmitter?

■ Adrenalin is transported in the blood stream to influence activity of target cells far away—this is the definition of a typical hormone (Book 1, Section 2.9).

A given substance can serve in both roles. The functional difference between a hormone and a transmitter may merely be one of distance between release and effect. In fact the transmitter released by all sympathetic postganglionic neurons is noradrenalin. Noradrenalin has similar effects whether released into the blood stream from the adrenal medulla or locally by a sympathetic postganglionic axon terminal. The transmitter released by the parasympathetic postganglionic neurons is acetylcholine. The transmitter released by both sympathetic and parasympathetic preganglionic axon terminals is also acetylcholine.

The opposing actions of the sympathetic and parasympathetic systems are illustrated well by their effects upon the heart. Stimulation of the parasympathetic nervous system slows the heart down, whereas sympathetic action on the heart speeds it up. While the parasympathetic system is normally concerned with maintaining the resting state of internal organs, the sympathetic system helps the animal respond to sudden emergencies.

As already mentioned, the hypothalamus plays an important role in the regulation of the ANS. Its links with the limbic system are responsible for many of the physiological changes that accompany emotional responses, such as sweating and a racing heart when excited or frightened. Such autonomic changes can occur when reading a really good thriller or ghost story, demonstrating the influence of cortical activity on autonomic function. Common outward signs of emotional states are the result of autonomic, especially sympathetic, activity.

There is an obvious link between the ANS and the endocrine system, so the main features of the endocrine system are described briefly in the next section.

**Figure 8.12** The pathways and target organs of the parasympathetic (on the left) and sympathetic (on the right) divisions of the ANS. The preganglionic axons are shown in black, and the postganglionic axons in red. Most of the sympathetic ganglia lie in a row on either side of the spinal column. Postganglionic axons from these to sweat glands, to the smooth muscle of blood vessels and around hair follicles are not shown. Splanchnic nerves do not synapse within sympathetic ganglia. Parasympathetic ganglia are found within the target organs themselves. Remember that although the parasympathetic and sympathetic systems are shown on one side only, they are actually on both sides of the body.

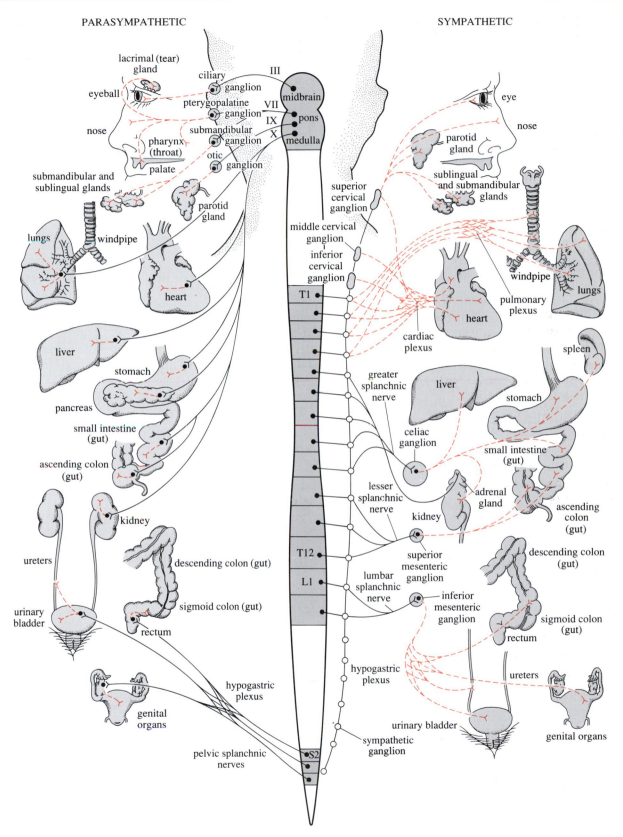

PARASYMPATHETIC

SYMPATHETIC

lacrimal (tear) gland
ciliary
ganglion
eyeball
pterygopalatine
ganglion
nose
submandibular
ganglion
pharynx (throat)
otic
ganglion
palate
submandibular and sublingual glands
parotid gland
lungs
windpipe
liver
stomach
pancreas
small intestine (gut)
ascending colon (gut)
kidney
descending colon (gut)
ureters
sigmoid colon (gut)
urinary bladder
rectum
genital organs
hypogastric plexus
pelvic splanchnic nerves

III
VII
IX
X
midbrain
pons
medulla
superior cervical ganglion
middle cervical ganglion
inferior cervical ganglion
T1
greater splanchnic nerve
lesser splanchnic nerve
T12
L1
lumbar splanchnic nerve
hypogastric plexus
S2

heart

eye
nose
parotid gland
sublingual and submandibular glands
windpipe
pulmonary plexus
lungs
heart
cardiac plexus
spleen
liver
stomach
celiac ganglion
small intestine (gut)
adrenal gland
ascending colon (gut)
kidney
superior mesenteric ganglion
descending colon (gut)
inferior mesenteric ganglion
sigmoid colon (gut)
rectum
ureters
urinary bladder
sympathetic ganglion
genital organs

## 8.6 The endocrine system

As you are now aware, many bodily functions are controlled by chemical messages released by cells (called **neurosecretory cells**) into the bloodstream. These chemicals or hormones bind with receptors on target cells and alter their activity in some way. This method of communication is ideal in situations where the target cells are widely scattered throughout the body and where responses need to be simultaneous, as in the preparation of the body for flight or fight discussed in the previous section.

The most important neurosecretory organs are the pituitary, the thyroid, the adrenals and the gonads. The pituitary is a composite gland lying beneath the hypothalamus, partly derived from the ventral part of the diencephalon and partly from the roof of the mouth. It releases hormones that regulate body growth, gonad function and the activity of other glands and organs, such as the kidneys which regulate salt and water balance in the body. It has very special and strong connections with the hypothalamus through both axons and a special blood vessel connection. The pituitary plays a pivotal role in controlling sexual behaviour in all vertebrates.

The thyroid and the outer part of the adrenal gland (the adrenal cortex) are involved in the regulation of basic metabolism, crucial in warm-blooded animals such as mammals and birds who generate their own heat. The adrenal medulla is part of the sympathetic nervous system discussed in the previous section.

The gametes (Book 1, Section 3.2.4) are formed in the gonads. The activity of the gonads is closely regulated by the pituitary. The gonads release hormones that regulate the production of eggs or sperm, and also the development of the embryo and reproductive behaviour (e.g. milk production in mammals).

## 8.7 A comparison of brains in different vertebrates

It would be quite possible to learn about the human brain without any knowledge of the brains of other animals. However, as there are so many structural and functional similarities between the nervous systems of different animals, models of brain function derived from other animals can be applied to humans. Moreover, looking at the structure of brains in a range of mammals can give an insight into the changes that have taken place in the evolution of the brain.

Figure 8.13 shows views of the brains of a frog, an alligator, a goose and a rat. The following sections discuss briefly the main differences in the structure of their brains and show how these variations relate to their different ways of life. Although the brains look rather different superficially, you should be able to see that they are all based on the same broad plan, which is shown most clearly in the fish brain, described in the following section.

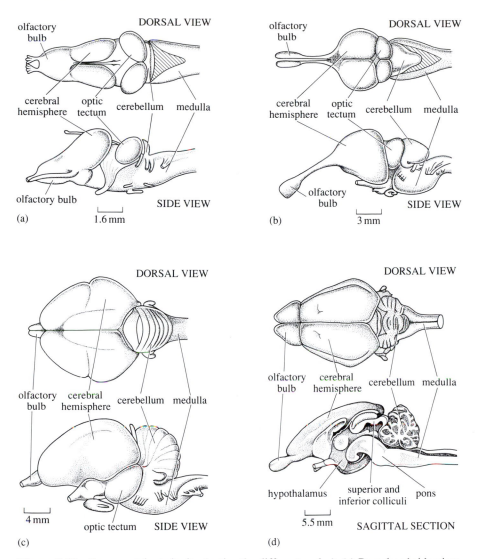

**Figure 8.13** Some vertebrate brains (notice the different scales). (a) Dorsal and side view of a frog brain. (b) Dorsal and side view of an alligator brain. (c) Dorsal and side view of a goose brain. The side view shows the lateral position of the optic tectum. (d) Dorsal and sagittal (cut down the midline) section of a rat brain. The sagittal section shows the position of the superior and inferior colliculi (see Section 8.4.4).

## 8.7.1 The fish brain

As you read through this description of the fish brain, remember that the CNS is a bilaterally symmetrical structure. Often you will find that the description refers to only one half while at other times it is describing both halves.

## The forebrain

The chemoreceptors in the nose are situated in the olfactory bulbs which are connected to the forebrain by the olfactory nerves (Figure 8.14). In an aquatic environment detection of substances in the water is important. Both predatory and reproductive behaviours depend on olfactory signals in many fishes. Migration of salmon back to the streams where they were born is controlled by olfactory cues, demonstrating the amazing sensitivity and refinement of this sense in these animals.

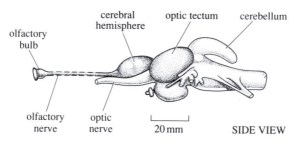

**Figure 8.14** Side view of the brain of a typical fish.

The rostral part of the forebrain seems to be involved in directing behaviour such as feeding and courtship. This region is sometimes referred to as the cerebrum, but cerebral hemispheres is a more accurate and less confusing word. (You might already begin to detect some important parallels between the fish and human brain.)

## The diencephalon

The diencephalon is the most caudal part of the forebrain, and connects the cerebral hemispheres with the rest of the brain. The dorsal part, the **thalamus**, receives sensory information primarily from the eyes, but it also has other inputs from vibration sense organs as well as projections from the spinal cord.

☐ What is the ventral part of the diencephalon called?

■ The ventral part of the diencephalon is called the hypothalamus.

The hypothalamus plays a very important role in the control of the internal environment through its connections with the ANS and the pituitary gland. The pituitary controls the function of many internal organs by secreting hormones which are transported in the blood to influence the activity of cells scattered throughout the body (see Section 8.6).

The forebrain in all vertebrates acts as an organizing centre for behaviour through its connections with the rest of the brain and with hormonal systems.

## The midbrain

The roof of the midbrain forms a paired structure containing layers of neurons called the optic tecta. The word optic is usually inserted in front of tecta here because, in many vertebrates, the tecta mainly receive a large and important input from the eyes. The optic tecta are composed of two symmetrical halves, as you saw in the human brain (Section 8.4.4). Each optic tectum receives optic axons from the opposite (contralateral) eye. The two tecta are connected together by large bundles of axons that cross the midline.

The tectum in fish, in common with many other of the simpler vertebrates, and colliculi in mammals, is an outer layer of cells outside the white matter of the brain core, and is the major control centre for the initiation of behaviour. The tectum directs movements via descending axons that connect with motor neurons in the spinal cord and the brain, such as those innervating the jaw and eye muscles.

Fish eyes, and those of all other vertebrates, are like those in the cephalopods (e.g. the octopus). They have a lens which focuses the light onto the light receptors. The light receptors are found at the back of the eye in the retina, which is composed of layers of neurons. As in all vertebrate eyes, the photoreceptors actually form the deepest layer of cells of the retina, the furthest away from the lens, unlike the receptors in the cephalopod eye which are situated in the layer nearest the lens. Axons from a particular kind of retinal neuron called retinal ganglion cells reach the brain along the optic nerve. The optic axons all cross over the midline at the optic chiasm and continue as the optic tract to the contralateral tectum where they synapse with tectal neurons (Book 3, Chapter 4).

The connections from each retina project in a precise topographic fashion onto the opposite tectum. This can be demonstrated by tracing the route of the axons from the retina to the tectum or vice versa (see Box 8.1).

☐   Can you recall from Section 8.4.3 what is meant by a topographic projection?

■   In a topographic projection the axons from neighbouring points on the sensory surface (e.g. the retina) influence neighbouring cells in the CNS. Such an arrangement provides the animal with an internal representation of the external world.

Each tectum also receives topographically arranged sensory inputs from touch and vibration receptors on the contralateral side of the body (fish do not have ears like mammals, but are very sensitive to vibrations and sound in the water). The reason why sensory inputs project to the opposite side of the CNS in vertebrates is obscure (there is no such crossing over in the invertebrates). It is possible that it could derive from the need for the first motor responses by young hatchlings to approaching danger to be bending of the body away from the site of stimulation. This is produced by contraction of the body muscles contralateral to the stimulated side.

The relative size of the tectum in many fish (and other vertebrates) reflects the importance of vision in their lives. The angler fish, for example, feeds on insects and can hit a fly accurately with a jet of water. It has a much larger tectum than fish living in murky, muddy water where olfaction is the more important sense. This difference between reliance on vision and reliance on olfaction is mirrored in brain structure. Figure 8.15 compares the brain of a shark, which relies principally on olfactory information, with the brain of a cod, that relies primarily on visual information.

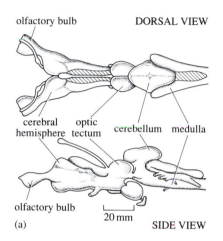

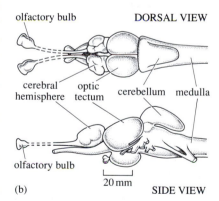

**Figure 8.15**   Dorsal and side views of the brain of: (a) a shark, a fish which relies on olfactory information, and (b) a cod, a fish which relies on visual information.

The connection between the eye and the optic tectum has been studied in detail using horseradish peroxidase (HRP, Box 8.1). If HRP is applied locally to the retina, it will be transported along the retinal axons in the optic nerve to their terminals in the optic tectum. The transport in this case is in the same direction as the conduction of action potentials and is therefore called **anterograde transport**. Figure 8.16 shows the presence of HRP seen as a dark area on the tectum following application to different regions of the retina as shown in the accompanying diagrams. In this experiment the brain was not sectioned but was left whole so that the overall pattern of the HRP-filled optic axons can be seen.

---

### Box 8.1  Tracing neural connections

One way of tracing neural connections is to inject (fill) a neuron intracellularly with a dye, as described in the previous chapter. However, this method only fills one neuron at a time and it is notoriously difficult to penetrate vertebrate neurons and then keep the microelectrode in place inside while the activity is recorded and the dye is injected.

The most common method of tracing pathways of axons between groups of neurons is to use their own transport system. Within living neurons proteins are continually being transported along the axons and dendrites, both to and from the cell bodies. This property of axonal transport has been utilized by neuroanatomists to trace the connections of neurons within the brain.

A dye injected into one part of the brain will be taken up by a small number of neuronal cell bodies and axon terminals close to the injection point. The dye will then be carried by axonal transport to the end of each axon, which may be in other parts of the brain. For this to be successful, the neuron and its axon must not be damaged by the dye, since transport will only occur in living cells.

The enzyme horseradish peroxidase (HRP) is frequently used as a dye to study the connections between different regions of the CNS. After injection of HRP into a local region of the brain, enough time is allowed for it to fill the neuron completely. The animal is then killed and selected brain regions fixed and sectioned (see Box 2.3). The HRP is made visible by treating the specimen with chemicals which turn the HRP into a solid substance that can be seen under the light or electron microscope.

HRP has proved to be very useful for detailed tracing of connections since the terminals and cell bodies are clearly visible, looking rather like Golgi stained preparations (Figure 8.17, *overleaf*). The drawing of a neuron in Figure 8.17 was made using a special attachment to a microscope (called a camera lucida) which has a system of mirrors so that whatever is viewed down the microscope can be drawn accurately.

In addition to HRP, there are a vast number of other dyes that anatomists can use for tracing connections between neurons, each with its own advantages and disadvantages.

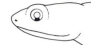

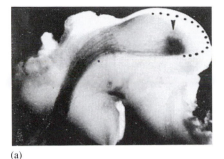

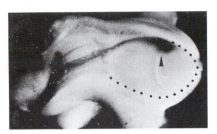

(a)

(b)

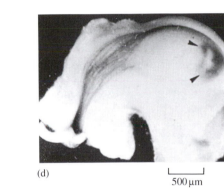

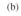

(c)

(d)

500 μm

**Figure 8.16**   Lateral views of tecta showing the position of stained retinal axons following local application of HRP to: (a) dorsal (D), (b) ventral (V), (c) temporal (T, next to the temples), and (d) nasal (N, next to the nose) regions of the retina, as shown in the diagram next to each photograph. The dots outline the optic tectum, the arrows indicate heaviest labelling. The experimental animals in this case were adult newts rather than fish, but the pattern of projection is similar in all vertebrates.

This kind of experiment has been repeated in many vertebrates, with similar results. The dorsal retina always projects to the lateral tectum, and the ventral retina to the medial tectum. Applying HRP to the part of the retina nearest the temples (the temporal retina) fills axons in the rostral tectum with dye, while HRP applied to the retina nearest the nose (nasal retina) gives dye in the caudal tectum. You need not remember this arrangement, only that there is a universal projection pattern from the eye to the brain in all vertebrates.

Axonal transport also occurs in the opposite direction, so that application of HRP at a localized site in the tectum will be taken up and transported back to the cell bodies in the retina. This is called **retrograde transport**. Figure 8.18a (*overleaf*) shows the bowl-shaped retina of a fish flattened out by making four peripheral cuts. The circle shows the position of retinal cells containing HRP following local injection into the caudal tectum.

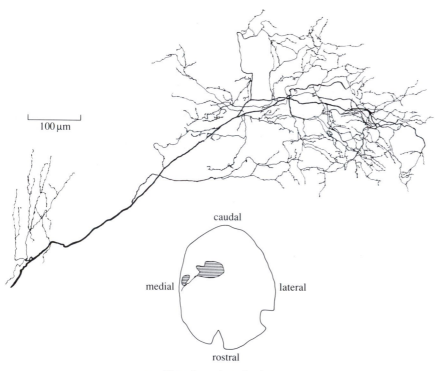

caudal

medial

lateral

rostral

position of axon branches in tectum

**Figure 8.17**  Drawing of the branching of single HRP-filled axon of a retinal cell in the frog tectum, and the position of these axon branches in the tectum. The small swellings on the finer branches are probably axon terminals.

The labelling patterns seen by retrograde and anterograde transport will not necessarily be the same. If the neurons at the application site have axon branches that terminate over a very wide area then the anterograde labelling pattern will cover a large area whereas cells filled retrogradely will be much more localized (Figure 8.19a). Conversely, if the axons from widely spread neurons converge onto a very localized target area, then a localized application of dye to this area will retrogradely fill many widely spread neurons (Figure 8.19b). Information about how much divergence and convergence there is in a pathway is valuable in trying to understand its function.

## The hindbrain

The sensory input from the vibration and balance organs enters the caudal half of the hindbrain, the medulla. Fish are very sensitive to vibrations in the water: if you jolt a fish tank (being careful not to let the fish see you move), all the fish will dart suddenly. The sensory receptors responsible for this reflex are specialized hair cells (Section 2.4.2) that sit in fluid-filled tubes which run down the middle of each side of the body. These are called the lateral line organs. Vibration information is important in shoaling fish, keeping them swimming together. In electric fish the lateral line organs have become further specialized for the detection of objects in the water. Here some of the muscles along the sides of the body emit pulses of electricity which bounce off nearby objects. The reflected signal that returns

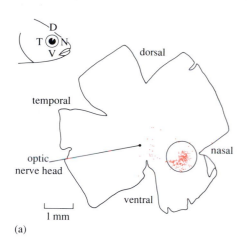

(a)

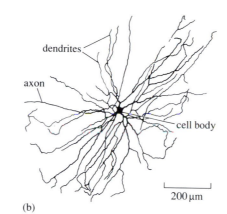

(b)

**Figure 8.18**   (a) Flattened retina of a goldfish showing the position of retinal cells filled with HRP (each small dot marks the position of a filled retinal cell) following local application to the caudal tectum. (b) The enlargement shows the appearance of a single filled retinal cell. The larger dot at the centre of the retina is the point at which the axons leave the eye, forming the optic nerve.

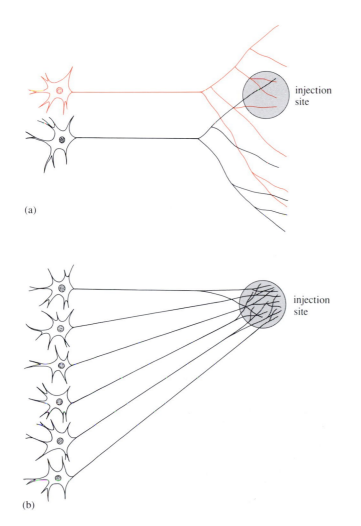

(a)

(b)

**Figure 8.19**   (a) Diagram showing two neurons with divergent axon branches. Application of HRP to the two cell bodies will fill the large area covered by their axon terminals, whereas application of HRP to the region of their terminals as shown will only fill the two cells. (b) Diagram showing many neurons with convergent axon branches. Application of HRP to a local region as shown will retrogradely fill many of the cells. Application of the dye to one of these cell bodies will only fill anterogradely a small area of branches from that particular axon.

199

provides the fish with information about those objects in the same way as submarine sonar detectors work. In some species of electric fish these signals are so powerful that they are also used to stun prey. Lateral lines are a speciality of an aquatic environment, and therefore are also present in tadpoles and aquatic newts, but not in adult terrestrial amphibians.

In the brief review of the invertebrate nervous system in Chapter 6 you read that all animals that actively swim have a specialized organ to detect gravity and movement (like the jellyfish, see Section 6.2.2). Vertebrates also have a system for detecting movement and position or orientation in space. This is called the vestibular apparatus and is coupled to the system for vibration detection. The vestibular apparatus is essentially similar in all vertebrates, consisting of three fluid-filled tubes arranged at right angles to one another. Movement of the fluid is detected by specialized hair cells. Input from the vestibular apparatus is conveyed to the brain along the eighth cranial nerve (vestibulocochlear), together with vibration information from the lateral lines. Notice the similarity of these receptors to those in jellyfish that signal orientation and movement.

Dorsal to the medulla, and just behind the tectum, is the cerebellum. A fish has to control its position in three dimensions and consequently the cerebellum is a relatively large structure (Figure 8.14).

### Summary of Section 8.7.1

This account of the organization of the fish brain has shown you how brain structure can be related to the function in the life of the animal. The brain is a bilaterally symmetrical enlargement of the hollow dorsal neural tube encased in the skull. The cerebral hemispheres in the rostral part of the forebrain receive chemical inputs from the olfactory bulbs. The midbrain optic tecta receive visual input from the retina, and the hindbrain receives vibration and orientation information. The optic tecta and cerebellum form a separate layer of cells lying outside the central core of the brain. This core contains many nuclei, such as the hypothalamus in the diencephalon, that are important in the regulation of general bodily functions.

The importance of the optic tecta and cerebellum in the initiation and execution of movements is reflected in the precise topographic organization of their sensory inputs. In the next section the brains of different vertebrates are compared to illustrate how brain anatomy is closely related to the animals' behaviour and lifestyle.

### 8.7.2  The amphibian brain

The amphibians (frogs, toads, newts and salamanders) are the descendants of the first land-dwelling vertebrates. The adult animals do not have gills like fish, but lungs like all terrestrial vertebrates. However, they are still very dependent upon an aquatic environment. All but a few return to water to breed, and the early stages of development are spent as aquatic, fish-like tadpoles. The frog brain is illustrated in Figure 8.20.

Adult frogs have good vision and their optic tecta are relatively large. Most do not have lateral lines, as fish do, but instead have an obvious eardrum behind each eye. The ear drum transmits sound vibrations mechanically, via a set of three small bones, to a part of the vestibular apparatus called the cochlea. (You will read more

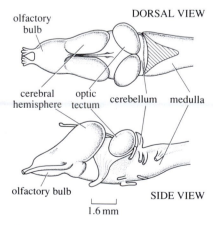

**Figure 8.20**　The brain of a frog.

about hearing in Chapters 2 and 3 of Book 3.) The fluid-filled space in the cochlea contains hair cells very like those in the fish lateral line system which respond to movements of the fluid. This ear design is common to all terrestrial vertebrates, including humans. Sensory axons from the cochlea, together with those from the vestibular apparatus, enter the brain as part of the eighth cranial nerve.

☐  Notice how small, relative to the rest of the brain, the frog's cerebellum is compared to that of a fish. How might this be related to their way of life?

■  The difference is related to their method of locomotion. Fish swim in three-dimensional space, whereas amphibians crawl or hop along the ground and cannot be described as fancy swimmers. Movement in two-dimensional space is simpler to coordinate.

### 8.7.3   The reptilian brain

Many reptiles (lizards, crocodiles, snakes, tortoises, etc.) have adapted to an exclusively terrestrial lifestyle, and do not require water to reproduce. They can be very good at conserving water, and consequently can live in very arid conditions. The brain of an alligator is illustrated in Figure 8.21.

Olfaction is an important sense for most reptiles. The darting tongue of the snake picks up chemical substances from the air or objects and conveys them to the olfactory receptors lying in a well protected sac within the skull. Most snakes also rely on vision and their optic tecta are quite large, but the scaly reptilian skin is not well supplied by sense organs. However, rattlesnakes have receptors on the head that are very sensitive to heat (infrared radiation). These receptors are arranged in a structure called the pit organ lying between the eye and the nostril which, like the eye, forms an image of the position of the heat source (Book 1, Section 2.7.2). It is this input that enables the rattlesnakes to strike accurately at warm-blooded prey in total darkness. The input from these infrared receptors is topographically arranged on each contralateral optic tectum in register with the visual map. This means that one point in space is represented at the same position in the tectum for both inputs.

☐  How would you expect the structure of the spinal cord in a snake to differ from that in an alligator?

■  All the segments of the spinal cord in the snake should be very similar, since snakes have no limbs and therefore there should be no obvious cervical or lumbar enlargements.

Notice how the relative size of the cerebral hemispheres is increased in reptiles, compared with amphibians, and in amphibians compared with fish. The evolution of the vertebrates is characterized by the increase in size of the cerebral hemispheres. In the more recently evolved vertebrates the cerebral hemispheres dominate the initiation and control of behaviour, integrating sensory information from the different sense organs.

### 8.7.4   The bird brain

Birds and mammals differ from the reptiles, amphibians and fishes in that they can maintain a fairly constant body temperature that is generally higher than the

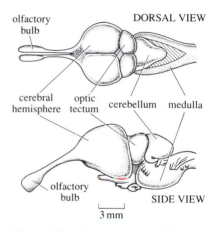

**Figure 8.21**   The brain of an alligator.

ambient temperature, using heat produced by chemical processes occurring within the body. Reptiles and amphibians that maintain a body temperature above the ambient temperature rely principally on external heat sources such as sunlight, and they regulate their body temperature by behavioural means.

An important consequence of high body temperature is that the rates of all cellular activity are increased. This means that action potentials are conducted faster, synapses act quicker, and activity in the whole nervous system is speeded up. The ANS plays a very important role in the regulation of body temperature (producing responses to cold such as puffing up the feathers in birds or shivering in mammals).

The brain of a goose is illustrated in Figure 8.22. The relative enlargement of the cerebral hemispheres noted in reptiles and amphibians is much more pronounced in birds, reflecting their increased importance in the initiation and control of behaviour such as courtship and feeding patterns. The enlarged cerebral hemispheres push the optic tecta out sideways, as you can see in Figure 8.22. Birds have rather a poor sense of smell, and small olfactory bulbs, but the ventral part of the cerebral hemispheres, the striatum, is enlarged. As you will learn in Book 4, Chapter 5, the bird striatum seems to be important in learning. In Book 1 you became acquainted with the importance of learning in the control of bird behaviour patterns such as feeding and learning to sing.

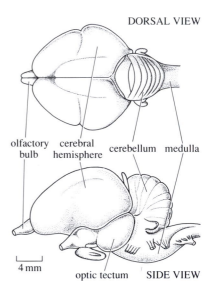

**Figure 8.22**    The brain of a goose.

☐    How is the size of the bird cerebellum related to its lifestyle?

■    The cerebellum is the part of the brain where the coordination of movement is carried out (Section 8.4.5). The large size of the cerebellum, relative to the rest of the brain, reflects the fact that coordination of flight is a complex process that involves movement in three rather than two dimensions.

The optic tecta are large in most birds. In many there is also a very elaborate topographically arranged map of sound space in register with the visual map. These maps are arranged so that a point in space is represented at the same position in the tectum for both sound and visual inputs. In birds such as owls, which locate their prey predominantly by sound, these maps are especially refined (Book 3, Chapter 4).

### 8.7.5    Comparisons with the mammalian brain

The mammalian brain looks quite different from the fish brain but, like the bird brain, it still has the same basic vertebrate brain organization. The midbrain tectum is no longer visible either from above or from the side: it is completely overlain by the cerebral hemispheres. As in birds the cerebral hemispheres exert overall control over behaviour. However, in mammals it is the dorsal rather than the ventral part of the cerebral hemisphere that has increased in size, ballooning out to form the cerebral cortex which covers most of the rest of the brain.

You should now realize that much of the increased complexity seen in the mammalian brain comes from the integration of the cortex with the rest of the brain. You should also be familiar with the names of the major structures in the brain and have some idea of what they do. There is more information about the anatomy and connectivity of the human brain in the videocassette *The Human Brain* and in later chapters of this and the other books of the course. In the next section the structure of the mammalian brain will be considered in greater detail and some of the methods used to study it will be described.

## 8.8  Studying the mammalian brain

At the start of Section 8.4, which introduced you to the structure of the human brain, you read that the most easily recognized landmarks were the cerebral hemispheres. In comparing brains from different groups of vertebrates (Section 8.7) you will be aware that there is a progressive increase in the relative size of the cerebral hemispheres in the evolutionarily more recent vertebrates. However, there are also differences in the cerebral hemispheres if comparisons are made within a group. In the mammals (Figure 8.23) you can see that, besides the difference in size, there is an obvious difference between the appearance of the rather smooth cerebral cortex in the shrew and the convoluted appearance of the cerebral cortex in primates (the group of mammals to which humans belong). The amount of convolution of the cat cortex is intermediate between the shrew and the monkey.

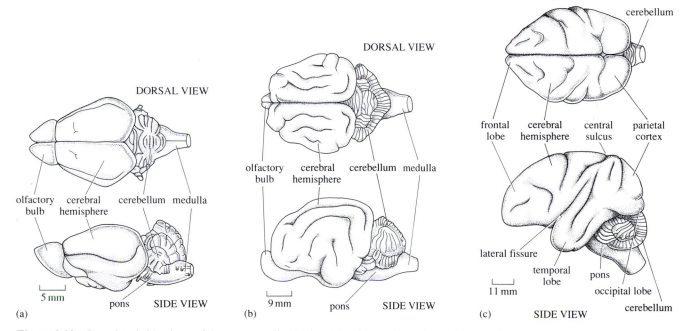

**Figure 8.23**  Dorsal and side views of three mammalian brains: (a) a shrew, (b) a cat, and (c) a monkey.

The convolutions arise because the sheet of layers of nerve cells forming the cortex has a much larger area than will fit easily into the relatively small skull; the area of the cortex in primates is enormously increased compared to other mammals. In humans it is composed of 10–15 thousand million neurons (plus four times as many glial cells). Spread out, it would cover an area of about $0.7\,\text{m}^2$ or the area of an average coffee table. Its size in primates and humans demonstrates its increased importance in the analysis of sensory information and the control of behaviour in these species, which is characterized by great flexibility and adaptability.

## 8.8.1 Anatomy of the cerebral cortex

The cortex in humans is about 3 mm thick; in mice it is 0.5 mm thick. There are six layers of cells identified by the sizes and shapes of their cell bodies, as shown in Figure 8.24. Each layer is conventionally referred to by number, with the lowest number at the surface. The largest cell bodies are found in layers 5 and 6; these neurons, most clearly seen in Golgi stained preparations (Section 2.3.1, Box 2.3), have a definite pyramidal shape. These pyramidal neurons have long dendrites that span most of the six layers and extend laterally along the cortex by as much as 0.5 mm, the longest pyramidal neurons being in layer 5. They are the principal output neurons of the cortex; their projection axons leave the cortex via the ventral white matter beneath to go to non-cortical parts of the brain. In layers 2 and 3 there are smaller pyramidal cells. Their axons also descend to the white matter, but go to other areas of the cortex rather than other regions of the brain. These cortico-cortical axons are usually referred to as **association axons**. Some of the longest association axons are found in the corpus callosum, the structure that links the two cerebral hemispheres together.

In addition to these two kinds of pyramidal cells there are a host of other neurons of different sizes and shapes whose axons remain within the cortex. The axons of these **intrinsic neurons** communicate vertically as well as horizontally through the cortical layers. The way in which the connections up and down between the different layers of the cortex are arranged suggests a columnar organization, the width of the columns being related to the lateral extent of the dendrites of the component cells. In the primary sensory areas the inputs (from the thalamus) form compact bushes in layer 4 (Figure 8.24b). The axons from other regions of the brain and also the association axons usually form divergent branching patterns, indicating a more diffuse influence on the cortical neurons.

In Section 8.4.3 the division of the cerebral cortex into primary sensory and motor areas was described. How did anatomists start to work out which regions were connected to what and what was their function? The first demonstration of localization of function in the cerebral cortex was made in 1870 by two Germans, G. Fritsch and E. Hitzig. They described how electrical stimulation of one region of the cortex (the motor cortex) in a dog produced movement of the limbs, while stimulation of the occipital region did not. Observations of loss of function in soldiers with head wounds sustained in the Franco–Prussian war confirmed that different regions of the cerebral cortex performed different tasks. Touching exposed regions of cortex with surgical instruments caused localized movements of the limbs or perceptions of tingling or flashes of light in conscious soldiers (there were no good anaesthetics in those days). In the early part of the 19th century Charles Brodmann published a detailed description of the cellular anatomy of the human cortex, dividing it up into 50 areas, each with its own distinctive anatomy (Figure 8.25). Subsequently, these primary sensory areas were studied using more sophisticated stimulation and recording methods (see Box 8.2). The position of the areas in relation to the ridges (gyri) and valleys (sulci), together with data obtained from patients and from animal studies, shows that these areas do in fact have different functions. Recently, nuclear magnetic resonance (NMR) imaging and positron emission tomography (PET) have provided less invasive methods of looking at the functional architecture of the cerebral cortex in health and disease (see Chapter 11 and Book 6). Positron emission tomography is an imaging technique which can be used to measure the minute fluctuations in blood flow through localized regions of the cerebral cortex associated with neuronal activity.

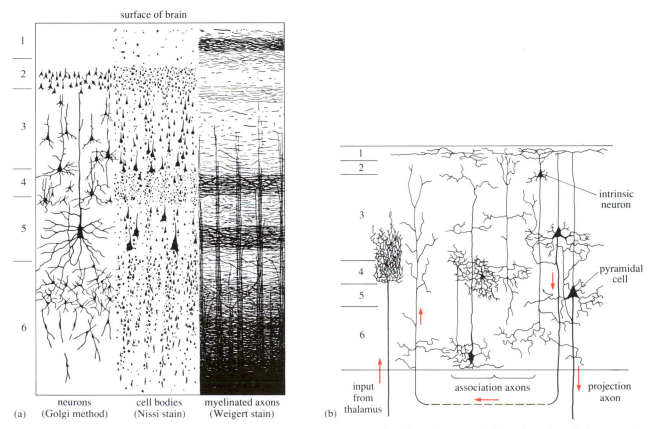

**Figure 8.24**   (a) Section through the human cerebral cortex that has been stained by various methods to show the cellular structure and the distribution of myelinated axons. (b) Diagram showing the shapes of some of the cells and the branching patterns of the axons from the thalamus and the association axons. Arrows show the direction of action potential travel.

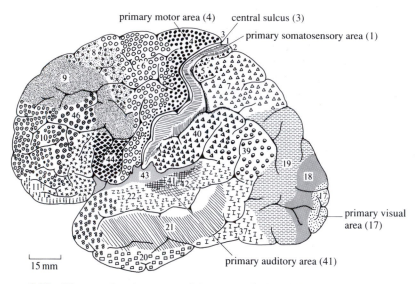

**Figure 8.25** Diagram showing some of the anatomically distinct regions of the human cerebral cortex identified by Brodmann. Different areas are given numbers. The symbols are used merely to indicate the extent of each area.

## Stimulating and recording from the brain

Over several decades neurophysiologists have mapped the brain extensively by using electrical recording devices to measure electric currents generated during neuronal activity. Experiments carried out on rodents, cats, primates and humans undergoing neurosurgery have allowed the mapping of visual, auditory and motor areas in the cerebral cortex. This has enabled the description of nerve pathways from the stimulus input, for example a flash of light, to the cortex and also from the primary motor area of the cortex to the muscular response evoked. The electrical activity of the brain can be monitored at different levels, from the whole brain (Box 8.2), recordings provided by electroencephalograms (EEGs), to multi-neuron recordings of groups of cells, and single-neuron recordings (Box 8.3, *overleaf*) monitoring the activity of one cell or axon only. As you will see, EEG recordings, despite the fact that they monitor a global brain process, can provide a lot of useful information about the function of areas of the cortex. In their turn, single-unit recordings have helped enormously in the investigation of the details of cortical function.

The activity in the surface layers of the cortex can be monitored by observing the changes in colour of voltage sensitive dyes with very sensitive TV cameras. Such methods, like the EEG recordings, provide information about general activity in the area rather than the activity of single cells.

## Box 8.2   Electrical recordings at the whole brain level

Disc shaped electrodes are placed on the surface of the scalp in order to measure small changes in electrical activity. Recordings of these changes are called electroencephalograms or EEGs. The EEG reveals spontaneous rhythmic fluctuations of voltage in various brain areas. Stimulation of the eyes with light flashes produces potentials that can be recorded from the visual cortex in humans. These are called visual evoked potentials.

EEG recordings are widely used to diagnose abnormal brain function in neurological and psychiatric contexts but the precise underlying mechanism for the production of an EEG is still unknown. However, EEGs are obviously related to the activity of the region of cortex closest to the electrode, as shown in Figure 8.26.

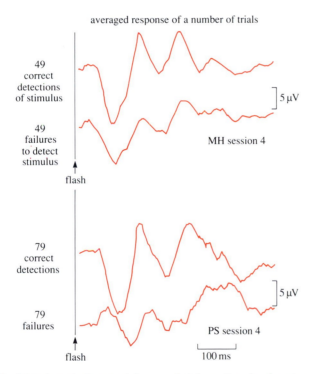

**Figure 8.26**   Visual evoked potentials recorded from the visual cortex of two human subjects, M.H. and P.S. Each subject was presented with a sequence of stimuli. The evoked potentials were averaged for equal numbers of trials in which the subject either detected, or failed to detect, the stimulus. The light intensity was dim so that the subjects did not always see the stimulus. The evoked response was smaller when the subjects did not see the light.

## Box 8.3   Extracellular recordings in the brain

A microelectrode inserted into the brain may come close enough to a neuron to detect its action potentials. The microelectrode usually consists of a very fine wire which is insulated except for the very tip (about 5–20 µm). The difference between the potential picked up at the tip of the electrode and a second electrode (which can be a large piece of metal) placed elsewhere on the body will be related to the activity of neurons near the microelectrode.

☐   What sort of size relationship would you expect to see between the recorded action potentials?

■   In accordance with the all-or-none principle of axonal transmission, each action potential from the same neuron is the same and the action potentials recorded from one cell are all the same size.

This fact provides a very useful way of being able to tell whether recordings are being made from a single neuron. With such a microelectrode in place, experimenters can study how different stimuli affect the firing rate of a neuron and thus how information is 'coded' by neurons and transmitted to and from the brain. In practice, when the electrode is first lowered into the brain, it picks up signals from several nearby neurons. The signals will be different sizes and shapes, because the neurons producing the signals will be at different distances from the electrode. This size difference enables the signals from different neurons to be distinguished from one another. Alternatively, the electrode can be moved slightly to increase selectively the signal from one neuron.

In order to be certain that the electrode is placed in the desired part of the brain a stereotaxic instrument is used. This consists of a head-holder which is fixed to the skull in a standard position. The position of the electrode is defined by coordinates which relate to specified positions on the skull. An atlas of the brain is used to relate the coordinates to the position of particular structures within the brain. The usefulness of stereotactic atlases depends on the fact that different brain structures have constant spatial relationships. Laboratory animal species are selected for their structural homogeneity and thus such atlases are quite accurate.

Stereotaxic instruments are also widely used for neuroanatomical tracing studies where tracers are injected into precise locations of the brain to discover their interconnections.

## The organization of the cortex

By recording from, and stimulating the brain, the layout of the cortex has been mapped. There are three primary sensory areas or cortices: the **somatosensory** cortex (receiving touch information) in the post-central gyrus just behind the central sulcus, the primary visual area in the occipital cortex, and the primary auditory area in the temporal cortex. The neurons in the primary somatosensory and visual areas respond to tactile or visual stimulation of localized regions of the skin or visual field. Just as for the visual projection to the optic tecta these inputs are topographically arranged so that neighbouring areas of the receptive surface project to neighbouring areas of the primary sensory cortex. The primary auditory area responds to sound stimuli, which are tonotopically mapped—low frequency (low-pitched) sounds stimulate one region and high frequency (high-pitched) sounds another.

Figure 8.27 shows the positions of the primary sensory and motor areas in a group of mammals. There is a lot of information on the organization of these areas in different mammalian groups as they are relatively easy to identify. While the positions of the primary sensory and motor maps are similar in the five mammals, the relative areas of cortex devoted to particular inputs vary greatly. For example, the proportion of the cortical area devoted to analysing auditory information in the rat, a nocturnal species, is much higher than in primates such as chimpanzees or humans, which are diurnal (active during the day). Notice that in primates the area of association cortex is greatly increased compared with the rat, especially in chimpanzees and humans. Similarly, the tarsier (bush baby), with its huge eyes, has a relatively large proportion of its cerebral cortex devoted to visual input. Such comparisons reveal the close relationship between cortical organization and the habitat and lifestyle of the mammal.

## 8.8.2 Variations in the organization of the primary sensory areas in mammals

Relative size is not the only way cortical organization varies between animals; the arrangement of the inputs within a sensory area can also be related to the relative role played by various sense organs in the animal's life. Rats and mice have relatively poor vision and a proportionately small primary visual area. They depend on their highly mobile whiskers to find their way about, using their sense of touch. A mouse or rat continuously sweeps the area ahead with its whiskers. This activity, called 'whisking', informs the animal about objects in its path.

☐ How do you find your way around a completely dark and unfamiliar room?

■ You probably extend your arms to search and feel your way around.

It is clear that you are using your hands in much the same way as a rat or mouse uses its whiskers, substituting tactile input for the more normal visual information. The mobile whiskers are the primary tactile organ for rats and mice and consequently have a large and specialized representation on the somatosensory cortex. In humans, the hands and lips are the primary tactile organs so there is a correspondingly large area of the sensory cortex devoted to them (Figure 8.10), with only an insignificant area receiving input from the immobile (but sometimes decorative) whiskers. The representation of the human body surface on the somatosensory cortex is called the homunculus or 'little man'. The representation of the whisker area of the face on the somatosensory cortex of the mouse is, therefore, relatively large and very elaborate, with afferents from each whisker projecting to a unique region of the map (Figure 8.28, *overleaf*).

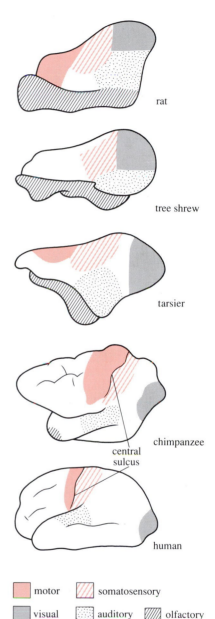

| ![motor] motor | ![somatosensory] somatosensory |
| ![visual] visual | ![auditory] auditory | ![olfactory] olfactory |

**Figure 8.27** The positions of the primary sensory and motor areas in a rat, a tree shrew, a tarsier monkey, a chimpanzee and a human. The unshaded regions are association cortex. The anterior/rostral part of the brain is towards the left.

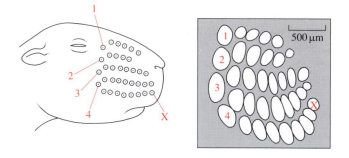

whiskers on muzzle —— project to —— layer 4 of somatosensory cortex

**Figure 8.28**   A schematic representation of the relationship between the whiskers on the mouse and the anatomy of layer 4 in the somatosensory cortex. The white areas are areas of lower cell density bordered by tightly packed cells. Each of these less dense areas, which look rather like a row of beer barrels, corresponds to a single whisker on the muzzle as indicated by the numbers. All cells within each of the 'barrels' respond only to movement of one whisker. The arrangement of the barrels is the same as the arrangement of the whiskers on the muzzle.

## 8.8.3   Inputs to the thalamus and to the primary sensory areas

The primary sensory areas of the cortex receive their topographically arranged inputs via the specific nuclei of the thalamus. The thalamus is not a uniform structure; it consists of nuclei, each of which is devoted to a particular part of the cortex and to particular kinds of sensory information. In addition to these specific nuclei, there are the non-specific nuclei that receive less organized inputs which are concerned with modulating cortical activity rather than relaying specific information. The difference in function between the specific and non-specific nuclei is reflected in the pattern of their terminations in the cortex. The terminals of thalamic axons relaying specific sensory information to the primary sensory areas are confined to layer 4 and are compact, while the non-specific afferent axons are much more diffuse. Neurons in the ventrobasal nucleus (also called the ventrobasal complex because it actually consists of a number of smaller nuclei) receive tactile inputs from the contralateral side of the body and send their axons to the primary somatosensory cortex. Neurons in the medial geniculate nucleus (MGN) receive auditory inputs and send their axons to the primary auditory area. Neurons in the lateral geniculate nucleus (LGN) receive optic axons and send their axons to the primary visual area.

☐   How would you expect the sensory projection to the specific thalamic nuclei to be arranged?

■   The specific thalamic nuclei all receive topographically organized sensory inputs.

The topography of the projections to the medial and lateral geniculate nuclei are especially interesting. The projection of auditory inputs to the primary auditory cortex is arranged tonotopically, giving information about the pitch of the sound. This tonotopic arrangement is also seen in the medial geniculate nucleus.

A great deal is known about the visual projection to the lateral geniculate nucleus and visual cortex. There are two reasons. The first is simply that vision is such an important sense in humans and so there has been a substantial amount of research carried out. The second is that it is relatively easy to plot the receptive fields of visually responsive cells to discover the topographic projections (see Box 8.1) or to trace connections from the retina to the LGN.

☐   Which sensory modality is arranged differently?

■   The olfactory input from the nose arrives via the olfactory bulb which projects directly to the olfactory cortex. (This illustrates the evolutionarily old nature of olfaction and the fact that you cannot make a topographic map using smells.)

Most mammals have what is known as **binocular vision**, meaning that the two eyes share an overlapping region of visual space. Binocular vision allows the distance to an object to be assessed more easily (Book 3, Chapter 4). The degree of binocular overlap depends upon the position of the two eyes in the head. Animals with laterally pointing eyes such as sheep or rabbits have a small degree of binocular overlap. Many predators or animals that need to gauge distance accurately (those that live in trees, for example) have forward pointing eyes and a large degree of binocular overlap, providing depth information over a wider area of the visual field.

☐   What are the destinations of optic axons in mammals?

■   The visual input to the brain arrives via the optic nerves. The optic axons synapse in the thalamus and the superior colliculus.

Figure 8.29 (*overleaf*) shows the arrangement of the optic axons from the two eyes to the lateral geniculate nucleus and the superior colliculus in a mammal with little binocular overlap (e.g. rabbit, rat, sheep) and one which has a large degree of binocular overlap (e.g. cat, monkey, human). You can see from this figure that the arrangement of fibres actually preserves the rule that sensory inputs from one side of the body (in this case, visual information from that part of the visual field on one side of the body) project to the opposite side of the brain. The proportion of optic axons that 'cross over' depends on the orientation of the eyes: only those axons receiving visual information from that part of the visual field that is on the same side of the body as the eye will cross over. Also notice that the field of view is much larger in the rabbit than in the cat or human.

The thalamus is not merely a relay station: it also processes and segregates different kinds of visual information (e.g. colour, shape and movement). The thalamus in addition receives a rich input back from the cortex. This connection in both directions allows the cortex to modify and control incoming information. Many parts of the mammalian brain are connected in this reciprocal fashion, with one centre receiving from another and in return regulating it. This reciprocity of connections makes descriptions of brain function very complex.

☐   What role does the superior colliculus play in behaviour?

■   It is involved with orienting the animal to relevant stimuli.

The visual information reaching the cortex via the thalamus is devoted to recognition of objects and patterns, while the collicular input is more concerned with how the visual field is moving relative to the animal. As you learnt in Book 1 (Section 2.3 on reafference) such information is very important; the animal must be able to distinguish between movement of visual stimuli produced by its own movements or by the movement of the stimulus itself. It can be seen here how the visual system deals with different sorts of information in different parts of the brain, bringing this information together at the cortex.

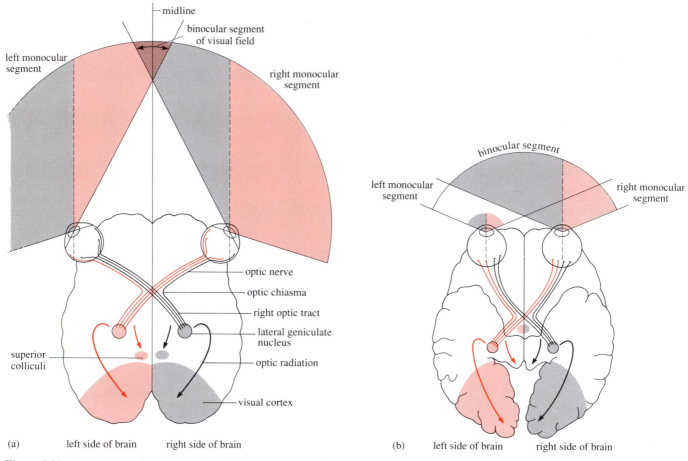

**Figure 8.29**   (a) A schematic representation of the arrangement of optic axons from the two eyes in a rabbit or sheep. (b) The projection of optic axons from the two eyes in a cat or primate.

## 8.8.4   Bilateral symmetry and the whole animal

As has been emphasized, the nervous system is a bilaterally symmetrical structure. In a sense there are two nervous systems which are joined down the midline. The animal, however, needs a representation of its environment that is continuous across the midline. Any discontinuities in the middle of visual space would seriously hamper the performance of a hunter chasing prey as it moves across the field of view. For the animal there cannot be a 'perceptual' seam.

Both visual cortices receive input from the region of binocular overlap in visual space in front of the animal—this can be a very large proportion of space for animals like the cat, or very small for the rabbit. The visual system solves the 'midline seam' problem through the interconnections between each visual cortex via the fibres in the corpus callosum. These connections must be very precise, with each point in binocular space being in perfect register for the inputs from each eye.

The visual space is not the only place where the two 'perceptual' halves of the animal must be joined. You are not aware of any discontinuities in the sensations produced by touch stimuli which cross the midline of your body, are you? In this case the continuity is simply established by overlapping and extension of receptive fields across the midline. (A receptive field is the area from which a sensory neuron receives its input.)

## 8.8.5    Primary motor cortex

The proportion of cortex devoted to the primary motor area does not show such a large variation between different mammals. This is probably because the size of these areas is related to the muscle mass they control. However, there are very great differences in the way different parts of the body are represented within the motor cortex in different animals. These differences can be directly correlated with the kinds of motor behaviour the animal can perform. The topography of the motor projection looks very much like that of the somatosensory projection. The cortical representation of those senses which have been elaborated in certain animals has a correspondence in the motor cortex as well as the sensory cortex. In the mouse and rat, the regions of the face in the motor cortex have an increased representation for the small muscles that move the whiskers. It was described previously how the sensory representation of the whiskers in the rat and mouse is very large and elaborate. The whiskers are not just used passively, but are actively moved by the animal during exploration, and so they also have an enhanced representation in the motor cortex. The muscle attached to each whisker is separately represented in a topographic map in the motor cortex, just like the sensory inputs for each whisker.

The somatosensory cortex in mammals that make extensive use of their forepaws for grasping or manipulating objects (monkeys, apes, raccoons, squirrels, etc.) shows an increase in the area taken up by control of the muscles in the hand. It is worth noting that the forepaw has become so important in some mammals that it has evolved into a hand. In Old World monkeys (i.e. those in Africa and Asia) and apes the thumb can also be moved opposite to the fingers, and this gives them an extremely important tool for manipulating objects. This is not the only interesting evolutionary development amongst the monkeys and apes: New World monkeys (i.e. those in North and South America) have a prehensile tail that can cling to branches, acting rather like a fifth limb. The South American capuchin monkey used by organ grinders in the last century can swing from its tail as well as grasp the begging bowl with it. Old World monkeys such as the rhesus monkey of India have very little motor control over the movements of their rather insignificant tails. As you might imagine, the area of the motor cortex devoted to the tail in Old World monkeys is tiny by comparison with that of the New World species.

The emergence of manual dexterity in both primates and raccoons is accompanied by changes in the way the motor cortex influences the motor neurons in the spinal cord. The motor output to the limb muscles, especially those in the hands or feet, is much more direct than to the muscles of the back; this direct pathway is called the pyramidal tract (also called the cortico-spinal pathway).

☐   From which neurons in the motor cortex does the pyramidal tract originate (see Section 8.8.1)?

■   The pyramidal tract contains axons from the pyramidal cells in layers 5 and 6 of the motor cortex, though motor output is really only from layer 5.

The name 'pyramidal' for the tract originates from the obvious pyramidal shape that the bundles of these axons form in the medulla just before they cross the midline. It is coincidental that the cells of origin in the cortex are also described as being pyramidal.

For most muscles the axons of the pyramidal tract synapse with interneurons in the ventral root of the spinal cord which, in turn, innervate the motor neurons. The pyramidal pathway to muscles of the primate hand is more direct; here the pyramidal tract axons contact many of the motor neurons directly, without the presence of an intermediate neuron. This direct and fast cortical control of motor neurons was once thought to be present only in primates, but it is now known to be present in racoons, animals famous for their manual dexterity.

## 8.8.6   Association cortex

The functions of the primary sensory and motor cortical areas are reasonably easy to study since they are related in an obvious way to externally applied stimuli or muscle movements, respectively. Figure 8.27 showed the sensory and motor regions in various mammals. The rest of the cortex, shown in white in Figure 8.27, contains the association areas (Section 8.4.3). As described in Section 8.4.3, the association areas do not receive direct sensory inputs or make direct contact with motor pathways: instead they are connected with other cortical areas. It was thought that these areas 'associate' or integrate information coming from or going to the primary sensory and motor areas. However, recent work has shown that many of the cells in the association cortex actually receive quite specific sensory inputs. Their responses suggest that these areas are concerned with the higher levels of interpretation of sensory stimuli and processing of motor commands. These areas also receive inputs from the non-specific thalamic nuclei.

The boundaries between the primary sensory and motor areas and the association areas are not sharp. Gradually, as the border is traversed, the specificity of the responses becomes more and more difficult to define. What seems to be happening is that the processing of sensory inputs becomes more complex as one moves away from the primary areas.

The much larger size of those areas devoted to the analysis of sensory information in primates reflects the greater importance of storage and sophisticated processing of sensory information in their lives (what humans like to distinguish as 'intellectual ability'). Much of this processing and analysis also involves referral to past events and present motivational states (Book 1, Chapters 6–8). The flow of information proceeds from the primary sensory areas to the association areas and finally to the limbic system before the output decision is made and the animal does something. In the next chapter you will learn that different regions of the association areas play important and unique roles in the functioning of the human brain.

## 8.8.7   Other regions of the cerebral hemispheres: the hippocampus

So far some aspects of the cerebral cortex have been considered. A less obvious part of each cerebral hemisphere is the hippocampus. The hippocampus is derived from the midline wall of the cerebral hemisphere. It lies beneath the cerebral cortex and forms the connection between the cerebral cortex and the rest of the forebrain (Figure 8.30).

The detailed structure of the hippocampus is similar in all mammals. It consists of three layers, rather than six as in the cerebral cortex, and looks like two interlocking horseshoes. The more dorsal horseshoe contains a central layer of large pyramidal cells similar in appearance to those in the cerebral cortex (this region is called Ammon's horn because it looks like the headgear of the Egyptian god of the same name), with their main dendrites pointing towards the centre of the horseshoe. The second horseshoe (called the dentate gyrus) consists of much smaller cells with their dendrites pointing outwards. A prominent pathway called the fornix connects the hippocampus at the apex of the dorsal horseshoe with other brain areas including the limbic system. The fornix also carries afferent axons to the hippocampus from the medial septum. If you trace round the swiss roll of the hippocampus from the dentate gyrus you eventually come to the cerebral cortex proper. The hippocampus receives many inputs from the cerebral cortex and also from the thalamus along this route. The hippocampi on each side of the midline are linked together via commissural fibres in the fornix.

The hippocampus seems to function similarly in all mammals since it is not noticeably different in either structure or relative size. The hippocampus is part of the limbic system and is involved in directing the way the animal responds to its environment and in learning. The importance of the hippocampus can be appreciated from the size of the fornix, which is as large as the optic nerve.

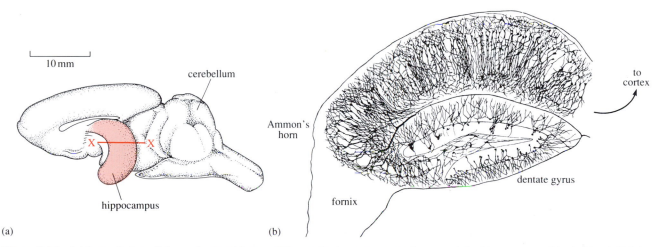

(a)

(b)

**Figure 8.30**   (a) Lateral view of the rat brain with part of the cerebral cortex removed to reveal the hippocampus (shaded in pink) lying beneath. The olfactory bulbs have been omitted for clarity. (b) A section across the hippocampus (slice shown by X—X in (a)) stained with the Golgi technique showing the layers of neurons.

### 8.8.8 The structure of the cerebellum

This brief survey of some of the details of mammalian brain circuitry would not be complete without a description of the anatomy of the cerebellum. As in all vertebrate brains, the mammalian cerebellum is important in maintaining posture and in the coordination of movements. The cerebellum varies in relative size between mammals, depending upon the importance and complexity of movements for the particular sort of mammal. Like the cerebral hemispheres, it is a deeply folded structure and has an outer cortex of cell bodies.

The details of the structure of the neurons in the cerebellar cortex and their connections are well known. This is chiefly because the structure has a high degree of order. A lot is known about how the neurons influence each other. However, next to nothing is understood about how it actually functions in the coordination and acquisition of skilled movements.

The cerebellar cortex is composed of three layers of cells (Figure 8.31). The most prominent are the large Purkinje cells (named after the anatomist Purkinje), which have elaborate, large, flat dendritic trees arranged in rows like a stack of playing cards. In humans there are about 15 million of them, with a combined dendritic area equivalent in size to two front doors. The axons of the Purkinje cells form the only output from the cerebellar cortex; they project to nuclei lying in the pons in the brain stem beneath the cerebellum. Cells in the cerebellar nuclei in turn influence motor neurons in the medulla and spinal cord, and also relay information back to the cerebral cortex via the thalamus.

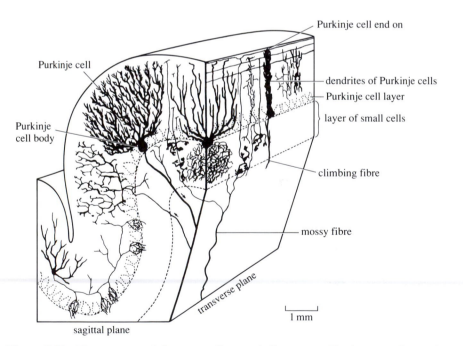

**Figure 8.31** The structure of the mammalian cerebellar cortex. The largest cells are the Purkinje cells, from the two views in the diagram you can see how their dendritic tree is very flat. The details of the other cell types are not relevant here. For clarity only one Purkinje cell is shown in detail; the cell bodies of other Purkinje cells are indicated with dotted lines.

☐   What kind of information would you expect to be relayed to the cerebellum?

■   Since the cerebellum controls movement and posture you would expect it to receive information from the muscles and from joint proprioceptors as well as from the vestibular system, touch receptors and also, of course, from the cerebral cortex, the source of motor commands.

Maintenance of posture and coordination of movements requires the integration of a large number of sensory inputs. Proprioceptive and vestibular inputs are routed directly to the cerebellum via the spinal cord and the medulla. Other inputs—such as touch, sight and hearing—arrive as projections from the appropriate regions of the cerebral cortex and superior colliculus.

These latter inputs, called *climbing fibres* because they 'climb up' and intertwine with the Purkinje cell dendrites, are extraordinary because one axon synapses with only one Purkinje cell—a rare one-to-one excitatory connection in the mammalian nervous system. The precision of the climbing fibre input contrasts with the other input which involves an intermediate cell whose axons run perpendicular to, and influence a huge number of Purkinje cells. Another remarkable feature of this cerebellar circuit is that the Purkinje cell axon is entirely inhibitory onto cells in the cerebellar deep nuclei, with GABA as its transmitter. Most major pathways in the nervous system are excitatory. Inhibitory synapses usually come from local intrinsic neurons rather than projection neurons.

## Summary of Section 8.8

Both the gross and fine structure of the brains of mammals are related to a particular animal's lifestyle. All areas of the brain seem to be connected directly, or indirectly, to practically every other part—an organization which will support extremely complex activity patterns. During evolution profound changes in brain structure have taken place.

# Summary of Chapter 8

The CNS contains millions of neurons, each one integrating information arriving at its synapses. In this chapter you have seen how the nervous system can be divided up into regions, each specializing in a particular function and each containing its own particular arrangement of neurons. Each region receives input and its output depends upon the nature of that input. In an analogous way the whole CNS receives information and produces appropriate motor responses.

Figure 8.32 (*overleaf*) is a very schematic diagram illustrating the flow of information from the sensory inputs to the motor outputs in the mammalian CNS. Remember that many of the connections between regions are reciprocal, and that some pathways pass straight through (e.g. the pyramidal tract from cortex to spinal cord). The reticular formation at the centre has connections with almost all other parts. The diagram is arranged hierarchically—the more complex the task the more structures are involved. The cortex is placed in the highest position, but some people would argue that the hypothalamus and limbic system exert such a strong control over the internal environment and behaviour that they should be at the top.

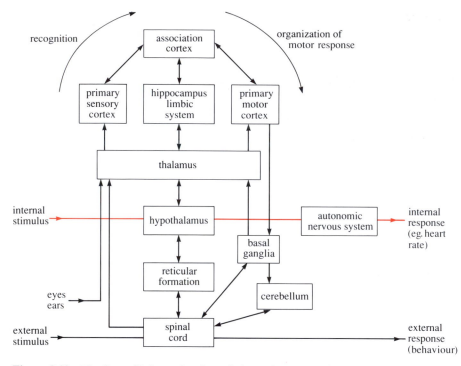

**Figure 8.32**    The flow of information through the various parts of the mammalian CNS.

At the bottom there are the inputs from the external environment. The olfactory input, which projects to the evolutionarily older ventral part of the cerebral cortex and which is closely connected to the centres concerned with motivation, has been omitted for clarity.

A sensory stimulus might produce a simple motor response localized to the spinal cord or a more complex series of activities. A series of 'loops' of increasing complexity can be seen, from simple reflexes confined to the spinal cord (straight across the bottom) to loops which include the cerebellum, then the cortex and the cerebellum, and finally to the involvement of all the structures shown in the diagram. As the loops involve more and more of the brain, the responses become less and less 'automatic' and more and more open to modification.

It is important to realize that this is a very static and serial view of what is happening. In the awake animal most information is being processed in several regions of the brain simultaneously. It may be shuffled to and fro, influencing the activity in other regions. One of the problems with trying to understand how it all works is that it is difficult to monitor the activity of populations of interconnected neurons. However, recent advances involving voltage sensitive dyes, the detection of local blood flow and nuclear magnetic resonance open the way to a more global view of neuronal activity in the brain. Certainly a great deal has been learnt from the careful analysis of activity in single cells, and the effects of various drugs upon those activities, but there is still a very long way to go.

# Objectives for Chapter 8

When you have completed this chapter you should be able to:

8.1   Define and use or recognize the definitions and applications of each of the terms printed in **bold** in the text. (*Questions 8.1 and 8.2*)

8.2   Explain, in terms that involve the expressions motor neuron, sensory neuron and axon, what is the distinction between white matter and grey matter in the spinal cord. (*Question 8.3*)

8.3   Describe the types of sensory inputs projecting to the vertebrate forebrain, midbrain and hindbrain, and their arrangement. (*Question 8.4*)

8.4   Show how brain structure is related to the lifestyle and habitat of the animal. (*Question 8.1*)

8.5   Explain the function of the mammalian cerebral cortex and how its increased prominence in the mammalian brain has affected the role of the midbrain optic tectum in the control of behaviour. (*Question 8.5*)

8.6   Recognize the input and output cell layers of the cerebral cortex. (*Question 8.8*)

8.7   Discuss the role and organization of the ANS in mammals.

8.8   Describe the role of the thalamus in the mammalian brain. (*Questions 8.6 and 8.7*)

8.9   Compare the differences in the topography of the primary somatosensory and motor cortex in mammals, with particular reference to behaviour and lifestyle. (*Question 8.9*)

8.10   Explain what is meant by binocularity and how this is reflected in the projection of optic axons to the mammalian brain. (*Question 8.10*)

8.11   Describe the roles of the cerebral and cerebellar cortices and the hippocampus in mammals. (*Question 8.11*)

# Questions for Chapter 8

### Question 8.1 (*Objectives 8.1 and 8.4*)
Label the optic tectum, cerebellum and cerebral hemisphere in the fish brain in Figure 8.33. What might be the lifestyle of this fish?

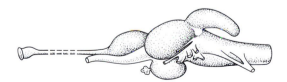

**Figure 8.33**   For use with Question 8.1.

**Question 8.2** (*Objective 8.1*)
Label the dorsal roots, ventral roots, grey matter and white matter, and sympathetic ganglia in Figure 8.34. In what region of the spinal cord would you find such structures? What do grey and white matter mean? Which neurons in the spinal cord have the largest cell bodies and what do these neurons do?

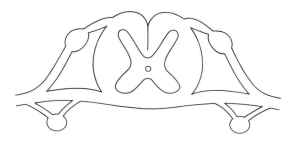

**Figure 8.34**   For use with Question 8.2.

**Question 8.3** (*Objective 8.2*)
Which of the following (a–d) is true of the butterfly-shaped central region of the spinal cord?

(a) It consists of grey matter containing mainly the axons of sensory neurons.

(b) It consists of white matter containing mainly cell bodies.

(c) It consists of grey matter containing mainly cell bodies.

(d) It consists of grey matter made up in large part of the cell bodies of sensory neurons, i.e. the dorsal root ganglia.

**Question 8.4** (*Objective 8.3*)
What is special about the arrangement of the projection from the eyes to the vertebrate brain?

**Question 8.5** (*Objective 8.5*)
Does the apparent reduction in the size of the optic tectum in mammals correlate with a decreased importance of vision?

**Question 8.6** (*Objective 8.8*)
'As he crept along the dark passage his heart was pounding, he thought he heard a noise and broke out in a cold sweat…'

Which part of the nervous system is responsible for these symptoms?

**Question 8.7** (*Objective 8.8*)
The thalamus has been described as the 'gateway to the cerebral cortex'. Explain what this description means.

**Question 8.8** (*Objective 8.6*)
In which layer of the cerebral cortex do thalamic inputs terminate, and how do terminals relaying specific sensory information differ from the rest?

**Question 8.9** (*Objective 8.9*)
In what ways would you expect the 'homunculus' to differ from the 'ratunculus', or the 'elephantunculus'?

**Question 8.10** (*Objective 8.10*)
What functional reason might explain the fact that 50% of the retinal axons cross the midline in humans, whereas in rats 90% cross over?

**Question 8.11** (*Objective 8.11*)
What are the roles of the cerebral cortex and cerebellar cortex in movement of mammals?

# CHAPTER 9
# MOTOR AND SENSORY SYSTEMS— THE INS AND OUTS OF THE BRAIN

## 9.1   Introduction

The major theme of this and the following chapter is: What does the vertebrate CNS do and how does it do it? In previous chapters, you have read about the evolution and diversity of nervous systems. As you followed the discussions, you should have gradually become better acquainted with the general structures of nervous systems. This should be particularly true of the mammalian nervous system, and by now the names of some of its prominent anatomical structures should be familiar. In Chapter 7 you worked through detailed physiological analyses of the way that apparently complicated invertebrate behaviour patterns were controlled through relatively simple neurophysiological networks. Chapter 9 will continue this analysis but with emphasis on the mammalian CNS. It will discuss key structures of the mammalian CNS, most of which you will have already encountered in this book, and describe the contributions they make to the functioning of the mammalian CNS.

After a general introduction to the divisions of the CNS and the terminology involved, the chapter starts with a look at the way that the muscles of the body are controlled to produce movement. The general descriptive term for the CNS structures involved in control of the skeletal muscles is the **motor system**. The introduction to the mammalian motor system starts in Section 9.3 with the structure of the spinal cord and its reflex organization, and then Section 9.4 turns to central structures that control the spinal cord organization to produce behaviour. In the discussions of motor control, some aspects of the sensory inflow from the body to the spinal cord and brain are introduced. Section 9.5 also introduces the organization of sensory systems in the brain and the way that information is represented in the CNS through the example of pathways that contribute to the sense of touch.

## 9.2   Divisions of the CNS: structures, systems and terminology

As a generalization, the path of the evolution of the vertebrates, particularly the mammals, is marked by the massive expansion of the forebrain regions. This expansion has produced a CNS structure characterized by the cerebral hemispheres, and parallelled by the development of more flexible behavioural control. That is, expressed in systems terms, the evolution of the vertebrates is characterized by an 'opening up' of behavioural control systems. By 'opening up' what is meant is behaviour that, earlier in evolution, took the form of 'reflex' or automatic responses, and that now shows flexibility. This development allows prior experience to make a more significant contribution to the selection of appropriate behaviour patterns. As a further generalization, this evolutionary trend to more open control of behaviour occurred in the context of an expansion and development of both sensory and motor structures and capabilities.

During this evolution, forebrain structures were not simply 'bolted on' to previously existing structures, and existing 'primitive' functions were not suppressed and replaced with new functions. Contrary to a sometimes still-expressed opinion and to early psychoanalytic theory, there is no evidence that the human cerebral cortex holds 'primitive centres' in check while imposing its more 'rational' control over human behaviour. Rather, in the evolution of the forebrain, integrated neural systems emerged that were both adaptations and enhancements of existing systems. The brains of mammals living today have evolved as integrated neurophysiological systems, rather than as 'primitive' systems suppressed and replaced by more recent ones.

The following sections will concentrate on motor and sensory systems of the brain to illustrate how CNS structures that are described anatomically as distinct entities form integrated systems. As you work through this chapter, you will find discussions about what systems in the brain and spinal cord do, the purpose of the chapter being to give an insight into how the brain and spinal cord work together as an integrated system. However, to do this, the chapter will start by 'pulling the brain and spinal cord apart' to give an idea of the organization of their constituent structures.

Figure 9.1 is a schematic representation of the mammalian CNS systems that will feature in this chapter. You have already been introduced to many of the structures of the CNS in Chapter 8.

Prominent in Figure 9.1 are connections from cortical regions to structures in the brain stem, and connections that travel down through the brain stem and spinal cord to terminate within the spinal cord. Also shown are the ascending pathways in the spinal cord that convey information from the body to the brain. Note also in Figure 9.1 the location of the cerebellum, a massive brain stem structure that plays an important role in motor control, and the basal ganglia, which are a collection of nuclei that are interconnected primarily with cortical regions. Figure 9.1 can be used to appreciate the dynamic nature of control over the muscles. It shows schematically the way that the consequences of muscular activity are fed back to spinal cord structures (as one of the inputs to the box labelled 'afferent input') and hence to the brain.

To put the following discussions in context, walking and running are examples of behaviour that involve rhythmic movements of the limbs, analogous to the rhythmic invertebrate behaviour discussed in Chapter 7. However, as you know from direct experience, such behaviour can be modulated without conscious involvement, in response to information fed back through the sensory systems of the limbs. In Figure 9.1, this would correspond to 'sensory consequences of movement'. This happens, for example, to compensate for sudden changes during walking that could upset the body's upright posture, with such compensatory responses occurring almost instantaneously without awareness or conscious involvement. The discussion of the neural organization of the spinal cord mechanisms will introduce the reflex pathways which act to maintain body posture and to organize the rhythmic muscular contractions that are involved in walking and running.

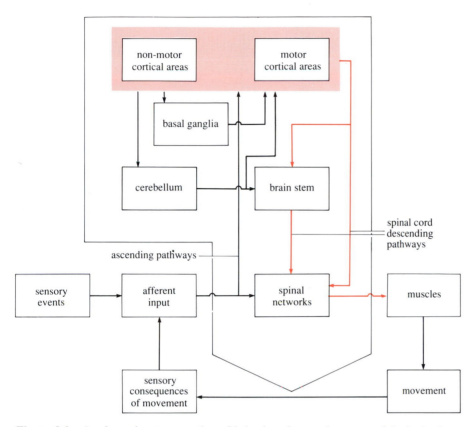

**Figure 9.1**   A schematic representation of behavioural control systems of the brain that influence the control of the skeletal muscles through the spinal cord.

As an example of other behaviour patterns in which brain stem and forebrain systems are involved, think about the activity that goes on when you pick up a cup of coffee. This is an apparently simple task that most people do, often without much thought, and yet it involves the integration of many 'items' of information. The individual has to be motivated to terminate some other activity to take a drink. The shape of the cup has to be recognized and distinguished from other objects, such as the saucer and the table top. The distance of the cup away from the hand has to be known along with the starting positions and dispositions of the hand and limbs. Once the hand reaches the cup, knowledge of its shape and weight is used to grasp the handle smoothly, lift the cup, and bring it towards the mouth.

Consider for a moment the facility and smoothness with which you carry out such voluntary operations as picking up a coffee cup, running and walking. This indicates that the movements are not carried out by performing a series of discrete and separately computed responses. Rather, there is an overall plan to the action, a plan that is compared with feedback on what movement has actually been effected and which guides any particular part of the action.

Starting at the level of the spinal cord and then continuing with brain structures, the following sections will describe neurophysiological structures that control the muscles of the body. They will emphasize the systems within which they are embedded that contribute to coordinated and integrated aspects of behaviour.

## 9.3    Spinal cord structure

As you have already learned, the spinal cord is a long, thin cylinder of nervous tissue contained within the spinal column, which is the backbone formed by the bony vertebrae. The neural tissue forming the spinal cord is physically continuous with the brain, the 'join' occurring at the posterior end of the brain stem (see Figure 9.2). Sensory inflow from the body (below the neck) occurs via sensory nerves that run from each part of the body to the spinal cord. Control over the muscles of the body occurs via motor nerves that run from the spinal cord to the various parts of the body (below the neck). These nerves are not arranged continuously along the length of the spinal cord but are bundled together in pairs, one on the left and one on the right. One left/right pair emerges from within each of the vertebrae that form the backbone. The sensory inflow and motor outflow between the spinal cord and the vertebrate body is organized on a segmental basis corresponding to the spinal column vertebrae. To get a picture of this, you should now compare Figures 9.2, 9.3 and 9.4.

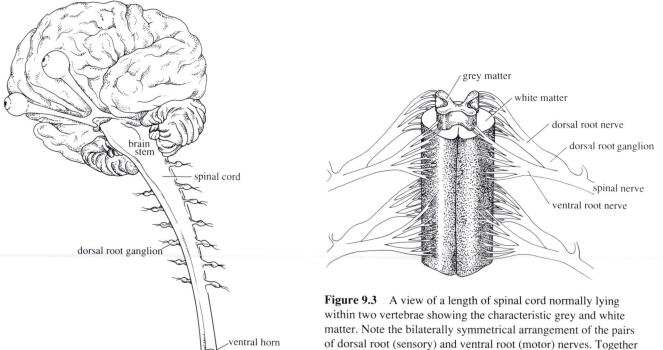

**Figure 9.2**    The human brain and upper part of the spinal cord.

**Figure 9.3**    A view of a length of spinal cord normally lying within two vertebrae showing the characteristic grey and white matter. Note the bilaterally symmetrical arrangement of the pairs of dorsal root (sensory) and ventral root (motor) nerves. Together these constitute what is known as a spinal nerve. Note also the dorsal root ganglion, where the cell bodies of the neurons that make up the dorsal root nerve are situated.

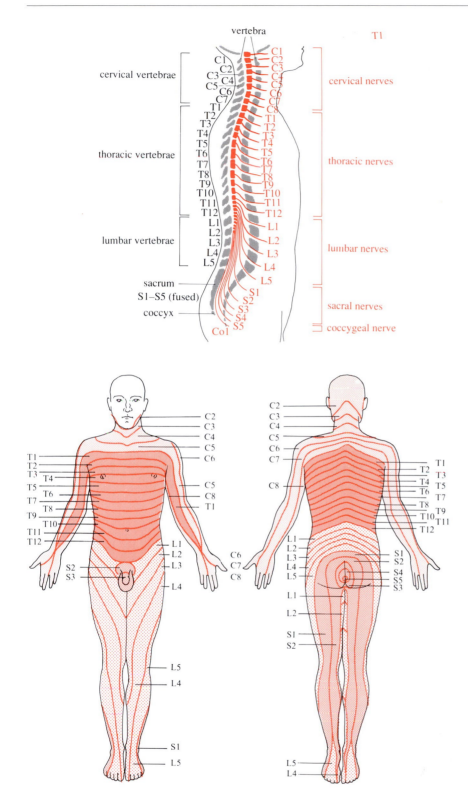

**Figure 9.4**   The dermatomes are regions of skin that correspond to the segmented structure of the spinal cord. Each dorsal root ganglion lies within a single vertebra of the spinal column and receives sensory information only from its corresponding dermatome. The prefix letters Co, S, L, T and C refer to the coccygeal (tail), sacral (hip), lumbar (lower back), thoracic (chest) and cervical (neck) regions of the spinal column, respectively. Within these regions each vertebra is numbered sequentially corresponding to its position (spinal nerve C1 does not have a dermatome). The dorsal root ganglia are labelled in red. From Carola, R. *et al.* (1990) *Human Anatomy and Physiology*, McGraw-Hill Inc.

The sensory inflow from the skin is arranged into areas called **dermatomes** (see Figure 9.4). Here, the sensory receptors in a particular band of the skin all connect with sensory neurons whose cell bodies lie in a single dorsal root ganglion within a single vertebra. In this context, the term 'segment' is used to describe the spinal cord tissue lying within a single vertebra, so sensory neurons from each dermatome project to a single segment of the spinal cord. Similarly, motor outflow to the body is arranged on a segmental basis with the motor nerves exiting via the ventral roots of the spinal cord, but the relationship between individual muscles and spinal cord segments is not as clear cut as seen in the dermatomes.

Control over the muscles of the head and sensory information from the head are not mediated by the spinal cord but by the cranial nerves that emerge from nuclei in the brain stem.

You will remember from Chapter 8 that the spinal cord is generally described as being divided into grey and white matter (Figure 9.3). The white matter consists of the pathways through which axons ascend and descend, to and from the brain. An example of one such (ascending) pathway is shown in Figure 9.5.

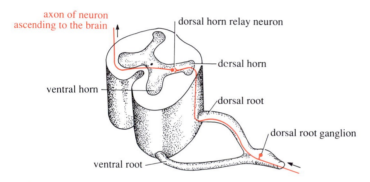

**Figure 9.5** Sensory information from the body enters the spinal cord via sensory nerves (the dorsal roots). A single representative sensory neuron is shown here. Many such sensory neurons constitute a sensory nerve. Synaptic contact is made with neurons in the dorsal horn of the grey matter of the spinal cord. Information is relayed to the brain via the ascending sensory pathways in the white matter. One ascending neuron is shown here as representative of an ascending pathway of neurons.

☐ What is the basis for the distinction between white and grey matter in the CNS?

■ The white appearance of some regions of nervous tissue comes from the whitish myelin coating that surrounds axons (Section 2.4.4). White matter contains a preponderance of axons. In contrast, neuron cell bodies and dendrites are unmyelinated. Tissue containing mainly neuron cell bodies is distinctively less white in appearance and is described as grey matter.

The cell bodies of spinal cord motor neurons, i.e. neurons whose axons synapse on muscle cells, are located within the ventral horns of the grey matter of the spinal cord. Their axons project via ventral root nerves (Figure 9.3) leading to the body.

## 9.3.1  Sensory input to the spinal cord

The sensory input to the spinal cord is via sensory neurons whose cell bodies are located outside the spinal cord proper, in the dorsal root ganglion. This is shown in Figures 9.2, 9.3 and 9.5. The sensory inflow to the spinal cord, via the dorsal root ganglia, conveys information about deformation of the skin (touch), temperature, joint position and movement, state of muscle stretch, as well as information about noxious stimuli and tissue damage. Noxious stimuli activate a class of sensory neuron termed nociceptors, introduced in Section 1.2, and discussed in detail in Book 3, Chapter 5.

In some cases, the axons of the sensory neurons whose cell bodies are located in dorsal root ganglia receive their sensory input from sensory receptors specialized in signalling information on touch, temperature, movement of the hairs on the skin, and deformation of the skin surface (Section 2.4.1). In other cases, the tip of the axon may itself be specialized to serve as a sensory receptor. Many of the details of the sensory receptors that detect and code information into action potentials are beyond the scope of this chapter, but will be discussed in Book 3. However, one example is looked at in detail in the next section. For the most part, the present chapter will concentrate on the way that the spinal cord is organized to respond to information.

The axons of the dorsal root ganglion cells enter the spinal cord grey matter at the dorsal horns. Most make synaptic connections with neurons located in the more dorsal regions of the grey matter. Some of the connections are with spinal cord neurons acting as relay cells, that is to say, cells whose axons project via the spinal cord white matter to the brain. Others will terminate on spinal interneurons—small neurons whose processes do not extend beyond the spinal cord. The axons of the spinal cord interneurons may terminate on motor neurons within the same segment of spinal cord, or they may terminate in other segments. In both cases, the influence of the spinal cord interneurons may be excitatory or inhibitory. Other sensory axons or axon branches project through the grey matter to terminate directly on motor neurons in the ventral horns at the same level of the grey matter.

Thus, some spinal cord motor neurons receive direct sensory input with no intervening interneurons. This direct connection in the spinal cord between sensory input and motor output is called a **monosynaptic reflex** (or monosynaptic reflex arc). Recall that a reflex response was featured in Book 1, Section 2.2 and Figure 2.1. Where a spinal cord motor neuron receives its synaptic input from interneurons, i.e. where interneurons are interposed between the sensory input and the motor neuron, the pathway is called a **polysynaptic reflex** (or polysynaptic reflex arc).

☐  Can you think of any features of synapses that will give monosynaptic and polysynaptic reflex arcs different characteristics?

■  The time required for an action potential to produce transmitter release at a synapse and to have an effect on the postsynaptic membrane is of the order of 1 ms. Thus, the responses of monosynaptic reflex arcs will be faster than those of polysynaptic reflex arcs. Importantly, with additional synaptic processing interposed between the sensory input and motor output, the polysynaptic pathway can be seen to be more open to influences other than the direct sensory input, and to be playing a more integrative role in the control of the muscles.

Axons from neurons in the motor systems of the brain project down the white matter of the spinal cord to terminate on interneurons and motor neurons in the spinal cord grey matter. This descending pathway acts through the motor neurons of the spinal cord to produce directed behaviour. In the following discussions, examples of the spinal cord reflex structure will first be described, followed by descriptions of the CNS structures that collectively act together with the reflex structure of the spinal cord to produce directed movement.

## 9.3.2  Muscles and muscle spindles

The previous section described some of the sensory neurons that convey information to the CNS. It considered the case where sensory neurons themselves serve as specialized receptors. One example of such a specialization is seen in the muscle spindle, which serves as a stretch receptor.

As its name suggests, the muscle spindle stretch receptor responds to changes in muscle stretch. Skeletal muscles consist of striated muscle tissue (Chapter 7), bounded in a membrane and connected to bone via tendons. Striated muscle, as well as the 'working' muscle fibres that generate the force that moves joints, contains specialized muscle cells called muscle spindles (see Figure 9.6). Like working muscle fibres, muscle spindle cells can contract. They can change their length independently of the working muscle cells but generate only a fraction of the force of working muscle. The working muscle cells receive their synaptic input from motor neurons in the ventral horns of the spinal cord. These motor neurons are called $\alpha$ *(alpha) motor neurons*. Muscle spindles receive independent motor input from a different class of ventral horn motor neurons called $\gamma$ *(gamma) motor neurons*. Action potentials in the $\gamma$ motor neuron cause the muscle spindle to contract and change its length independently of the working muscle. As you will see, this allows the muscle spindle to measure accurately the amount of stretch in the working muscle, regardless of the length of the working muscle.

Wrapped around the muscle spindle is the distal tip of an axon from a sensory neuron. The cell body of this sensory neuron is in a dorsal root ganglion of the spinal cord. When the tip of the sensory neuron is stretched, ion channels embedded in its membrane change shape. This modifies the flow of ions across the membrane and changes the rate at which it generates action potentials.

☐   What will cause the muscle spindle to change its length?

■   The amount of stretch in the membrane will be influenced by two factors. First, changes in the length of the working muscle as it contracts or is stretched will change the degree of stretch in the muscle spindle. Second, activity in the $\gamma$ motor input to the muscle spindle will also modify its length. Either factor will result in a change in the rate of action potential generation in the sensory axon attached to the muscle spindle.

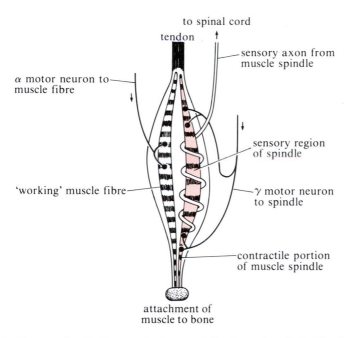

**Figure 9.6**   The muscle spindle receptor is a specialized muscle cell that lies in parallel with working muscle fibres. Wrapped around the centre section of the muscle spindle is the ending of the axon of a sensory neuron. As the working muscle fibre is stretched, the muscle spindle elongates, increasing the activity in the sensory neuron.

The muscle spindles are able to change their length relative to their host working muscle fibres through changes in the activity in the γ motor neurons that activate them. One function of this γ motor system is to fine-tune the muscle spindles so that they are kept at the length where they are at their most sensitive to small changes in the amount of stretch. Also, during the initiation of movements by descending activity from the brain, α and γ motor neurons are activated together.

### 9.3.3   The stretch reflex

Figure 9.7 shows an example of the most basic spinal cord reflex mechanism, the monosynaptic stretch reflex. The figure is a schematic representation of the pathway underlying the so-called knee-jerk reflex. If you have ever visited your GP for a check up, you may have had your knee-jerk reflex tested. A brisk tap on the tendon below the knee produces a reflex contraction of the thigh muscle with a corresponding jerk of the lower limb, mediated by the pathway shown in Figure 9.7. This stretch reflex starts with a sensory neuron whose axon is activated by stretch in the thigh muscle caused by the brisk tap (Figure 9.6).

☐   What will be the result of stretching the muscle?

■   The effect will be first to activate the stretch receptor(s). In turn this will activate the α motor neuron and thereby cause the muscle to contract, thus opposing the stretching.

Let us now look more closely at how this system works. Each stage in this loop is excitatory. First, muscle stretch produces activity in the stretch receptor. This activity is conveyed as action potentials in the sensory neuron. Activity, in turn, excites the α motor neuron which, in turn, excites the muscle.

The tap stretches a number of stretch receptors. This results in the generation of receptor potentials in the sensory neurons whose tips constitute the detectors of the stretch. In turn, this causes action potentials in the motor neurons associated with these sensory neurons and thereby muscular activity in the leg, which is revealed as a jerk.

However, the stretch reflex did not evolve as a diagnostic tool for the medical profession! The stretch reflex is a basic negative feedback mechanism (Book 1, Section 7.2.2). You will recollect that a negative feedback loop operates to maintain the state of a system, e.g. the thermostat negative feedback loop that maintains the temperature of a room close to a preset value. Similarly, the stretch reflex in the various limbs of the body acts to resist stretch to maintain the length of muscle when it is stretched by extraneous factors. This stretching can be the result of external forces such as gravity. To take another example, a sudden gust of wind will not normally blow you over. Any stretching or compression in the muscles caused by starting to fall over causes automatic compensatory action on the part of the muscles to restore the *status quo*. The overall effect of the activity of stretch reflexes is to maintain a body's posture, and so the stretch reflex is classed as a postural reflex.

Figure 9.8 illustrates stretch reflexes working in 'real life'. The poor horse's back does not buckle under the load of the rider even though the loading on the back muscles increases almost instantaneously. Stretch in the horse's back muscles activates their stretch reflexes which increases the muscle tension to oppose the loading imposed by the rider. The rider jumping onto the horse also loads the horse's limbs causing the joints to start to close. The horse remains standing and its limbs brace against the increase in load almost instantaneously.

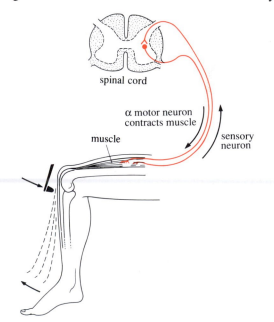

**Figure 9.7** The knee-jerk reflex—an example of a monosynaptic stretch reflex. The sensory neuron synapses with an α motor neuron located in the grey matter of the spinal cord. The axon from this α motor neuron lying in the ventral region of the grey matter makes synaptic contact with muscle cells in the same thigh muscle that signalled the stretch.

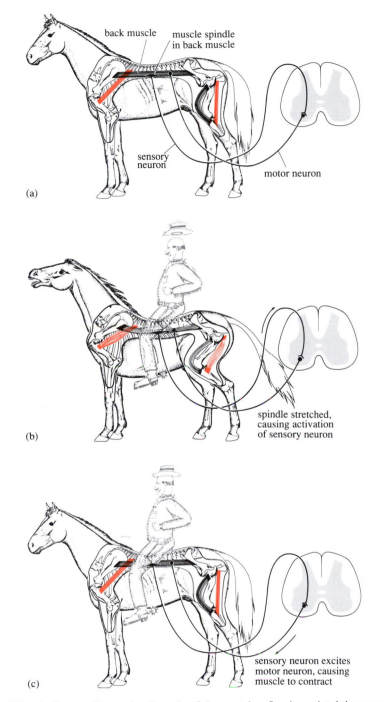

**Figure 9.8**    A diagram illustrating the role of the stretch reflex in maintaining muscle at constant length. (a) The horse stands still with the muscle length maintained. (b) An additional load lands on the horse's back and the muscles supporting the spine are stretched, along with other muscles keeping the horse erect against gravity. (c) Stretch reflexes in the various stretched muscles are activated, contracting the muscles to maintain the horse's posture.

Such responses to disturbances in the limbs that maintain posture are very fast, too fast for the brain to be involved in the control system directly. Here, the stretch reflex can be seen to play a major role in initiating the response of the limbs to change in external forces but it is part of a much more complex neuromuscular system of postural control.

Movement of joints such as the horse's knee and ankle joints involves changes in the lengths of sets of muscles that control the opening and closing of the joints. Each joint will have a set of muscles that act to open it, and another set that closes it; muscles that open the joint are called extensor muscles, and those that close the joint are called flexors. Flexors and extensors act in opposition to each other. Movement of joints is mediated by additional reflex mechanisms 'superimposed' on the stretch reflexes to ensure that the activation of the extensor muscles, and the flexor muscles, is coordinated.

☐ Why is it necessary to coordinate the extensor and flexor muscles that control the movement of a joint?

■ It is necessary to prevent the simultaneous activation of extensor and flexor muscles to avoid possible physical damage to muscles and tendons and for efficient limb movement.

☐ What feature of neuronal interactions could be exploited to prevent simultaneous activation of opposing muscles?

■ Inhibition of one muscle system by the opposing muscle system through inhibitory interneurons could prevent simultaneous activation.

The spinal cord reflex mechanism that prevents simultaneous activation of opposed sets of muscle is called **reciprocal antagonist inhibition**, and is shown schematically in Figure 9.9, using the example of the human elbow joint. This is a more accessible example than the horse's knee joint but the principles of operation of the reflexes are the same. Figure 9.9 shows a schematic arrangement of muscles in the upper arm which move the elbow joint. Here, the biceps and triceps muscles oppose one another. Contraction of the biceps muscles closes the joint while contraction of the triceps muscles opens it. Due to their opposite effects on the joint, the two muscles are said to have an antagonistic relationship.

☐ Imagine that a subject is asked to bend their elbow and hold the forearm out horizontally, as shown in Figure 9.9. Suddenly an unexpected weight is applied to the arm. How will the two opposed stretch reflexes respond to loading the forearm?

■ First, the biceps muscle will be stretched. Activity in its stretch reflex pathway will have the effect of increasing the activity of the biceps muscle to oppose the opening of the joint produced by the weight. Second, activation of the inhibitory connection from the biceps sensory fibre to the triceps α motor neuron will decrease the activity in the triceps motor neuron. This will stop the triceps stretch reflex from opposing any restorative movement produced by the biceps.

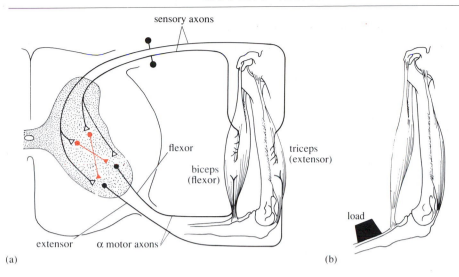

(a)

(b)

**Figure 9.9**   Reciprocal antagonist inhibition. (a) A schematic representation of inhibitory connections between the stretch reflex systems in two opposing muscles. In both muscles, the sensory neurons make synaptic connections both with their α motor neuron and with an inhibitory interneuron that inhibits the α motor neuron of the antagonist muscle. (b) This shows the forearm being loaded. The weight increase starts the joint opening, which stretches the biceps (flexor) muscle and releases the tension on the antagonist triceps (extensor) muscle.

To return to the example of the horse, a similar reciprocal inhibitory relationship exists between the sets of antagonist muscles that control the position of the leg (and other) joints. This helps explain how the horse almost instantaneously maintains its posture when loading on its limbs changes, e.g. when a rider mounts.

Reciprocal antagonist inhibition provides a general illustration of how spinal cord mechanisms provide control over body posture that is mediated locally in the spinal cord and which does not depend upon the motor systems of the brain for its action.

☐   What measurements would show that the control systems contributing to postural control act locally at the level of the spinal cord, and are not under direct control of motor systems involving the brain?

■   Measurements of the latency of onset of the muscular responses to a change in the external forces should (and do) show that they occur too quickly for them to be mediated by the brain.

☐   What factors are important in calculating how long it would take for the brain to contribute to postural adjustments?

■   First, the distance between an affected muscle group and the spinal cord, and the speed of conduction of action potentials in the sensory nerve will allow calculation of the time the sensory information will take to reach the spinal cord. Second, calculations can be made for the time sensory information takes to reach motor structures in the brain and to return down the spinal cord and to the muscles. Third, the number of synapses involved will limit the speed of response.

In contrast to the relative simplicity of the connections described so far, brain sensory and motor systems involve many interconnections, as you will read later in this chapter. Central processing of information through the activity of complex brain pathways involving many synaptic junctions takes relatively long periods of time. Experiments on human reaction times show that voluntary responses take about 100 ms to start. By contrast, reflexes that involve single synapses in the spinal cord start in a fraction of this time. However, both in structure and function, spinal cord reflexes can be more complex than the stretch reflex and reciprocal antagonist inhibition just described.

The stretch reflex is an example of a monosynaptic reflex (described earlier); that is, there is only one synapse in its central path within the spinal cord. Within the spinal cord, there are numerous examples of reflexes which have more than one synapse in their pathway and whose basic functions are to maintain body posture. Here, sensory input (from dorsal root ganglion cells) synapses on interneurons in the dorsal region of the grey matter, and the motor neurons then receive their input from the network of interneurons within the spinal cord. The next section gives an example of integration of reflexes across a wider region of the spinal cord.

## 9.3.4 Spinal control: supra segmental organization

The stretch reflex is a local reflex that acts to maintain the state of specific individual muscles. In reciprocal antagonist inhibition, the underlying neural connections were shown located within a single segment of the spinal cord. The reflex organization of the spinal cord is not, however, restricted to single segments.

Protective reflexes are very complex, involving the coordination of functionally related muscle groups whose motor outflow derives from several segments of the spinal cord. You must have had experience of stepping on a sharp object with your bare foot, as represented in Figure 9.10. Leg withdrawal in response to noxious stimulation of the foot is the result of coordinated reflex activity of many muscle groups in the affected and opposite leg. Sensory input to one segment can produce activity in motor neurons from other segments through ascending and descending branches of the sensory axon and/or activation of ascending and descending interneurons. Figure 9.10 shows a simplified representation of the situation where the sensory axon sends out ascending and descending branches. The spread of activity then activates patterns of reflexes based on reciprocal antagonist inhibition and other processes to produce organized protective behaviour. Frequently, such noxious stimulation results in abrupt involuntary withdrawal of the entire leg, accompanied by compensatory activity in the other leg and in other parts of the body—activity that has started even before you experience any pain.

The organization imposed by networks of interneurons from several segments within the spinal cord goes beyond the production of protective reflexes. As a dramatic example of the extent of the organization mediated by the networks of reflexes in the vertebrate spinal cord, the stories of headless chickens running around farmyards after they have been decapitated *en route* to the pot are more than apocryphal. After a chicken's head is removed in this way, its legs display running movements. Also, for a short period, the headless torso can 'run' around, albeit in a non-directed way. The CNS structures that remain after decapitation, i.e. the spinal cord, clearly must have the capacity to control the muscles of the limbs to produce coordinated movements.

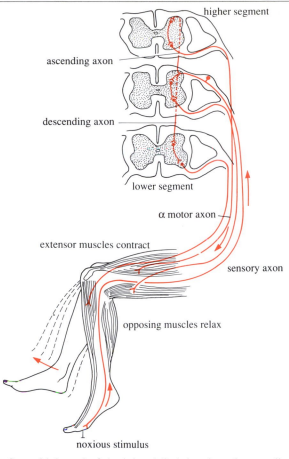

**Figure 9.10**   Reflex withdrawal of the injured limb involves the coordinated activity of muscles, controlled in several segments of the spinal cord. The sensory axons to the central segment synapse on interneurons in the ventral horns of the spinal cord, but also send out ascending and descending branches, activating α motor neurons in higher and lower segments. Note that single representative ascending and descending interneurons are shown.

In four-legged animals, the activities of the four limbs are linked through a network of interneurons extending across many spinal segments. Evidence for the extent of mammalian spinal cord organization is provided by early experiments in cats in which ascending and descending pathways between the brain and spinal cord were cut. When the cats were supported with their feet in contact with a moving surface (a moving belt) the limbs, after being initially dragged by contact with the belt, took up a typical but rudimentary walking pattern. As the moving belt is speeded up, the limbs switch from the walking pattern, in which diagonally opposed limbs move together, to the running pattern, where fore- and hindlimbs move together. Here, recordings of the activity of the motor nerves driving the individual limbs showed that bursts of neural activity were produced corresponding to the activity of the limbs.

This experiment shows the extent of the functional organization of the mammalian spinal cord. The limb movements induced by the initial movement of the belt activate the reflex networks in the spinal cord. The basic spinal cord reflex structures, acting within single segments, are linked through suprasegmental networks of interneurons. These networks are brought into play when they are given sensory information from the soles of the feet and from movement in muscles and joints. The reflex organization of the spinal cord then acts to superimpose 'order' on the movements to coordinate the activity in the four limbs. The locomotory movements that are produced are rudimentary and lack the force and directedness of normal locomotion but display the form of normal walking and running movements.

## Summary of Section 9.3

The α motor neurons receive direct and indirect sensory input from receptors in muscles and from nociceptors, respectively. The discussions in the previous sections have emphasized the automatic activity of the spinal cord, the control over the muscles that is imposed by the reflex organization of the cord. At the simplest level, monosynaptic reflexes act to maintain the length of muscles. Examples of polysynaptic reflexes were then described which coordinated the activity of opposed sets of muscles that flex or extend a joint.

In addition to motor neurons (the α and γ motor neurons) and sensory neurons (the neurons that relay sensory information to the brain), the spinal cord contains a large population of interneurons. These make synaptic connections with α and γ motor neurons and interneurons in the same segment of the spinal cord and also in other segments higher and lower in the spinal cord. Spinal interneurons receive their inputs from sensory axons entering at the spinal cord dorsal roots and from pathways descending from the brain, as well as from other spinal interneurons.

Evidence from animals in which the descending influences from the brain have been removed indicate that the reflex organization of the spinal cord contains sufficient neural 'machinery' to organize and coordinate the contraction of the muscles to produce running and walking movements.

The 'picture' of the spinal cord painted by the discussions in this chapter is of a network of interacting reflexes, organized to sequence limb movement, that is placed between two sources of input. These are sensory input from the limbs and body, and the stream of descending 'motor' commands from the brain. On the one hand, spinal cord mechanisms act to maintain the dispositions of the body and limbs at rest and also in response to unpredictable changes, such as a loss or change of footing during movements which could compromise any on-going movement. On the other, the descending influences from the brain motor system structures act mainly upon spinal cord interneurons to produce directed movement.

# 9.4   Central motor systems

Section 9.3 looked at the maintenance of the *stability* of the body. For example, a horse is standing still and then a disturbance occurs that threatens that stability. Automatic action is taken to counter the disturbance. However, as you might well be thinking, life involves somewhat more than just maintaining stability and protecting the body against noxious stimulation. It is also about *initiating directed action*. In humans, this is often described as voluntary action. Whereas the spinal cord has considerable autonomy to effect postural and protective reflexes, it is commands from the brain that initiate directed action. How is such action effected? This is the question addressed in this section.

Although protective reflexes are organized at a spinal level and voluntary movement involves commands from the brain, the muscles that effect action are the same in both cases, as are the motor neurons that activate these muscles. Thus a given motor neuron can be activated either by local sensory neurons in its own segment of spinal cord (e.g. in maintaining stability or as part of a protective reflex) or by descending influences from the brain (e.g. as part of voluntarily initiated behaviour).

The details of the way that voluntary motor control is superimposed upon reflex action are very complex and it is sufficient to note that it involves a very sophisticated control system. As you saw in Section 9.3, an externally applied disturbance to a muscle evokes compensatory action (e.g. the knee-jerk reflex). Initiation of a voluntary movement also involves a change in the length of working muscle. However, what clearly does not happen is that the stretch reflex triggers compensatory responses to voluntary actions. In the production of movement, both $\alpha$ and $\gamma$ motor neurons are active. One function of the $\gamma$ activity is to control the stretch reflexes so that they are used to facilitate movement rather than to oppose it.

This section will identify the major brain systems that act upon the spinal cord mechanisms in the initiation of directed movements.

## 9.4.1   Brain stem pathways

Figure 9.1 shows a schematic representation of the pathways that descend from the brain to the spinal cord. These influences on the spinal cord are highly complex. In the discussions that follow, the specializations of different components will be teased out. In the final analysis, however, you should recognize that, even though different structures contribute to different aspects of behaviour, the motor system acts as a coordinated whole.

In terms of their evolutionary history, the pathways from the brain stem are the 'oldest' motor pathways and are found in all living vertebrate species. The brain stem pathways have their origins in four groups of nuclei: the reticular formation, the vestibular nuclei, the tectum and the red nuclei, as shown in Figure 9.11 (*overleaf*).

The reticular formation is a system that has been associated with a variety of functions, and it plays a role in maintaining or changing the general level of arousal of the CNS. The arousing function is more typical of the superior regions of the reticular formation which make extensive connections within the cortex and generally throughout the forebrain. The caudal regions of the reticular formation in the lower brain stem make synaptic connections within the spinal cord and have been implicated in the organization and control of behaviour patterns, which will be discussed in more detail in the next chapter.

The tectum is a region in the upper brain stem which in mammals includes the superior and inferior colliculi (Section 8.4.4). These play a role in the analysis of visual and auditory information and in the location of sources of visual and auditory information relative to the eyes and ears.

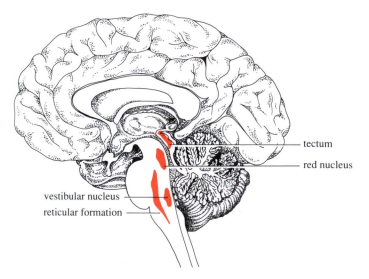

tectum

red nucleus

vestibular nucleus

reticular formation

**Figure 9.11**   The four groups of nuclei from which the descending brain stem pathways originate.

The vestibular nuclei play a role in the processing of information from the vestibular apparatus in the ear, which is important for the sense of balance.

Finally, the red nucleus provides motor output for systems including the cerebellum. These systems receive information ascending in the spinal cord about the movement of joints and about the length of muscles. The cerebellum has a very regular, ordered structure, which is important for the sequencing of movement. Damage to the cerebellum results in a disturbance to the coordination of movements. The brain stem influences on the spinal cord thus originate from brain systems concerned with the location of objects in space (tectum), with the balance of the body (vestibular), and with the level of arousal (reticular formation), as well as with information about the state of the limbs and muscles (red nucleus).

The four sources of brain stem influence onto the spinal cord take different routes to the spinal cord, where they synapse with two distinct groups of α motor neurons. The pathway from the red nucleus influences α motor neurons that control the distal muscles, i.e. the limb muscles. The other three pathways influence the axial muscles, i.e. the trunk and neck muscles. Further details of the descending brain stem pathways are beyond the scope of this course.

In some vertebrates the brain stem pathways are the major source of motor control. In others, evolutionary changes in the motor regions in the cerebral cortex are associated with changes in motor capabilities, particularly in bipeds where voluntary control over the forelimbs becomes more specialized. The next section looks at the pathways originating in the cortex.

## 9.4.2   Pyramidal tract pathways

From Chapter 8 in this book and the videocassette *The Human Brain* you will recall that stimulation of a motor region of the cortex called the pre-central gyrus results in muscular contraction in discrete regions of the body.

☐ What is the 'representation' of the muscles in the motor cortex (pre-central gyrus) called?

■ The motor homunculus, which indicates the different regions and volumes of cortical tissue devoted to control of the muscles in the motor cortex (see Figure 9.12).

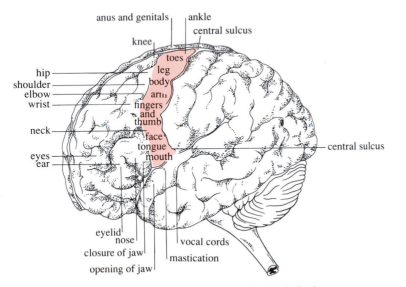

**Figure 9.12**  The representation of the regions of the body in the motor cortex.

Having identified the motor homunculus, the next question is: What are the normal influences upon the muscles that are reflected in the motor homunculus?

The starting point for an answer to this question comes from the neuroanatomical connections of the motor cortex. Figure 9.1 shows that the motor cortex and associated pre-motor cortical areas make connections with brain stem structures (discussed in previous sections). Activity in the motor regions of the cortex then influences the way that brain stem structures control the spinal cord. Importantly, though, there is also a pathway running directly from the motor cortex down the spinal cord. This is the pyramidal tract (Section 8.8.5). Axons from the motor cortex on each side of the brain meet at the level of the medulla in the brain stem and cross over the midline to continue on down to make connections within the spinal cord.

☐ What is the effect of the crossing over of pyramidal axons?

■ The result is that each of the motor cortices controls muscles on the contralateral (opposite) side of the body.

Axons in the pyramidal tract pathways mainly synapse upon interneurons and, in regions of the spinal cord concerned with control over the distal muscles, particularly the hands, directly upon α motor neurons. Here, the pyramidal tract pathway is complementary to the pathway from the brain stem, which controls the muscles of the limbs rather than the fingers. In humans, a sizable proportion of the population of the cortical cells that contribute to the pyramidal tract are very large and terminate directly on α motor neurons in the spinal cord rather than onto interneurons. These cortical cells are called Betz cells after their discoverer, and are found in regions of the motor cortex that control the muscles of the arms, hands and fingers. Betz cells also occur in other primates and in racoons, but the difference between the human cortex and other primates in Betz cell populations is thought to contribute to the greater human ability to control the use of the fingers independently of each other and, therefore, to human manual dexterity.

☐  What is the advantage of direct termination onto α motor neurons in the spinal cord?

■  This gives the Betz cells faster communication to the muscles of the hands. If the pathway included interneurons interposed between the descending spinal afferents and the α motor neurons, additional synaptic delay would be imposed.

In the evolution of the mammals, the brain stem pathways to the spinal cord evolved first and then persisted with relatively little change across the range of mammalian species living today. In contrast, the pyramidal tract is an evolutionarily newer feature which shows great variation. In some mammals, such as the hedgehog, the pyramidal tract is relatively undifferentiated. During the evolution of the primates, the relative numbers of connections from the pyramidal tract directly onto α motor neurons increased progressively. In modern species of primates, bush-babies (*Tarsius*) have some Betz cells, monkeys have more, and the apes have the greatest numbers. Humans have the highest proportion of Betz cells of all primates (see Figure 9.13). This development parallels the development of both the cerebral cortex and manual dexterity.

### 9.4.3  Central organization

The cortical motor regions influence the muscles, through direct connections with the spinal cord interneurons and α motor neurons and by influencing the brain stem motor structures. Consider again the previous example of the voluntary behaviour of picking up a coffee cup.

☐  What components of the action necessary to pick up a coffee cup might be controlled via those pyramidal tract neurons that synapse directly onto α motor neurons?

■  Those actions that need to be controlled quickly and which require manual dexterity, such as grasping the cup.

Figure 9.1 indicates that two other major structures, the basal ganglia and the cerebellum, are also implicated in the control of behaviour; it is to these structures that the discussion now turns.

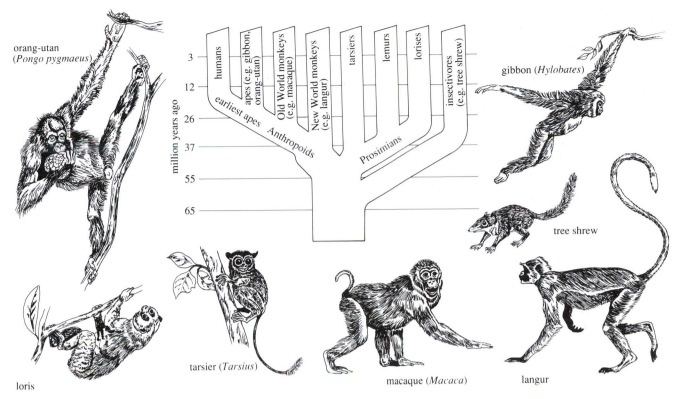

**Figure 9.13**   The evolutionary relationships of the primates.

## The cerebellum

The importance of the cerebellum (Section 8.8.8) is indicated by the fact that it contains more neurons than the cerebral cortex. It has several distinct nuclei, but the details of its structure are beyond the scope of this discussion, which concentrates on the general contribution this structure makes to the control over movement.

The cerebellum (Figure 9.14, *overleaf*) receives input from sensory pathways, transmitted via the spinal cord, giving it information about the state of muscles, joints and stretch receptors. It also receives input from sensory regions of the cerebral cortex and information about balance from the vestibular system in the ear. A conspicuous feature of the cerebellum is its highly regular and repetitive neuronal structure (Section 8.8.8) which appears to be suited to the generation or representation of temporal patterns of neuronal activity and, by implication, to the sequencing of muscular contractions.

As Figure 9.1 indicates, output from the cerebellum goes to the motor cortex and to the brain stem. In the brain stem, the cerebellum's major output structure is the red nucleus, which is one of four brain stem nuclei that make direct synaptic connections with the spinal cord (Figure 9.11). Damage to the cerebellum can result in poor coordination and lack of precision in movement. A patient with damage to the right lobe of the cerebellum reported 'The movements of my left arm are done subconsciously, but I have to think out each movement of the right arm.' The cerebellum, unlike the motor cortex, influences the muscles on the ipsilateral (same) side of the body.

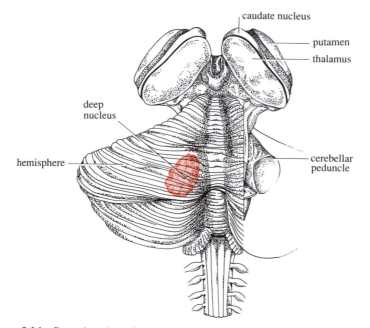

**Figure 9.14**    Posterior view of the cerebellum and thalamus in the human brain.

Sir John Eccles, who spent much of his research career studying the cerebellum, suggests that cortical centres give general commands to carry out movement, leaving the computation and execution to subcortical, notably cerebellar, mechanisms. One aspect of behaviour to which the cerebellum makes a contribution is in the production of *ballistic* responses. Ballistic responses are learned sequences of behaviour that are carried out too fast for the brain to use any sensory feedback from the muscles to sequence and structure the behaviour. That is, a ballistic response is 'programmed' as a temporal sequence of muscular movements. Examples of ballistic sequences are the spectacularly high-speed passages beloved by concert pianists and the so-called 'instinctively' accurate responses of champion tennis players and cricketers that are acquired with much practice.

Of course, the cerebellum did not evolve in the context of piano playing, or even cricket or tennis. The ability to produce ballistic sequences of muscle control is important in sustaining movement without involving the CNS in excessive levels of computation, which would be necessary if the sensory consequences of every muscle movement had to be processed before the next was initiated. In this context, the cerebellum has been implicated in motor learning: that is, in learning sequences of muscle movement so that the activity becomes 'automatic'.

## The basal ganglia

The basal ganglia are a collection of four structures: the caudate nucleus, putamen, globus pallidus and the substantia nigra (see Figure 9.15). The caudate nucleus and putamen are often collectively described as the striatum. Like the other motor system structures described above, the basal ganglia are bilaterally symmetrical and are located close to another large structure that is composed of several subdivisions, the thalamus. The anatomical locations of the basal ganglia and thalamus are shown in Figure 9.15.

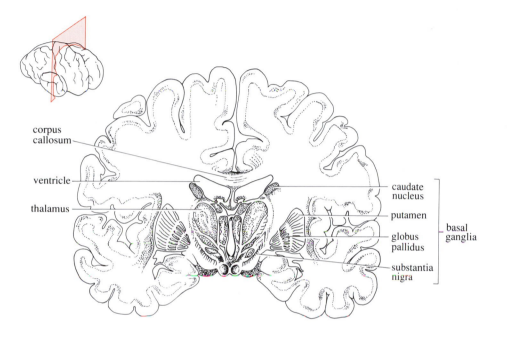

**Figure 9.15**   A coronal section through the human brain. The tail of the caudate nucleus can be seen adjacent to the lateral ventricle, and the putamen and globus pallidus lying laterally from the body of the thalamus.

The interesting feature of the basal ganglia are their interconnections with other parts of the brain. These are extensive and point to the basal ganglia having a unique integrative role. Figure 9.16a (*overleaf*) illustrates the anatomical connections of the basal ganglia. It shows a loop involving structures in the thalamus, motor and somatosensory cortex and wide regions of surrounding cortex, and a midbrain structure called the substantia nigra (literally meaning 'black substance'). The basal ganglia receive inputs from regions of the cortex that carry out detailed processing of somatosensory and visual information (discussed in Chapter 4 of Book 3).

Figure 9.16b (*overleaf*) shows the anatomical connections made by the cerebellum. Compared with the basal ganglia, the cerebellum receives a more restricted input from the regions around and including the motor and somatosensory cortex. Importantly, unlike the cerebellum, the basal ganglia do not have access to the motor systems of the brain stem.

245

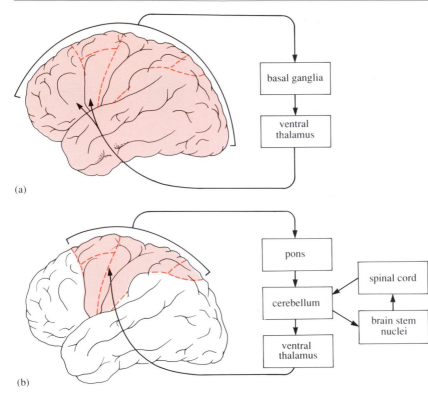

(a)

(b)

**Figure 9.16** (a) The basal ganglia receive input from a very wide region of the cerebral cortex extending beyond the motor cortex and somatosensory cortex. (b) The cerebellum receives input indirectly from a more restricted region of the cerebral cortex and participates widely in evolutionarily 'old' sub-cortical systems.

☐ How do the patterns of connectivity of the basal ganglia and cerebellum differ?

■ The basal ganglia are implicated more in cortical systems and less with the evolutionarily older brain stem structures.

At first sight, the implications of the differences in connectivity of the basal ganglia and cerebellum suggest that the functions of the basal ganglia are likely to relate to the functions of forebrain and cortical systems in *planning* behaviour. Clues to the basal ganglia's role here are given from people suffering from the condition called Parkinson's disease. In Parkinson's patients, cells in the substantia nigra die off. These cells, which synthesize a transmitter substance called dopamine, make extensive synaptic contact within the caudate and putamen (the striatum). This pathway is called the nigro-striatal pathway. Parkinson's disease has a number of symptoms. First, there is a basic tremor of the limb muscles, particularly the hands, when the patient is at rest and not concentrating on carrying out some activity with the hands. Secondly, there is increased muscle tone and rigidity. Thirdly, there is a slowness both in the initiation and execution of movements.

Disturbances of control over the distal muscles is characteristic of damage to the basal ganglia in humans. Depending on the extent of the damage to the basal ganglia, patients exhibit rhythmic involuntary movements such as writhing movements of the limbs and hands, and sometimes uncontrollable flailing movements.

Broadly, the symptoms of Parkinson's disease fall into two categories: (1) those that influence basic muscular coordination, and (2) those that influence a 'higher' function in the planning and initiation of movements. The first category includes the tremor and increased muscle tone and rigidity. The second is inferred from the Parkinson patient's slowness to act and inability to carry out particular tasks.

The comedian Terry Thomas was forced to give up his career after developing Parkinson's disease in his later life. Before his death, he spoke very eloquently and movingly about the difficulties it brought and the solutions he had to adopt to carry out what were previously trivial tasks. At one point in his illness, Thomas found that he could no longer move about normally and found it particularly difficult to negotiate doorways. Thomas said that the appropriate walking movements 'just would not come'. Instead, he found that he had to move in a different rhythmic way, such as by waltzing, to get through the doorway. An intuitively plausible explanation is that Thomas was substituting another well-learned pattern of behaviour for the central plan for walking which had become unavailable.

## Summary of Section 9.4

The final common pathway of the motor system is made up of the α motor neurons of the spinal cord. These are the final route to the muscles.

The spinal cord is a structure that 'sits' between the motor systems of the brain and the muscles. Activity from the brain's motor system descends via the pyramidal tract and brain stem pathways to 'drive' the organization of the spinal cord to produce movement. The organization of the spinal cord, which has the capability to sequence the activity of antagonistic muscle sets, sequence limb movements and to maintain body posture, is exploited by the central motor systems.

For rhythmic behaviour patterns, such as running and walking, the central motor systems do not control each muscle precisely. These 'details' are handled by the organization of reflex networks in the spinal cord, leaving the central systems to modulate the activity of the spinal cord networks to produce movement. The spinal cord organization also acts as a 'front line' defence against potentially damaging events. Sensory information about sudden muscle stretch or noxious stimulation can trigger protective reflexes that interrupt on-going activity to maintain posture or prevent damage almost instantaneously, leaving the central systems to respond over a longer time period.

In the control over voluntary non-rhythmic behaviours, such as the example of lifting a coffee cup to take a drink, the cortically-connected structures of the motor system are more involved in the direct control of muscles, such as control of the fingers.

The two central motor structures, the cerebellum and the basal ganglia, play different roles in the organization of behaviour. The cerebellum acts within its cortical loop organization and has access to information about the muscles and joints from ascending spinal cord pathways and from vestibular, visual and auditory systems. It is involved in programming behaviour by generating the sequencing or patterning of muscle contractions and in their integration within the general control of the disposition of the body. Damage to the cerebellum can result in loss of coordination, with individual movements losing their 'flow' as the movements have to be constructed laboriously by other motor system structures.

Evidence from disorders such as Parkinson's disease suggest that, in contrast to the cerebellum, the basal ganglia play a 'higher', more executive role in the control of behaviour. One symptom of Parkinson's disease is that the victim has difficulty in *initiating* behaviour, as if the plans for the action become inaccessible. Here, the absence of any *direct* connection to either the motor cortex or the brain stem motor systems, and the presence of connections from the cortical areas involved in sensory processing and with the pre-motor cortical areas (Figure 9.16) suggest such an executive role.

This scheme, in which the basal ganglia are given an 'executive' role in the control of directed behaviour, is both highly speculative and a gross oversimplification. Nevertheless, it does provide a convenient starting point for an understanding of how individual structures in a complex and interconnected system contribute to the control of the final common pathway—the motor neurons. One virtue of such speculation is that it does help to pull together the information presented in previous sections and provide a context for understanding how different regions of the CNS contribute differently to ordinary behaviour.

The facility and smoothness with which you carry out operations such as reaching out for a coffee cup to take a drink indicates that they are executed as a well-learned overall plan. From the previous descriptions and discussions of unique features of central motor system structures some inferences about the involvements of particular structures seem reasonable.

For example:

☐ Given the connections of the pyramidal pathway, what involvement will it have in the task of retrieving a coffee cup?

■ The pyramidal tract is involved in the fine control of the hand and fingers, so it is reasonable to suppose that it is more crucially involved when the cup is being grasped and less heavily involved during the reaching movements.

☐ How might the cerebellum be involved in the task of lifting the coffee cup?

■ The cerebellum has been implicated in the organization of ballistic sequences of movements, and it is a reasonable proposition that it will be heavily involved in programming the sequence of arm movements required to get the hand smoothly to the cup and back to the mouth, and also in programming the sequence of finger movements to grasp the cup. Here, the cerebellum will be involved in organizing the activity in both the pyramidal and brain stem pathways through its anatomical connections with these systems.

☐ What role might the motor systems involving the basal ganglia play in the task of retrieving the coffee cup?

■ It is a reasonable assumption that the basal ganglia play a key role in planning the activity by bringing together information from the vision and touch systems with previously stored experience of cups, such as their expected weight. It would then pass the general specifications of the movement to the cerebellum, leaving it to organize the detail of the necessary muscle movements.

# 9.5   Sensory systems of the brain

The previous section described some of the motor systems that evolved and became 'refined' during the evolution of the mammalian brain. However, the mammalian motor systems did not evolve in isolation. Fine control over the muscles requires appropriately sensitive sensory information about the state of muscles and joints. In parallel with the evolution of more flexible motor control, particularly over the limb muscles, was an evolution of sensory systems that better supported the motor capabilities. The massive expansion of the cerebral hemispheres that marks the mammalian line of vertebrate evolution was accompanied by an increasing emphasis on cortical structures in the processing of sensory information.

An objective of this section is to introduce sensory information processing through a discussion of the system that codes and represents touch stimulation to the skin. The section will follow the flow of information along the spinal cord, then through the brain to the somatosensory cortex. It will look at the way that the pathways represent the body surface and process information about touch. This discussion will use the central representation of touch to introduce general principles of sensory information processing and the representation of stimuli in the brain. In this way the present chapter sets the scene for Book 3, which will describe the neuroanatomy, neurophysiology and perceptual phenomena of vision and pain.

## 9.5.1   Spinal cord structures

Generally, information from sensory receptors in the body is transmitted via sensory neurons whose cell bodies are located in the dorsal roots of the spinal cord (see Figure 9.17).

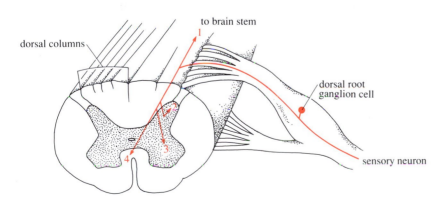

**Figure 9.17**   The sensory neurons from the skin enter the spinal cord via the dorsal roots and ascend in the dorsal columns (well-defined pathways in the white matter of the spinal cord) to the brain stem or higher segments (1). Branches of the sensory neurons may also activate local spinal reflexes (termination on dorsal horn interneuron (2), termination on ventral horn (motor) interneuron or $\alpha$ motor neuron (3)), or descend to the lower spinal cord segments (4).

You will recall that sensory inflow from the body is organized into dermatomes, whereby sensory information entering through the dorsal roots of a particular vertebra originates from a local well-defined region of the body (see Figure 9.4).

Axons of dorsal root neurons enter the spinal cord and then branch, with each branch following one of three routes.

1 It synapses with interneurons or α motor neurons locally within the spinal cord.

2 It ascends within the white matter of the spinal cord to project to the brain.

3 It ascends or descends within the white matter of the spinal cord to synapse on interneurons and/or α motor neurons in higher or lower segments.

You have already learned about the direct effects of sensory information on behaviour. Section 9.3.3 described the stretch reflex and illustrated how it functioned to withdraw the limb automatically in response to a sharp tap to the knee. Here, sensory receptors (the muscle spindle receptors in the muscles) feed their information via their sensory neurons to the spinal cord, where they act through reflex pathways within the grey matter.

However, information that allows the brain to organize responses over the longer term also ascends within the spinal cord. Axons of the dorsal root neurons project via well-defined pathways within the white matter of the spinal cord to the brain. These pathways are collectively known as the *dorsal columns*. Essentially, dorsal column pathways convey information to the brain about touch, joint position, the degree of stretch in muscles signalled by muscle spindle receptors—information that the brain needs to have to formulate its instructions to 'work' the body in an integrated way.

As this chapter concentrates on how the brain 'represents' sensory information, the details of the different ascending pathways and the nature of the information they contain are not important. Chapter 5 of Book 3, which deals with touch and pain, will fill out details of spinal cord organization. Figure 9.18 is a schematic representation of the passage of sensory information about touch on the skin ascending via the dorsal columns. Axons ascending from the spinal cord first synapse at the level of the medulla in structures called the dorsal column nuclei (DCN). Axons from the neurons in the DCN cross the midline at the level of the medulla and then continue, synapsing in a part of the ventrobasal nucleus in the thalamus called the ventro-posterior lateral (VPL) nucleus. Axons from cell bodies in the ventrobasal nucleus then terminate in the somatosensory cortex.

## 9.5.2  Topographic organization within the spinal cord and brain

Figure 9.4 shows the arrangement of dermatomes, by which each dorsal root ganglion receives sensory input from a localized area of the body. It also shows how, in effect, the spinal cord itself constructs a 'map' of the body. Sensory information from lower regions of the body is represented in lower segments of the spinal cord, upper regions in the higher segments and the trunk in the middle regions. In this way, the grey matter within each segment of the spinal cord is concerned with processing information from a specific region of the body, with the

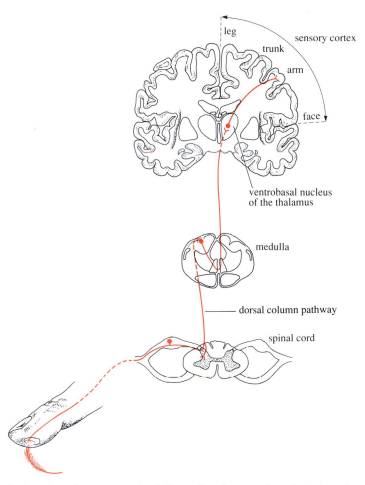

**Figure 9.18**   The pathway conveying information about touch on the skin to the cortex.

entire body represented sequentially in adjacent 'snapshots' along the length of the spinal cord. You have already met this type of organization, topographic representation, in Chapter 8.

Looking at the finer detail of the topographic map of the body surface within the spinal cord, what is to be seen? Electrical recordings from the sensory neurons in a dorsal root ganglion indicate that individual neurons respond only to stimulation of one small patch of skin within a relatively small area of that root's dermatome. For any such sensory neuron, the small region of skin from which it can be influenced is called its **receptive field**. Significantly, adjacent sensory neurons have adjacent, and often overlapping, receptive fields.

☐   In terms of the activity of the sensory neuron, what will be the evidence for a receptive field?

■   The only time that the rate of discharge of action potentials rises above the spontaneous rate of discharge will be when a very localized region of skin is being touched or stroked. This region of skin is the receptive field for that individual sensory cell.

☐ From your understanding of sensory neurons, how is the receptive field likely to be 'constructed' (Section 2.4.1)?

■ Sensory neurons are activated in one of two ways—either through specialized cells called sensory receptors, or by specializations of the sensory neuron's own distal membrane that allow the sensory neuron to be excited when the membrane is stretched or deformed. The local region of skin where all the receptors that synapse with one particular sensory neuron, or where all the neuronal endings of a particular sensory neuron are located, constitutes the receptive field of that neuron.

Figure 9.19 shows two types of the second kind of sensory neuron. The neuron on the right has the peripheral end of its axon wound around the base of a hair. When the hair is moved, the membrane of the axon is deformed, producing action potentials. In non-hairy skin, such as the fingers, the tips of the axon branches themselves are the receptors. Here, deformation of the skin deforms the axonal membrane and produces action potentials in the sensory axon. Such a sensory neuron is shown on the left of Figure 9.19.

The receptive field of a single dorsal root ganglion cell will be defined by the branching pattern of its axon. Stimulation within the area of skin containing the branches of a single dorsal root ganglion cell will result in activity in that neuron. Obviously, stimulation outside that region will not have any effect on that particular dorsal root ganglion cell but will activate other dorsal root ganglion cells whose receptors *are* stimulated. The number of branches the peripheral axon of a sensory neuron makes depends on the region of skin it innervates. This variation in branching plays a crucial role in the differences from one region of skin to another in the ability to discriminate fine detail.

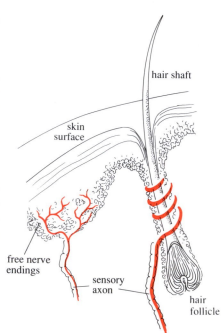

**Figure 9.19** A sensory neuron ending in association with a hair follicle responds to movement of the hair (right). The endings of a sensory neuron interposed with skin cells form touch receptors (left).

☐ Think for a moment about your own experience of differences in your ability to discriminate objects by touch. In which regions of skin would you expect to find marked differences in the degree of branching of sensory peripheral axons?

■ The finger tips and the back stand in sharp contrast. The finger tips are very touch-sensitive and can make fine discriminations. For example, if you touch two sharp points simultaneously onto your finger tips, you can discriminate between two points that are only a few millimetres apart. If the tips are closer, you can only feel a single point even though two are present. If you do the same experiment on the skin of the back, the points have to be separated by a centimetre or more before you can reliably say that there are two points.

☐ What differences in the branching of peripheral axons might you expect to occur in the finger tips and in the skin on the back?

■ Axons branch less in the finger tips.

In the finger tips, there is a high density of neuron endings but little divergence (as in Figure 9.20a), so that each peripheral axon is connected to only a very small area of skin. Here, activity in a peripheral axon signals touch in a very localized region. In the skin on the back, there is a lower density of receptors, so they are spread out more with a high degree of divergence (as in Figure 9.20b). Receptors over a relatively wide area form part of each peripheral axon.

One result of having receptors in a wide area of skin associated with a single peripheral axon is that the neuron will give the same response to stimulation anywhere in its receptive field. Thus it will give only 'coarse-grained' information to regions of the CNS to which it is connected. In Figure 9.20a, tactile stimulation at point 1 is detected by neuron A but not B. Stimulation at point 2 is detected by neuron B but not A. Thus the pattern of activity in A and B can discriminate between locations 1 and 2. In Figure 9.20b, two sensory neurons with larger and overlapping receptive fields are shown. Stimulation at either points 1 or 2 will excite activity in both A and B. Therefore A and B are unable to discriminate between stimulation at these two locations.

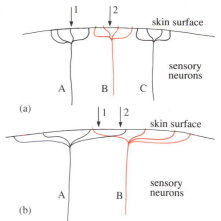

□ Which of the two systems, those shown in Figure 9.20a or b, would be described as providing fine-grained and which coarse-grained information?

■ The system in Figure 9.20a provides relatively fine-grained and that in Figure 9.20b relatively coarse-grained information.

□ Consider the information signalled by a single peripheral axon of a sensory dorsal root ganglion cell. What can be deduced about the way that the region of skin forming a particular dermatome is represented in the spinal cord?

■ Essentially, sensory information about events occurring on the skin within a dermatome is conveyed as a series of independent 'snapshots'. That is to say, each dorsal root ganglion cell will convey information about activity within its receptive field, its own little patch of skin.

**Figure 9.20**   Diagram showing endings of sensory neurons and how they provide receptive field properties. (a) Three non-overlapping receptive fields provided by three sensory neurons, A, B and C. Simultaneous stimulation at points 1 and 2 can be discriminated. (b) Two overlapping receptive fields provided by two neurons, A and B. Simultaneous stimulation at points 1 and 2 cannot be discriminated.

Figure 9.21 (*overleaf*) shows the difference in size of receptive fields located in the fingers, palm and wrist of a monkey.

□ On the basis of the receptive fields shown in Figure 9.21, which regions will be the best at tactile discrimination?

■ The fingers, because two closely separated points are more likely to produce activity in adjacent non-overlapping receptive fields. On the arm, two points at the same separation would tend to lie within a single receptive field.

Collectively, the population of receptive fields of dorsal root ganglion cells within a segment of the spinal cord represents the entire dermatome, with any particular small region of skin represented many times in receptive fields that to some extent overlap one another. Such overlapping was shown in Figure 9.20b. Also, adjacent dorsal root ganglion cells have adjacent or overlapping receptive fields. In this way, the population of dorsal root ganglion cells represent the entire surface of the skin.

□ From what you have learned so far in this book, what information could activity in a single sensory neuron in the dorsal root ganglion convey?

■ Logically, it could give information about: (1) position of the stimulus within the dermatome, and (2) the timing of the stimulation, such as onset and duration; (3) the rate of the action potentials could also code for the intensity of the stimulus.

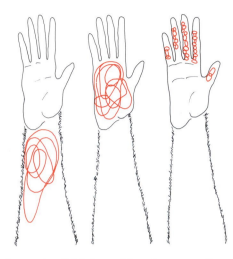

**Figure 9.21** Typical receptive field sizes of dorsal root ganglion cells of a monkey with receptive fields in the forearm, palm and fingers. Each cell has a single receptive field and the sizes of the receptive fields are an indication of the tactile sensitivity of the region of the body.

The receptors in the skin that respond to mechanical deformation can be divided into two types. One group responds to low levels of mechanical stimulation, and are called low-threshold mechanoreceptors. The other group, the high-threshold mechanoreceptors, respond to greater levels of mechanical stimulation. It is the low-threshold mechanoreceptors that contribute to the sense of touch. (The roles of the high- and low-threshold pathways will be described in more detail in Book 3, Chapter 5.) The two categories of information about mechanical stimulation of the skin are kept separate. Similarly, information about skin temperature does not, for example, get mixed up with information about touch.

### 9.5.3   The central representation of touch

The sensory information that ascends from the body via the spinal cord does not all go to the same place in the brain. Information from the muscles and joints, temperature receptors and from receptors that contribute to the sensation of pain travel in different pathways from the touch pathway. However, in all cases, the ascending nerves cross over the midline either in the spinal cord itself or in the medulla, so that sensory events on one side of the body are represented contralaterally in the brain. The subject of this section is the central representation of touch. We will concentrate on the pathway that runs ipsilaterally (on the same side) from the dorsal root ganglia through the dorsal column nuclei (DCN) and then crosses over to the contralateral ventrobasal nucleus of the thalamus.

The thalamus is a large forebrain structure subdivided into a large number of nuclei (see Figure 9.22). This section concentrates on the ventrobasal nucleus, which receives synaptic input from the touch system. You are not expected to remember the names of thalamic structures, other than the ventrobasal nucleus, or their relative positions. It is important to recognize, though, that the thalamus is not solely concerned with relaying and processing sensory information. In the next chapter you will encounter thalamic nuclei that have functions in motor control and, in later books, thalamic nuclei that have been implicated in memory systems.

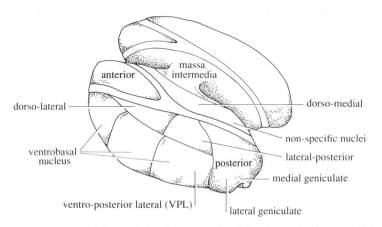

**Figure 9.22** The subdivisions of the thalamus. The thalami from both sides of the brain are shown.

Figure 9.23 shows responses recorded from a cell in an area of the ventrobasal nucleus that 'deals with' the right forearm. The receptive field of this cell shows a different form from the receptive fields found in dorsal root ganglion cells, as discussed in Section 9.5.2. The first point of difference to note is that the field has a concentric organization, that is to say, it has two regions which have different response properties, one lying within the other and both being roughly circular. The inner region is marked by crosses and the outer by triangles on Figure 9.23a.

Trace 1 in Figure 9.23 represents the neuron's electrical activity, the neuron having a certain spontaneous firing rate. If the skin in the centre of the receptive field is stimulated during time $t_1$, by, for example, touching it with a fine probe, there is an increase in the rate of production of action potentials. Trace 2 shows what happens when the outer region of the receptive field is stimulated during time $t_1$.

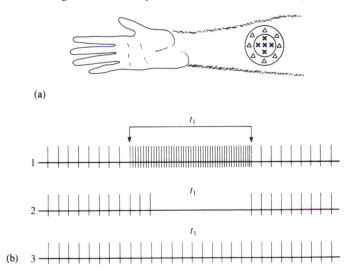

**Figure 9.23** (a) Concentrically organized receptive field of a neuron in the ventrobasal nucleus. (b) The responses of ventrobasal nucleus cells to stimulation of their concentrically organized receptive fields by a tactile stimulus. Trace 1 shows the stimulation of the centre, trace 2 the stimulation of the outer area, and trace 3 the simultaneous stimulation of both regions.

☐ How would you characterize the response shown when the outer region of the receptive field is stimulated?

■ The activity of the neuron is inhibited so that the frequency at which it shows action potentials is reduced to below its spontaneous level.

Note that in trace 1 the increase in frequency of firing following application of the touch stimulus is almost immediate. In trace 2 the inhibition occurs following a slight latency.

☐ How might you explain this difference in latency?

■ The longer latency of the response in trace 2 is attributable to extra synaptic delays in the pathway mediating the response from the periphery. That is, extra synaptic processing is necessary to produce the inhibitory effects.

Trace 3 in Figure 9.23b shows the effect of simultaneous stimulation of the centre and outer regions of the receptive field. Here, the inhibitory effects of stimulation of the outer area cancel out the excitatory effects of stimulation of the centre. For this reason, the centre and surround regions are said to have a mutually *antagonistic* relationship.

A schematic representation of the organization within the neural pathways that produces the concentrically organized receptive field with an antagonistic relationship between centre and outer area is shown in Figure 9.24. The activity of a small number of receptors in the skin (×, △) is conveyed via the axons of sensory neurons in the dorsal root ganglion (DRG). For clarity, just one axon receiving input from the central region and two axons receiving input from the outer region are shown.

The three ascending axons project via the dorsal columns and each synapses on a different single neuron in the dorsal column nuclei (DCN). In turn, the axons of the DCN neurons synapse on neurons in the ventrobasal nucleus. Ventrobasal neuron A receives an excitatory input from the neuron that is activated (via the DCN) by touch in the centre of the receptive field. Note the way that the ventrobasal neurons receiving information from the outer area of the receptive field are connected to inhibitory interneurons, shown in red. Further, these inhibitory interneurons are shown synapsing on neuron A, the ventrobasal neuron receiving input from the centre region of the receptive field.

☐ While recording the activity of cell A in the ventrobasal nucleus, what would be the effect of stimulating the centre region of the field in the forearm?

■ Dorsal root ganglion sensory neurons that are associated with the receptors that are stimulated will be activated (as represented by one of the crosses associated with one neuron). This activity will be transmitted to the DCN where it will activate the cell which is shown connected to neuron A in the ventrobasal nucleus. Thus the ventrobasal neuron A will be activated (see Figure 9.23b, trace 1, period marked $t_1$).

☐ What will be the effect of stimulating a region in the outer area of the receptive field in the forearm, associated with the representative neuron b? (This sensory neuron influences neuron B in the ventrobasal nucleus.)

■ There will be a similar sequence of events leading to the excitation of neuron B with the same time course as shown for neuron A.

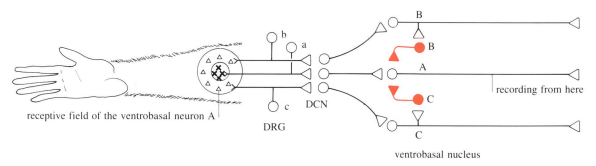

**Figure 9.24** The concentrically organized receptive field of a ventrobasal neuron is 'constructed' from an arrangement of the activity in many dorsal root ganglion sensory neurons (only a representative three being shown here) relayed through the dorsal column nuclei (DCN) to the ventrobasal nucleus. Within the ventrobasal nucleus, inhibitory interneurons produce an inhibitory relationship between inner and outer regions of a ventrobasal neuron's receptive field.

The significance of the inhibitory interneurons in the ventrobasal nucleus for the 'construction' of the receptive field of ventrobasal neuron A should now be clearer. When ventrobasal cell B (or C) is activated by stimulation of the outer region of the field in the forearm, it activates an inhibitory interneuron, which in turn inhibits ventrobasal neuron A.

☐ From the standpoint of ventrobasal neuron A, how will stimulation of the centre and peripheral regions of the field in the forearm differ?

■ Stimulation of the central region will produce an excitatory response in cell A. Stimulation of the peripheral region will result in inhibition of the activity of cell A but with a delay introduced by the synaptic delays occurring in the activation of the inhibitory interneuron.

Trace 2 in Figure 9.23b shows the response of ventrobasal neuron A to stimulation of the outer area of its receptive field. The spontaneous activity of the neuron is inhibited with a delay resulting from the extra synapses in the inhibitory pathway through the interneurons B and C.

Trace 3 in Figure 9.23b shows the response of ventrobasal neuron A to simultaneous stimulation of the centre and outer area of its receptive field. In the figure the inhibitory and excitatory responses 'balance out'. In 'real life' tactile stimuli are unlikely to balance out completely, so that a 'blip' of activity may occur at the onset of the tactile stimulus.

This type of organization, involving antagonistic relationships between the outer and centre areas of concentrically organized receptive fields, is called **lateral inhibition**. It is found in most sensory systems, including the mammalian CNS, and is a fundamental neural mechanism for processing sensory information that you will encounter again in later books in this course.

☐ What is the physical stimulus that would maximize the rate of action potentials in ventrobasal neuron A?

■ A tactile stimulus that covers the entire centre region of the receptive field but does not invade the inhibitory outer region.

With a concentrically organized field, once the stimulus extends beyond the centre region it affects the inhibitory outer area and the response starts to get smaller and may be cancelled out completely. In this way, as well as signalling the position of a stimulus on the body, a concentrically organized receptive field can give information about the physical size of the area stimulated.

Output axons from the thalamus project to the cortex to synapse in the somatosensory cortex. Here, the entire body surface is mapped onto the cortex. The relative areas of different regions of the human body represented in the somatosensory cortices in the left and right hemispheres are shown in Figure 9.25. This grotesque representation is called the sensory homunculus (see Figure 8.10b for the motor homunculus).

The orderliness of the sensory representation of the body in the various nuclei *en route* to the cortex indicates an orderliness in the anatomical connections between the successive structures. The simplest explanation of this phenomenon is that, during the development of the brain, the axons extending from the neurons in the dorsal root ganglion to the DCN, those extending from the DCN to the thalamus, and those from the thalamus to the cortex keep in fixed positions with their neighbours. In this way, the topographic relationship is maintained. In fact the picture is a little more complex than this and will be described in more detail in Book 4.

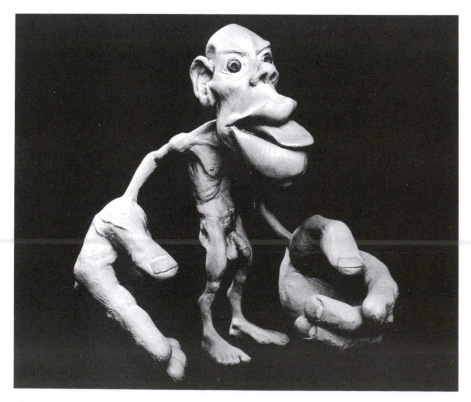

**Figure 9.25** A reconstruction of the distorted representation of the human body surface in the two somatosensory cortices.

The grotesque appearance of the homunculus in the somatosensory cortex (see Figure 9.25) reflects the amount of cortical tissue devoted to processing information from the different regions of the body. Look at the difference in representation of the fingers and the trunk. The disproportionately large amount of cortical tissue devoted to the fingers is parallelled by a high density of touch receptors in the fingers. Corresponding to these receptors, there is a relatively large number of neurons in the dorsal root ganglia that carry information from the receptors in the fingers. In turn, there is a proportionately large number of neuronal axons in the ascending pathways through the brain. A disproportionately large representation in the homunculus implies a disproportionate amount of cortical processing for that region of the body surface and a high sensitivity to sensory stimulation.

Notice the large areas of sensory cortex devoted to regions of the head in Figure 9.25. Using this convention, Figure 9.26 compares the sensory representations of four different mammals: human, rabbit, cat and monkey. The comparison indicates a different balance in the representations of the limbs, trunk and head regions, reflecting different evolutionary pressures acting during the evolution of these species.

☐   Can you suggest why the rabbit may have such a relatively large representation of the head?

■   A speculative answer is that the rabbit is very sensitive to touch on its head because it has evolved to navigate in restricted conditions in dark burrows where tactile rather than visual information is more important.

Sensory input from the head to the CNS does not enter via the spinal cord. Instead, sensory input (and motor output to muscles in the head) flows via the cranial nerves (Figures 8.6 and 8.12). The details of the cranial nerve pathways are not important for the purposes of this chapter.

In a similar way to that by which convergence within the ventrobasal nucleus in the thalamus produces 'higher order' receptive field properties, convergence within the somatosensory cortex also produces receptive fields with complex properties. Figure 9.27 (*overleaf*) shows how responses of neurons in the hand region of the somatosensory cortex respond to touch. The complex feature of these neurons is that they do not respond to a stationary stimulus. The stimulus has to be moving in a particular direction across the receptive field for the neuron to respond. It is possible to hypothesize complex circuit diagrams with inhibitory interconnections between cortical cells which can explain such complex features. The responses shown in Figure 9.27 indicate that the sensory cortex is a region in which complex processing of information provided from the thalamus takes place. More details of cortical sensory processing will appear in Book 3.

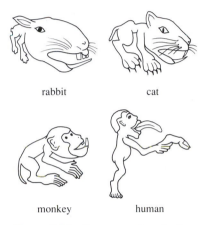

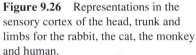

**Figure 9.26**   Representations in the sensory cortex of the head, trunk and limbs for the rabbit, the cat, the monkey and human.

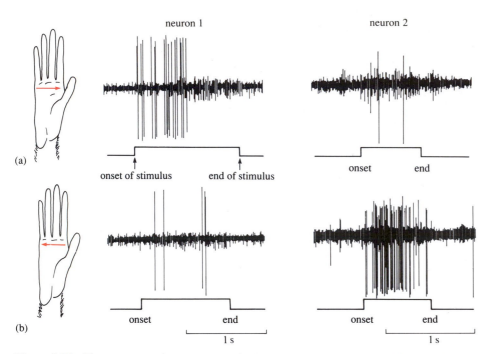

neuron 1

neuron 2

(a)

onset of stimulus    end of stimulus

onset    end

(b)

onset    end

onset    end

1 s    1 s

**Figure 9.27**   The responses of some neurons in the somatosensory cortex are directionally selective. Neurons 1 and 2 have receptive fields in the same position in the hand but have opposite directional preferences. (a) Neuron 1 responds when a stimulus is brushed towards the thumb, but neuron 2 does not respond. (b) Neuron 2 responds when the movement is in the other direction, but neuron 1 does not respond.

## Summary of Section 9.5

Section 9.5 has introduced a number of features of the central representation of information about touch to the skin. These are examples of basic strategies of information representation used generally in sensory systems in the CNS. An important feature of the touch system is that the information entering the spinal cord is represented in a topographically organized way. Here, each sensory neuron entering the dorsal roots conveys information about only a limited region of skin called its receptive field. Furthermore, the neurons entering the dorsal roots are organized along topographical lines. Each dorsal root only receives information from a restricted area of the skin surface called a dermatome and dermatomes are arranged serially so that adjacent dorsal roots receive information from adjacent dermatomes, as shown in Figure 9.4.

In addition, within each dorsal root nerve, sensory neurons are organized so that neurons with adjacent and/or overlapping receptive fields are adjacent to one another. The consequence of this arrangement is that activity in an individual neuron signals not only that a touch stimulus has been detected but it also signals the position on the body at which it occurred.

When the sensory neurons carrying information from touch receptors in the skin terminate within the ventrobasal nucleus of the thalamus they synapse upon projection neurons and upon inhibitory interneurons. Section 9.5.3 described the arrangement of inhibitory and excitatory connections within the ventrobasal that produces a transformation of the information conveyed by the inputs from the DCN to the ventrobasal nucleus. This type of arrangement of excitatory and inhibitory inputs to ventrobasal cells, called lateral inhibition, produces a concentric organization in which there is an antagonistic relationship between centre and outer areas of the receptive field. One feature of the concentrically organized receptive fields of ventrobasal neurons is that they can signal information about the size of a stimulus. If the stimulus encroaches on the inhibitory surround, the response of the ventrobasal neuron decreases.

Section 9.5 has shown how neuroanatomical and neurophysiological information can be used to understand how a complex neural structure can function as an information processing device. The structure of the touch pathways themselves produced a topographic representation of the body surface within the CNS. In this way, activity in a particular subset of neurons in the touch pathway signals the location of a stimulus on the body surface.

Furthermore, convergence of information within the sensory pathway through inhibitory interneurons 'extracts' and represents higher-order features of a touch stimulus, such as its size and direction of movement. The mechanisms described here provide models for a general understanding of sensory information processing within the CNS, which will be extended in later books in this course (particularly Book 3). They provide a start to understanding how CNS structures extract information about objects and events in the external world from the constant sea of information that is continually bombarding its sensory receptors.

# Summary of Chapter 9

This chapter has given a brief introduction to the ins and outs of the mammalian brain. You are now aware of the role that sensory information plays in the elicitation of spinal reflexes and of the way that the brain extracts information about the location, nature, intensity and movement of stimuli that touch the skin. In the processing of sensory information within the CNS, you can appreciate the role that inhibitory interneurons play in extracting stimulus features from the activity of adjacent receptive fields. The mechanism of lateral inhibition introduced in this chapter is a fundamental feature of most sensory systems.

The evolutionary development of adding extra levels of processing into simple pathways extends sensory processing capability and, through enhanced sensory discrimination, allows more 'sophisticated' responses to stimuli. CNS motor systems have evolved greater responsiveness in a similar way. The system of reciprocal antagonist inhibition, for example, produces an integrated reflex system that provides automatic postural control and compensation for unexpected events such as the occurrence of potentially damaging stimuli.

The evidence from 'spinal' animals indicates that the spinal cord reflex structure alone is sufficient to organize coordinated running and walking movements. In the evolution of the primates, which involved the transition from four-legged locomotion to two-legged locomotion, significant developments occurred in the organization of the motor cortex. The increasing capability for fine control of the fingers was achieved through direct access by the finger region of the cortex to the α motor neurons in the spinal cord controlling the finger muscles.

The primate motor cortex, through the pyramidal tract, provided the fine control over the forelimbs that is associated with voluntary behaviour. However, this cortical system acts in conjunction with other forebrain and brain stem structures that also act upon spinal cord structures. One feature of the organization of the supra-spinal motor structures is the complexity of the loop pathways they form. The cerebellum is primarily involved in pathways with the brain stem structures. Its contribution is to organize the sequencing of muscle contractions which produce movements. In contrast, the basal ganglia, which are primarily involved in loop pathways with the forebrain structures, play a role in the planning and initiation of movements.

# Objectives for Chapter 9

After you have completed this chapter, you should be able to:

9.1 Define and use, or recognize definitions and applications of, each of the terms printed in **bold** in the text. (*Question 9.1*)

9.2 Explain the anatomical and neurophysiological relationships between a dermatome and a dorsal root ganglion. (*Question 9.1*)

9.3 Describe how muscle spindles can serve as stretch detectors and explain the knee-jerk reflex in these terms. (*Questions 9.2 and 9.3*)

9.4 Describe, with the help of a diagram, what is meant by 'reciprocal antagonist inhibition'. (*Question 9.3*)

9.5 Give a brief account of the role of the pyramidal tract, basal ganglia and cerebellum in the control of behaviour. (*Questions 9.4 and 9.5*)

9.6 Explain how the receptive field property of a dorsal root ganglion sensory neuron depends upon its axonal branching. (*Question 9.6*)

9.7 Describe the organization of the inflow of sensory (tactile) information to the CNS in such a way as to explain the meanings of the terms dermatome and receptive field. (*Question 9.6*)

# Questions for Chapter 9

**Question 9.1** (*Objectives 9.1 and 9.2*)
What is meant by the term dermatome? Select the appropriate description(s) from the following statements (a–d).

(a) A dermatome is a segment of the spinal cord.

(b) A dermatome is an alternative term for dorsal root ganglion.

(c) A dermatome is the receptive field of a single dorsal root ganglion sensory neuron.

(d) A dermatome is the area of skin innervated by a single segment of the spinal cord.

**Question 9.2** (*Objective 9.3*)
Which of the following (a–d) are appropriate descriptions of the muscle spindle?

(a) The muscle spindle lies in parallel with working skeletal muscle.

(b) The muscle spindle contracts to exert the force that moves joints in protective reflexes.

(c) The muscle spindle monitors the stretch of working skeletal muscle.

(d) The muscle spindle activates the distal region of an associated sensory neuron.

**Question 9.3** (*Objectives 9.3 and 9.4*)
Which of the following statements (a–g) are true?

(a) Cell bodies of $\alpha$ motor neurons are located in the ventral horns of the spinal cord grey matter.

(b) Cell bodies of $\gamma$ motor neurons are located in the dorsal horns of the spinal cord grey matter.

(c) A monosynaptic reflex has only one synapse in its pathway.

(d) A polysynaptic reflex has only one synapse in its pathway.

(e) Cell bodies of sensory neurons that carry information from the skeletal muscle stretch receptors are located in the dorsal horns of the spinal cord grey matter.

(f) The interneurons of the spinal cord connect intra-segmental reflexes to provide integrated postural control and protective reflexes.

(g) Directed locomotory behaviour in vertebrates results from an interplay between descending influences from the brain and the organization of reflexes in the spinal cord.

**Question 9.4** (*Objective 9.5*)
Complete the sentence 'Ballistic movements are…' with one answer selected from the following statements (a, b).

(a) those that involve carefully computed negative feedback at each stage to ensure successful completion of the movement.

(b) those that are performed so rapidly that there is not time for negative feedback to modify the response.

**Question 9.5** (*Objective 9.5*)
Which of the following statements (a–h) are correct?

(a) The pyramidal tract is the descending pathway from the motor cortex to the brain stem motor neurons.

(b) The pyramidal tract controls the limb muscles.

(c) One difference between the pyramidal tract and the brain stem pathways to the spinal cord is that the former makes direct connections with $\gamma$ motor neurons.

(d) The cerebellum does not have direct connections with the motor system structures of the brain.

(e) The descending pathways from the motor cortex cross over the midline at the level of the spinal cord to control the contralateral muscles.

(f) One function of the cerebellum is to control ballistic sequences of muscle movements.

(g) In Parkinson's disease the dopaminergic pathway from the substantia nigra to the cerebellum degenerates.

(h) One way of characterizing the differences in function between the basal ganglia and the cerebellum is that the former is involved in planning activity and the latter in the organization of muscle control to carry out the activity.

### Question 9.6 (*Objectives 9.6 and 9.7*)
Which of the following statements (a–i) are correct?

(a) The dorsal root sensory neurons carry sensory information from the body to the CNS.

(b) The relationship between the dermatomes and the spinal cord is an example of topographic representation.

(c) A receptive field of a sensory cell can be defined as that region of the sensory surface from which responses in the cell can be evoked.

(d) The concentric inhibitory outer areas of ventrobasal nucleus cells are part of their receptive fields.

(e) The concentric organization of the receptive fields of ventrobasal nucleus cells is an example of lateral inhibition.

(f) The concentric organization of the receptive fields of ventrobasal nucleus cells is produced by inhibitory interneurons. These interneurons are driven by neurons ascending from dorsal root ganglion cells with receptive fields in the peripheral region of the ventrobasal nucleus cell's receptive field.

(g) Stimulation of the outer (inhibitory) region of a receptive field will not be able to influence the frequency of action potentials in a neuron if the excitatory region is stimulated simultaneously.

(h) One factor determining the sensitivity to touch of a region of the body is the amount of cortical tissue devoted to its processing.

(i) The higher order features of stimulus processing found in cells in the somatosensory cortex can be explained by convergence of inputs from cells with lower order stimulus processing features.

# CHAPTER 10
## FROM REFLEXES TO ADAPTIVE BEHAVIOUR

## 10.1  Introduction

Chapter 7 in Book 1 introduced the concept of **species-typical behaviour**. This is behaviour that is shown in an almost identical manner by all members of a given species. The example discussed was lordosis—the mating posture of the female rat that facilitates mounting by the male. In contrast to such species-typical behaviour, other aspects of behaviour can show a wide variation amongst members of the same species, and this was also described in the chapter. Consider, for example, the very different means a dog might utilize in order to escape from a house. Similarly, tales of the tricks exhibited by rats in getting to food are part of country folklore, as well as being subject to experimental investigation.

Much of what would be described as species-typical behaviour is a stereotyped response to a particular identifiable stimulus.

☐   Cast your mind back to Book 1, Chapter 2. The definition 'A totally stereotyped and specific response to a specific stimulus' was given. To what did this definition refer?

■   A reflex.

In this chapter it is necessary to qualify use of the term 'reflex'. In some cases, for example, the knee-jerk reflex to a tap on the leg, a reflex is invariably shown to a given stimulus. If it fails to occur, pathology is indicated. In other cases, the term reflex is still used but there are conditions when a response to the particular stimulus does not occur. For example, in some cases, reflexes only appear at a certain developmental stage, and in other cases, they only appear when the internal environment is appropriate. For instance, the lordosis reflex only occurs when oestrogen levels are sufficiently high. However, when reflexes do occur they have the characteristic described in the definition of Book 1; they are a stereotyped response to a particular stimulus. For instance, lordosis takes the same form in all female rats. The present chapter will look at reflexes of this kind.

In the previous chapter, you became acquainted with some examples of the neural processes underlying a few reflexes. The reflex organization of the spinal cord was introduced, and was described in terms of reflexes that both protect against noxious stimuli and ensure immediate and automatic maintenance of body posture. In this role, such spinal reflexes act as a 'front-line' defence against potential damage or postural disturbance before the central systems can respond. The spinal cord reflexes were also described as organizing basic rhythmic locomotor movements such as running and walking. However, such reflexes are not enough to produce locomotory movements that are correctly directed and have the appropriate intensity. To achieve this, the brain modulates spinal cord reflex pathways, by means of descending pathways from the brain to the spinal cord.

Explanations of mammalian behaviour consist of much more than accounts in terms of locomotor movement and the maintenance of body posture. In explaining behaviour, factors that determine the timing of, and decision-making involved in, an animal's activity are usually discussed in terms of motivation (Book 1, Chapter 7) or learning (Book 1, Chapter 6). In this chapter, continuing the exploration of the relation between structure and function of the brain, the emphasis will be on the motivational aspects of the neurophysiology underpinning the expression of such behaviour patterns. The underlying processes involve brain systems that rely on sensory information about the state of the external world and about the internal state of the animal. They act through the motor systems to produce behaviour that is appropriate for the animal's immediate internal and external environments. In other words, this chapter is concerned with the factors implicated in the *selection* of particular behaviour patterns.

☐ Chapter 7 in Book 1 discussed motivational systems in the context of four properties of behaviour. What are these four properties?

■ (1) The changing responsiveness of animals to a constant external stimulus (e.g. a hungry animal responds to food by ingestion whereas a satiated one will not ingest the same food).
(2) The flexibility of some behaviour patterns (e.g. a novel route can be employed to reach a given goal).
(3) The decisions between different activities made by animals (e.g. whether to eat or copulate).
(4) The species-typical behaviour patterns shown in a particular motivational context (e.g. a sexually motivated female rat displays a mating posture termed lordosis).

Species-typical behaviour patterns are usually the end points of more flexible behaviour. For example, animals explore and forage for food and water in a rich variety of ways and such behaviour is terminated by species-typical behaviour patterns such as biting, chewing, sipping and swallowing. In the laboratory, they can be taught such 'tricks' as running mazes and pressing levers to obtain food. These flexible behaviours are terminated by species-typical ingestive behaviour. While it is characteristic of species-typical behaviour that it is relatively stereotyped, it does not follow that stereotypy is diagnostic of species-typical behaviour. For example, you will recall from Book 1, Section 2.4.1 that animals in zoos and farms commonly develop frequently repeated, stereotyped patterns of behaviour called stereotypies. These are highly specific to individuals, and thus clearly cannot be termed species-typical.

Close experimental analysis of behaviour patterns such as biting by cats indicates that biting movements are released by stimulation of the skin around the mouth. However, anyone watching a cat stalking a mouse or a bird does not have the feeling that this is a 'clockwork' animal responding in a reflex way. Up to the end-point, the whole animal is engaged in what appears to be a very flexible and purposeful exercise.

Such descriptions lead to a classification of two classes of behaviour, called **appetitive behaviour** and **consummatory behaviour**. The relatively flexible appetitive behaviour leads to, and is terminated by, the less flexible and more reflexive species-typical consummatory behaviour. As a broad generalization, appetitive behaviours are based on locomotion, e.g. walking, running, accompanied by exploration of the environment.

When an animal is motivated to perform a particular behaviour pattern, changes will usually be observed in the physiology of its body. These changes are appropriate for the behaviour in question. For example, at a time of attack or fleeing, the body is ready for action. The heart rate is high and relatively large amounts of blood are pumped to the skeletal muscles to provide them with the oxygen and energy that they need in order to contract. In contrast, at a time of quiet rest, energy reserves are conserved and heart rate is slowed. As was described in the previous chapter, this 'internal housekeeping' of the body is the responsibility of the ANS. However, the ANS derives an input from the same brain systems that are involved in motivation and species-typical behaviour. Thus, these processes give integration to behaviour and, as part of getting an overall picture, this chapter will also consider the role of the ANS in adjusting the physiology of the body.

The present chapter will therefore look at some of the brain processes that have been shown to be implicated in: (1) the appetitive phase of behaviour, (2) the species-typical behaviour shown at the end-point, and (3) the reactions of the ANS. It will emphasize the integrated nature of these three aspects. However, it will concentrate upon the production of species-typical behaviour in particular motivational states. The reason for the emphasis upon this aspect is that the understanding of the brain processes underlying species-typical behaviour is relatively good. The chapter will also return to a consideration of *cognitive maps*, that is, a spatial representation of the environment (introduced in Book 1, Chapter 8). The animal's ability to show flexible behaviour, directed towards a goal, requires the nervous system to construct and utilize a cognitive map. This has been the topic of intense theoretical speculation and experiment at a neural level, and some of the results of such experimentation are described in Section 10.6.

First, the discussion turns to the brain mechanisms involved in species-typical behaviour.

## 10.2   The role of the limbic system

The major CNS structures that have been implicated in the control of an animal's activities are interconnected in a system in the forebrain called the limbic system (Figure 10.1, *overleaf*). Limbic system structures include the hippocampus, amygdala, septum, thalamus and hypothalamus. Also important in the control of behaviour are the brain stem reticular formation and related structures such as the central grey matter of the brain stem (which consists of a diffuse network of neurons surrounding the ventricles in the centre of the brain stem).

The discussion will turn later to the role of structures in the limbic system in the organization of appetitive behaviour, which does not involve the activation of reflexes but which can be 'programmed' in different ways by the CNS. First, it is necessary to focus upon one part of the limbic system, the hypothalamus, whose role in motivation has been well established by experimental evidence.

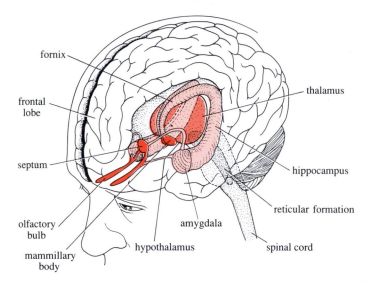

**Figure 10.1**   The limbic system (the main limbic system structures are shown in red).

# 10.3   The hypothalamus

The hypothalamus (Figure 10.2a) is a bilaterally symmetrical collection of nuclei bordering on the third ventricle (Figure 10.2b). These nuclei make extensive bidirectional contacts with other limbic system structures and with a variety of brain stem structures, including the reticular formation and the associated central grey matter. Through its close connection with the pituitary gland, the hypothalamus controls the release of certain hormones into the bloodstream and, through neurosecretory cells in the walls of the ventricle, it controls levels of hormones circulating in the ventricles of the brain.

The hypothalamus is a complex region which receives information about the general state of the animal's physiology; for example it 'knows' about factors such as fluid levels and sugar concentration in the blood stream (introduced in Book 1, Chapter 7). Thus, the hypothalamus is in a position to play a central role in the homeostatic mechanisms regulating, for example, nutrient and fluid levels. The hypothalamus is also sensitive to the concentrations of hormones circulating in the blood and ventricular systems. Its sensitivity depends upon the location in the hypothalamus of specialized receptors that 'monitor' the bloodstream and the cerebro-spinal fluid in the ventricles. The hypothalamus thus plays a central role in those behaviour patterns that are greatly influenced by hormones, such as copulation and maternal behaviour. Furthermore, information concerning immediate environmental events and stimuli reaches the hypothalamus through the olfactory and cortical inputs to the limbic system.

Figures 10.3 and 10.4 (*overleaf*) are simplified schematic representations emphasizing the focal nature of the hypothalamus within the CNS. They illustrate the interconnections of the hypothalamus with the limbic system and also with the thalamo-cortical system, its access to information about the internal states of the animal and its control of the body's physiology and musculature through the pituitary and brain stem.

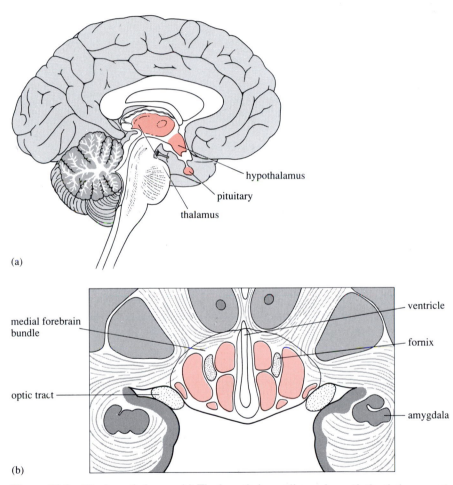

(a)

(b)

**Figure 10.2** The hypothalamus. (a) The hypothalamus lies underneath the thalamus and above the pituitary gland. The pituitary secretes hormones into the bloodstream under the control of the hypothalamus. (b) A coronal section through part of the brain. The hypothalamus is a collection of nuclei (shown in red) grouped together around the third ventricle. Coursing around and between the hypothalamic nuclei is the medial forebrain bundle, a fibre tract which connects the hypothalamic nuclei with many other brain stem and midbrain structures.

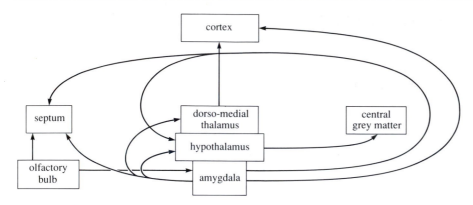

**Figure 10.3** A schematic representation of the hypothalamus in relation to other brain regions.

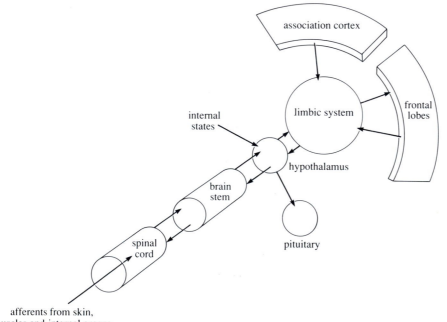

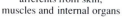

**Figure 10.4** A schematic representation of the focal position of the hypothalamus in the CNS illustrating its interconnections with the forebrain limbic and cortical systems and its output pathways via the pituitary and the brain stem.

The hypothalamus participates in four classes of input–output relationship, as shown in Table 10.1. These relationships can be understood in terms of (a) the collection of nuclei that make up the hypothalamus and their interconnections with other brain structures and (b) the capacity of the hypothalamus, on the one hand to stimulate the release of hormones and, on the other, to monitor hormone levels.

**Table 10.1**   Classification of hypothalamic input–output relationships.

| | |
|---|---|
| Class 1 | Involving neural input and output |
| Class 2 | Where the input is neural and the output is hormonal |
| Class 3 | Where the input is hormonal and the output is neural |
| Class 4 | Where both input and output are hormonal |

The neural output of the hypothalamus exerts immediate influence over the activity of limbic system brain structures and, through its descending connections with the brain stem, the hypothalamus is involved in the control of motor output. Not shown in Figures 10.3 and 10.4 are the connections between the hypothalamus and the ANS. These are via brain stem structures which activate cranial nerves and specialized autonomic neurons in the spinal cord.

## 10.3.1   The hypothalamus and the ANS

The ANS, introduced in Chapter 8, has two divisions.

☐   What are they called?

■   The sympathetic and parasympathetic divisions.

☐   What is the role of the sympathetic division?

■   Generally, activation of the sympathetic division prepares the body for action (discussed in detail in Book 5, Chapter 5). Under conditions of fear or anger, the sympathetic nervous system increases the rate at which the heart beats and the rate of blood flow to the skeletal muscles. Glucose levels in the blood are increased, body temperature and sweating are increased, and the pupils of the eyes are dilated.

Inputs to the ANS from the hypothalamus are an important source of such activation. The adrenal glands are activated to release adrenalin and noradrenalin into the blood stream through the action of the sympathetic nervous system, under the influence of the hypothalamus. The sympathetic nervous system has the converse effect on the digestive system and reduces the mechanical and secretory functions of the stomach and intestines, thus reducing their need for blood to remove the products of digestion.

☐   What are the effects of the parasympathetic nervous system?

■   In general, these are the opposite of the sympathetic system, preparing the organism for more sedentary activity.

The level of activation of the body's physiology will depend upon the balance of activities in the sympathetic and parasympathetic nervous systems. They are thought to function independently of one another so that parasympathetic and sympathetic could both be high, both low or one high and the other low, with the balance of activity controlled by the hypothalamus.

Its variety of control systems give the hypothalamus a strategic role in the integration of an animal's behavioural and physiological responses to environmental stimuli, that is, in the way that the animal as a whole responds and behaves. The hypothalamus influences the body's physiology through the ANS and through hormonal release into the ventricles and bloodstream. The physiological changes produced by the ANS prepare the body for the changes in its activity that are also being simultaneously programmed through the hypothalamus.

The present section and the next both consider relationships between hormones and behaviour. However, whereas the ANS provides an example of hormones released under hypothalamic control, the following section gives an example of where the hypothalamus is influenced by circulating hormones. Both sections serve to illustrate the pivotal role of the hypothalamus as a mediator between the CNS and the endocrine system.

## 10.3.2 Lordosis: a case study for explanations of hypothalamic control

For a number of species, fertilization can only occur during certain periods of time (during that part of the female's reproductive cycle known as *oestrus*). Obviously, it is of adaptive value for a female's sexual motivation to be aroused and reflexes that facilitate copulation to be exhibited at those times when fertilization is possible (Book 1, Sections 2.9 and 9.1). An example of the correlation between, on the one hand, hormonal state and, on the other, sexual motivation and receptivity was given in Book 1, Section 7.2.3. Sexual motivation and receptivity have both appetitive and consummatory phases. This section looks at an example of consummatory behaviour which is species-typical: the lordosis reflex in female rats.

Lordosis is a reflex response which facilitates sexual mounting of the female rat by a male. The stimulus for lordosis is tactile stimulation of the female's rump, usually by the male rat's belly. The lordosis reaction consists of the female raising her hind quarters, accompanied by a characteristic body posture (Figure 10.5).

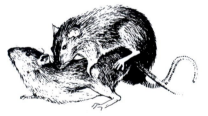

**Figure 10.5** Lordosis is the female's reflex response of raising the rear quarters in response to tactile stimulation of the hind quarters from the male.

☐   Lordosis does not occur if the spinal cord is cut. What does this indicate about the control of this reflex?

■   It indicates that central structures are involved in the mediation of the reflex.

This reflex is strongly influenced by oestrogen. During oestrus, when oestrogen levels are high, the chances of fertilization are greater. The lordosis reflex is also relatively easy to trigger by the appropriate tactile stimulus when oestrogen levels are high.

A study by Donald Pfaff and coworkers, at Rockefeller University in the 1980s, into the mechanisms mediating lordosis in the female rat is very illuminating. They were able to tease out the contributions made by brain and spinal cord structures underlying the reflex. The neural control circuit for the lordosis reflex identified by Pfaff is shown in Figure 10.6. They identified that the basic neural mechanism controlling the pattern of motor activity is present at the spinal level, as indicated schematically by the pathway 1–2–3 in Figure 10.6. Tactile stimulation by the male at X triggers activity in sensory neurons (1) which through interneurons (2) make contact with motor neurons (3). However, at times when the female is *unreceptive* to the male, the afferent input to the spinal cord is *insufficient* to activate the spinal cord motor neurons driving the back muscles.

The afferent sensory input is also conveyed via the spinal cord to brain structures, as represented by the dotted pathway (4) in Figure 10.6. This pathway terminates in three brain stem structures, the reticular formation, the central grey matter and the lateral vestibular nucleus. For the purposes of this discussion, the individual roles of these structures are not important: what is important to note is the descending pathway from these structures to the spinal mechanisms underlying the reflex (the solid lines in Figure 10.6). When the female is unreceptive, the descending contributions from these structures on to the spinal cord motor neurons are insufficient to facilitate the motor neurons to produce lordosis in response to tactile stimulation of the female's rump.

Pfaff's investigation revealed that the 'key' that unlocks the lordosis reflex is a pathway from the hypothalamus to the central grey matter (the red pathway (5) in Figure 10.6). When circulating levels of oestrogen are sufficiently high, the hypothalamus is sensitized by oestrogen. As a result, the pathway from the hypothalamus facilitates activity in the central grey matter. In turn, the brain stem reticular formation is facilitated via pathway 6 (shaded pink). The result is that the descending influences from this structure onto the spinal cord facilitate the reflex pathways for lordosis, making them able to be activated by appropriate tactile stimulation.

This analysis indicates how the hypothalamus acts to make available selective neural circuits, and so plays a role in determining the behaviour patterns that are available. The type of response involved in lordosis is typical of the organization of species-typical behaviour involved in mating, fighting and submissive behaviour, maternal and social behaviour. Such species-typical behaviour, as the name implies, is typical of the behaviour of individuals (female individuals in the case of lordosis) of the same species and usually of closely related species, and appears with similar forms from individual to individual.

The organization of such species-typical reflexes is under the 'supervision' of the hypothalamus and typically involves extensive spinal cord and midbrain circuitry. Although such species-typical behaviour is classed as reflexive, because its appearance depends upon both an appropriate environmental stimulus such as the tactile (touch) stimulation from the male and events taking place in the brain, the control of such behaviour is not as rigid as in reflexes such as the knee-jerk reflex (Section 9.3.3). Rather, the reflexes typified by the lordosis reflex are integrated into sequences of behaviour patterns, where such sequencing depends, second-by-second, on the responses of the targets of the behaviour.

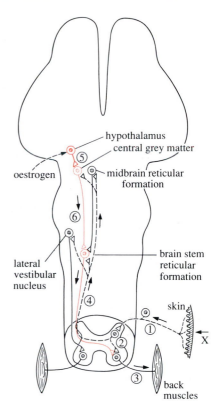

**Figure 10.6**   Schematic diagram of the rat brain showing the neural organization underlying the lordosis reflex in female rats (see text for details).

### 10.3.3   Hypothalamic neural input–neural output relationships

In the brain stem neural circuit that mediates lordosis, the facilitatory influences from the hypothalamus that are 'switched on' by oestrogen play a critical role. In the absence of oestrogen, tactile stimulation of the rump does not produce the reflex, and lordosis does not appear. Pfaff's analysis of the neural circuitry underlying the lordosis reflex gives important insights into the way that the hypothalamus works more generally in the selection of behaviour, by showing how it switches particular reflex pathways on and, by implication, in withdrawing the facilitation, how it switches them off.

Thus in the presence of oestrogen the hypothalamus acts to make a particular reflex pathway available by facilitating regions of the reticular formation that act on the spinal cord to organize the reflex. By the criteria of Table 10.1 this is an example in class 3—hormonal input and neural output.

With its extensive neural interconnections with other limbic system structures and with brain stem nuclei, the hypothalamus is well situated to relate neural input to neural output (a class 1 relationship in Table 10.1). Class 1 relationships give immediate control over behaviour, allowing it to be changed abruptly without the delays involved while hormones circulate in the bloodstream and ventricular system. Evidence supporting the existence of such a relationship is found from experiments in which regions of the hypothalamus and brain stem are stimulated electrically.

In cats, electrical stimulation of lower regions of the brain stem containing the reticular formation and the central grey matter elicit fragmented reflex activities. These are commonly isolated reflexes such as snarling, hissing, biting movements or arching of the back, and erection of hair. The interpretation of these findings is that, as with lordosis, the brain stem provides an input that facilitates the appearance of these components of species-typical behaviour.

☐ Could the lordosis example help to understand how these reflexes are elicited?

■ From Pfaff's analysis of lordosis, it is likely that the hypothalamus acts in a similar way to facilitate some brain stem mediated reflexes; in other words, to make them available.

Experiments by J. P. Flynn and coworkers at Yale University in the 1960s and 70s indicate how electrical stimulation of the hypothalamus can switch an animal's response. In 'relaxed' laboratory conditions, if the facial regions around a cat's mouth are stimulated using a pencil-shaped object, the cat turns its head away from the rod. However, when localized regions of the hypothalamus are stimulated simultaneously with stimulation of the face, then the cat reliably turns towards the rod and attempts to bite it.

☐ What is a possible explanation of the change in the cat's response to the tactile stimulation, which is induced by hypothalamic stimulation?

■ A reasonable interpretation is that the hypothalamic stimulation 'switches on' or makes available a different set of reflexes. In the condition where there is no hypothalamic stimulation, the 'irritating' stimulation of the facial region produces a defensive response. During the hypothalamic stimulation the cat responds with an attack response.

Electrical stimulation is, of course, an abnormal stimulus and extrapolation needs to be made with caution. However, it is possible that it mimics aspects of the processes underlying normal behaviour. In this particular case, it might mimic a central motivational state that makes the cat more likely to attack. In fact, the change in the cat's behaviour is intuitively plausible. Surely everyone has had the experience of responding quite differently to similar situations in a way that is related to states often described as moods. A good example of this is a provocative joke by family or friends. On a 'good' day, a joke might be accepted as such, but on a 'bad' day it can elicit a quite different response.

## 10.3.4   Localization of function within the hypothalamus

As well as modifying behavioural responses, in experimental animals electrical stimulation in many regions of the hypothalamus produces changes in bodily states mediated through the ANS.

Localized electrical stimulation of the hypothalamus indicates that activation of the sympathetic and parasympathetic divisions is mediated by different regions of the hypothalamus. Also, electrical stimulation of these different regions produces behaviour patterns that are appropriate for the autonomic responses. In the 1930s, the German neurophysiologist W. R. Hess reported that stimulation of regions of the hypothalamus that produced sympathetic autonomic activity also produced integrated sequences of 'fight' or 'flight' behaviour: attacking or fleeing from objects. He described the behaviour elicited from parasympathetic regions of the hypothalamus as 'frolic', due to it being relaxed and playful in nature.

More recently, studies in cats, rats and monkeys have confirmed differences in the role of medial and lateral regions of the hypothalamus. Flynn and coworkers carried out experiments in which they stimulated lateral and medial regions of the hypothalamus in cats in the presence of a rat. Stimulation of the medial hypothalamus produced an 'affective' (meaning 'emotional') attack with an accompanying emotional display characteristic of intense activity of the sympathetic division of the ANS: hissing, growling, arching of the back and erection of the hair on the back. During the attack, there was intense hissing and the cat clawed at the rat but did not bite it unless the stimulation was prolonged.

Stimulation of more lateral areas of the hypothalamus produces a quieter form of attack which is not 'emotional' but is more reminiscent of the normal behaviour of the cat when stalking and killing prey for food. Here, the cat does not vocalize or show any emotional arousal but captures the rat in a way that is typical of cats catching small animals.

☐   What is an explanation of the change in the cat's behaviour when changing between lateral and medial hypothalamic stimulation?

■   Stimulation of the two areas in the hypothalamus results in the activation of different sets of reflexes, so that similar environmental stimuli produce different forms of response.

An interpretation of the differences in the cat's behaviour during medial and lateral hypothalamic stimulation is that stimulation of the lateral hypothalamus activates reflex pathways for predatory behaviour while medial hypothalamic pathways activate reflex pathways for behaviour patterns used as threats in social interactions involving the establishment of dominance or the defence of a territory. Such behaviour would normally be elicited by another cat or by a large predator such as a dog that had cornered the cat. Here, a possible explanation is that the effect of the electrical stimulation of the medial hypothalamic region is to restrict the animal's available behavioural repertoire. All that it can do is to behave towards the rat in a way that would normally be elicited in response to, for example, a predator or another cat in a territorial dispute.

## 10.3.5  Hypothalamic control: integration of reflexes

The preceding discussions have painted a picture of the hypothalamus as playing a crucial role in the selection of appropriate behaviour through the integration of the body's physiology with its behavioural control systems. At its focal position in the CNS, the anatomical connections of the hypothalamus involve it in receiving information about both limbic and cortical forebrain systems and about the physiological state of the body. By its output, the hypothalamus also exerts a controlling influence upon other neural structures. The hypothalamus plays a crucial role in the control over the body's physiology through the ANS and pituitary and in the control over behaviour through the brain stem reticular formation.

Activation of different regions of the hypothalamus by hormones circulating in the bloodstream or ventricles, or by neural activity impinging on the hypothalamus from limbic system structures, results in the sensitization of different sets of reflexes. However, these do not occur in isolation, and are accompanied by appropriate activity in the ANS. For example, during behaviour in which the animal has to be active, under the influence of the ANS, heart rate is increased, and the circulation of blood controlled so that the flow to the gut is decreased, while the muscles get an increased supply to prepare for the potential demands of activity. The control of related physiological and behavioural responses is localized in particular regions of the hypothalamus, giving an integration of physiological and behavioural responses.

In lordosis, the role of the hypothalamus is not one of directly eliciting behaviour. Rather, it *primes* or, in other words, sensitizes sets of reflexes which are then available to be elicited by appropriate environmental stimuli. Thus, lordosis does not appear simply when oestrogen first acts on the hypothalamus to sensitize the brain stem pathways. Rather, such sensitization is a necessary (but not sufficient) first condition for lordosis to appear, but the appropriate tactile stimulus also has to be present. It is reasonable to extrapolate an understanding of lordosis to other motivational systems: in doing so, one would assume that different combinations of neural and/or hormonal influences on the hypothalamus activate it to make different sets of reflexes, e.g. sexual, maternal, aggressive, social and exploratory, available to be elicited.

By means of such sensitization from the hypothalamus, discrete reflexes become available and a series of reflexes can then become organized into a behavioural sequence by appropriate environmental stimuli. For example, the influence of pheromones may activate the male rat's hypothalamus to prime copulatory reflexes, i.e. to make them available. Then a combination of visual and tactile stimuli trigger and sequence the mounting, thrusting and ejaculatory reflexes. Such reflexes can be elicited independently of one another by electrical stimulation of the brain stem but it is only with appropriate visual and tactile stimuli from a female that they appear in the normal sequence and lead to insemination. Similarly, elements of cat fighting behaviour, e.g. snarling, hissing and biting, can be elicited independently by midbrain stimulation but in real life appear in sequences that are dictated by the behaviour and responses of the target animal.

Although the discussion has focused upon the central role of the hypothalamus, you should not interpret this as meaning that the hypothalamus is *the* centre in the brain that controls an animal's behaviour. Rather, it is *a* region that exerts a role in interaction with other brain regions and external stimuli. A similar logic, i.e. seeing the hypothalamus in the context of associated brain regions, is usually applied to interpreting the effects of artificial electrical stimulation of the hypothalamus. In such terms, the interpretation is that the electrical stimulation is in some respect mimicking the effects of influences upon the hypothalamus from other limbic system structures. In this view, the hypothalamus is responding as it would under natural conditions to 'information' it receives from other limbic system regions.

Now, having identified a role for the hypothalamus in selecting and integrating behavioural and physiological responses to stimuli, the next section will look at the hypothalamus in the wider context of the limbic system and the influences of specific limbic system structures and brain stem structures upon it.

# 10.4  Wider brain stem and limbic system influences

The discussion so far has emphasized the hypothalamus as a focal point for the integration of bodily states with behaviour and for sensitizing reflexes. As indicated by the previous discussion, the hypothalamus does not act in isolation but as a focal point within a more widely distributed behavioural control system. Accordingly, the next sections will briefly introduce anatomical structures that influence the activity of the hypothalamus.

## 10.4.1  Interactions with the hypothalamus

### The medial forebrain bundle and hypothalamic integration

The collection of nuclei forming the hypothalamus is surrounded by a pathway called the medial forebrain bundle (Figure 10.2b). As well as containing fibres that descend from the hypothalamus and forebrain structures, at the level of the hypothalamus the medial forebrain bundle contains ascending fibres that originate in brain stem structures. These ascending influences have both general and specific influences in maintaining the level of arousal of the brain. The ascending reticular formation has been implicated in maintaining the second-by-second level of arousal of the brain and in 'alerting' the sensory structures to process sensory information. Both the raphe nucleus and locus ceruleus (nuclei in the brain stem) have been implicated in the control of phases of sleep.

### The amygdala

The amygdala is a complex nucleus that is interconnected within the limbic system and with the cortex. An important feature of the amygdala is that it receives a major projection from the olfactory system, providing a direct route from the sense of smell (Figure 10.7). This is significant in the present context because the sense of smell is an important determinant of the kind of species-typical behaviour that has been discussed here. Figure 10.7 shows a schematic representation of the major interconnections made by the amygdala with other limbic system structures and with the cortex (you do not need to know the details).

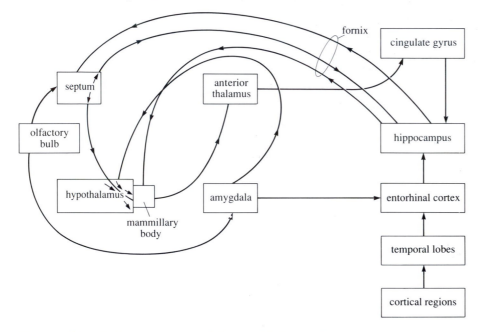

**Figure 10.7**    A further development of Figure 10.3 showing the relationship between the hypothalamus and other brain structures. The entorhinal cortex is an area of olfactory association cortex next to the primary olfactory cortex.

Experiments in which the amygdala has been damaged have shown that it has a variety of effects on behaviour. Frequently, animals (usually cats) in such experiments are described as being hyperactive and restless, and overly responsive to stimuli. The intensity of sexual and aggressive behaviour is also increased and is sometimes directed toward inappropriate objects. In the context of the previous discussions of the focal role of the hypothalamus, a possible interpretation of these findings is that the amygdala normally inhibits the hypothalamus. In this way the amygdala would restrict the hypothalamus in its role in activating brain stem reflex pathways.

However, experiments by Flynn (described in Section 10.3.3), in which the amygdala and hypothalamus were simultaneously stimulated electrically, indicate a more complex relationship between these two areas. In experiments in which the hypothalamus was being stimulated to produce the predatory behaviour of a cat toward a rat, simultaneous stimulation of the lateral amygdala made the attack less likely to occur. Stimulation of the medial region had the opposite effect and facilitated the attacks.

## 10.4.2   The limbic system and appetitive behaviour

The discussions of the role of the hypothalamus in the selection of behaviour have so far concentrated on its functions in potentiating species-typical reflexes: here, the examples were of biting, predatory and sexual reflexes. However, as noted in the introduction to this chapter and in Book 1, Chapter 7, mammals in general display flexibility in the appetitive phase of behaviour. How does the hypothalamus play a role in activating such appetitive behaviour?

Perhaps, the role of the basal ganglia under the influence of the substantia nigra (which itself is influenced from the hypothalamus) is to activate 'plans' for locomotor activities. This line of speculation is prompted by the symptoms of Parkinson's disease, in which the cells projecting from the substantia nigra to the other structures of the basal ganglia degenerate, leaving the patient with a variety of symptoms, one of which is the inability to initiate locomotory behaviour.

This speculative analysis then points to a further possible role of the hypothalamus in behavioural control, as follows. As well as activating sets of brain stem reflexes, the hypothalamus also activates appropriate appetitive behaviour through its influence upon the motor system via the basal ganglia. This is a role that fits with its known roles in integrating autonomic reactions and those reflexly organized behaviour patterns that are the end points of appetitive behaviour. Logically, the hypothalamus might be expected to play a central role in appetitive behaviour. For instance, from functional considerations, times of foraging for food would be expected to take account of nutrient levels. The timing of courtship would be similarly influenced by hormone levels. In fact, there is supporting evidence for a role of the hypothalamus in appetitive behaviour, described in the next section. This comes from studies of electrical stimulation of the hypothalamus, where new appetitive behaviour patterns are added to the animal's behavioural repertoire.

# 10.5   Electrical stimulation of the brain and self-stimulation

Normally, behaviour that, for example, regularly leads a food-deprived animal to food will be learned. Such behaviour has consequences for hypothalamic activity. Laboratory experiments indicate that both the sensory consequences of eating and the longer term effects upon blood sugar level have central effects in terminating the eating behaviour and that this is mediated by the hypothalamus. In fact, a region of the hypothalamus appears to act as a 'satiety centre' to turn off the facilitation that other hypothalamic regions exert on eating behaviour. Insight into the role of the hypothalamus in such normal behaviour has been gained from a fascinating discovery that forms the topic of this section.

Rats with electrodes implanted in some hypothalamic and medial forebrain bundle sites will learn to press a bar in a Skinner box (Book 1, Section 6.3.4) to receive a brief electrical shock to the brain (ESB) through the electrode. This phenomenon is called **electrical self-stimulation**.

Rats display high levels of curiosity and will explore a novel environment. Sooner or later during the exploration of the Skinner box chamber, a rat with such an implanted electrode will press the bar accidentally by leaning on it or bumping into it. After the first occasion that the bar is pressed, the rat's exploratory behaviour starts to change. It spends more time in the vicinity of the bar and will eventually press it again. This process continues until the exploratory activity stops and the rat repeatedly self-administers ESB. In some stimulation sites, rats will learn complex patterns of bar pressing and make many hundreds of bar presses to receive ESB. They will also ignore available food and water in order to self-stimulate.

The interpretation of the phenomenon of self-stimulation is not without controversy, but there is general agreement that such energetic responding is not just a bizarre quirk unrelated to normal motivational processes and behaviour. Rather, it might reflect in exaggerated form aspects of the normal functioning of hypothalamic and related systems in the selection of appetitive behaviour. Evidence that electrical self-stimulation is tapping into normal hypothalamic functions comes from findings that at some sites, such as in the lateral hypothalamus, the rats have to be hungry or thirsty to bar press. Also the experimenter can stimulate the same sites as those at which the rat self-stimulates. When this is done, it can often cause satiated rats to eat or drink. However, in some hypothalamic self-stimulation sites, satiety reduces or abolishes self-stimulation. Such findings indicate that self-stimulation involves the activation of pathways normally involved in the mediation of hunger/feeding or thirst/drinking.

An important feature of self-stimulation is that an animal will learn a behavioural response, such as bar pressing or maze running, to obtain it. Having learned the task, the animal will continue to work to obtain such stimulation. In behaviourist language, the brief electrical shock to a self-stimulation site provides the *reinforcement* to learn a behavioural sequence. In instrumental or operant learning (Book 1, Section 6.3.4), the reinforcing event makes the behaviour pattern that occurred immediately before it more likely to occur in that environment in the future. Here, the idea is that behaviour patterns that lead to a reinforcement become incorporated into the animal's behavioural repertoire. In terms of an understanding of the principles of motivation (Book 1, Chapter 7), the *motivation* for this behaviour is provided by the brief shock to the brain. The significance of the concepts of motivation and reinforcement will be discussed further in Book 5. For the purposes of this discussion, the important feature of the phenomenon of self-stimulation is that it identifies a further role for neural systems in the hypothalamus and related systems in the control of behaviour.

Previously in this chapter, the hypothalamus was described as making available sets of reflexes that are organized at the level of the brain stem. The phenomenon of self-stimulation indicates that the hypothalamus and related structures also provide a mechanism for incorporating new behaviour into the animal's repertoire. Bar pressing in a Skinner box might seem a very simple example of behaviour but this restricted environment is useful for studying the characteristics of the learning and behavioural modification that occurs through self-stimulation.

To summarize, the hypothalamus, in conjunction with other limbic system regions, acts to prime, or make available, reflexes that are appropriate for the immediate needs of the animal. Factors such as sexual pheromones or food deprivation determine the varieties of reflexes that are facilitated. Later discussions on electrical self-stimulation indicated that, as well as making reflexes available, hypothalamic mechanisms for reinforcement act to incorporate appetitive behaviour into the animal's behaviour repertoire. In the case of electrical self-stimulation, it is assumed that the appetitive behaviour of lever-pressing is reinforced by the electric current in the brain. In some way, this mimics the effects of, say, the reward of food to a hungry animal. While this is an overly simplified description of the functions of the hypothalamus and limbic system, it has served to illustrate how these systems act to tailor and extend an animal's behaviour by allowing the animal to adapt to its environment through the incorporation of successful (i.e. adaptive) behaviour patterns into its repertoire.

Appetitive behaviour (e.g. searching for food, laying down scent trails for a mate) as well as, for example, escape behaviour in response to a predator involves the animal forming an internal representation of its environment. This is the topic of the next section.

# 10.6   The hippocampus and cognitive maps

The hippocampus, a prominent limbic system component, is a structure lying beneath the temporal lobes and close to the amygdala. It receives its input from two sources: the temporal lobes via the entorhinal cortex and the septum via a structure called the fornix (Figure 10.7). By means of the input from the entorhinal cortex, the hippocampus receives information from wide regions of the cortex derived from all sensory systems. The hippocampus also sends fibres via the fornix to the septum and mammillary body. Via its septal inputs the hippocampus forms part of a limbic system loop which then feeds back into the hypothalamus via both the septum and mammillary body (Figure 10.7).

The hippocampus has long been known to be associated with memory functions. In rats, hippocampal damage impairs the ability to learn to run through a maze to obtain food. Here, the impairment of ability has been shown not to be related to a general memory deficit as such. Rather, the rats seem to forget information about the maze, such as which arm in the maze they have visited recently. Specifically, the deficit is in the animal's capacity for **place learning**. In other words, the animal is deficient in terms of its construction and updating of a spatial, or cognitive, map of its environment.

The concept of a cognitive map was introduced in Book 1, Section 8.2.1: Figure 10.8 (*overleaf*) shows a well-known experiment in this area carried out by Richard Morris. A rat is placed in a tank containing opaque liquid (water with milk added), with a platform placed just below the surface of the liquid. The rat is unable to detect the platform visually, and initially finds it by trial and error. Over a series of trials, however, it becomes more proficient at swimming directly towards it. The animal is able to extrapolate where the platform is, based upon cues that it can detect visually, e.g. locations and objects in the room and their location, or by means of other senses. Consider the neural processes underlying such place learning. The assumption is that neurons are able to code the location of the platform within a nervous system structure that constitutes a cognitive map of the environment. Logically, it might be expected that specific sets of neurons would be activated when the rat is swimming towards the platform and at the location of the platform.

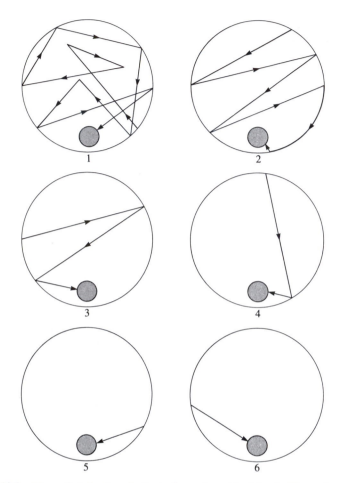

**Figure 10.8**  The rat's behaviour in the tank employed by Morris. The rat's route over six trials is shown. At first (1) the rat takes a while to locate the submerged platform. Over trials (2)–(6), the improvement in performance is clear. Note that, irrespective of where the rat starts off, it finally comes to swim directly to the platform.

In the 1970s and 80s, work by John O'Keefe and his collaborators at University College, London, helped in an understanding of the way that the nervous system underlies such place learning. O'Keefe made painstaking studies of the activity of single neurons in the rat hippocampus while the rat is exploring a complex maze (Figure 10.9a). Neurons in specific regions of the hippocampus seem to respond only to particular features of the environment. Figure 10.9b shows the behaviour of a single hippocampal neuron, called a **place cell**, while a rat is moving about in a multi-arm radial maze of the kind shown in Figure 10.9a.

☐   Examine Figure 10.9b. When is the neuron active?

■   There is the occasional background action potential wherever the rat is, but the neuron shows reliable activity above this level only when the rat is in arms 2 or 3.

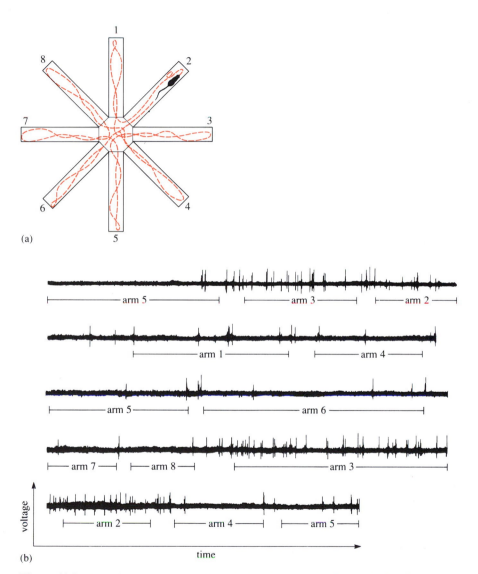

(a)

(b)

**Figure 10.9**   Experiment on place cells and place learning. (a) The kind of path generally taken by a rat in a multi-arm radial maze. (b) Response of a single cell in the hippocampus as the rat moves from arm to arm in the radial maze. The continuous recording from the cell has been divided into five sections for ease of presentation.

In O'Keefe's experiments, the rat could see the laboratory through the open tops of the arms, and there were distinctive visual stimuli arranged on the laboratory walls. The assumption that the neurons under study form part of a cognitive map implies that they are activated as a result of the rat being located in a particular place within its environment.

☐ How might you investigate whether the hippocampal cells were responding to the position of the arms of the maze relative to the visual cues in the laboratory outside the maze or to other cues, such as smell, in the arms of the maze itself?

■ One solution, the one used by the researchers, was to rotate the maze between trials (see Figure 10.10).

Suppose that a hungry rat is placed in the maze and that each arm contains one small pellet of food. The optimal strategy, i.e. the most efficient way of gathering the food, is to visit each arm only once. Now suppose that the rat has eaten the food in seven of the arms (1–7 in Figure 10.10a). The rat is removed for a while and then put back into the centre area of the maze. In between removing the rat and replacing it, the maze is turned through an angle, as shown in Figure 10.10b.

☐ If the rat is working on the basis of visual cues outside the maze, which arm would you now expect it to visit?

■ Arm 7.

☐ If the rat is working on the basis of cues within the maze (e.g. it only visits arms that have not been recently scented), which arm would you now expect it to visit?

■ Arm 8.

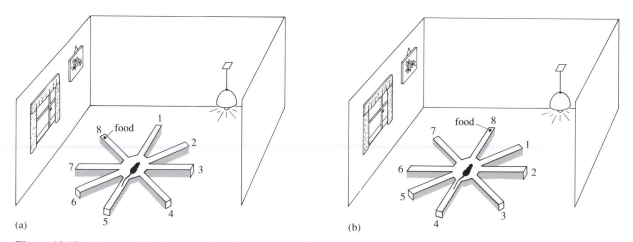

(a)

(b)

**Figure 10.10**  Maze used for demonstrating the existence of a cognitive map. (a) The rat depletes arms 1–7 of food. It is then removed from the maze for a short while. (b) The maze is rotated and the rat is returned.

In fact rats tend to take arm 7 in such a situation. In this way, O'Keefe was able to show that it was not simply features of the arms themselves, such as olfactory cues, that were important in determining the behaviour of the hippocampal cells. Rather, when the maze was rotated, cells responded when the rat was in arms that were in a particular position relative to specific visual stimuli in the laboratory. These experiments strongly suggest that hippocampal cells respond to specific 'geographic' features of the environment and collectively create a spatial map of the animal's 'world'.

In the light of these findings, the effect of hippocampal damage on a rat's ability to learn a maze is not that the rat's memory in a general sense is damaged. Other tasks are unimpaired. Rather, the animal is hindered in its ability to utilize information about environmental cues that normally are represented in a cognitive map.

# Summary of Chapter 10

Previous chapters in Book 2 introduced structures and systems in the brain that process sensory information and those that control the musculature of the body to produce behaviour. The discussions in this chapter have presented complementary information and have introduced structures and systems that play a role in the *selection* of behaviour. That is to say, placing an animal in a given environmental context will not always be associated with the same response. Behaviour depends upon the internal state of the animal, e.g. the presence of a male rat will typically elicit lordosis in a female whose hypothalamus has been sensitized by oestrogen, but not in a female not in oestrus. While the chapter's initial focus on the hypothalamus and its role in sensitizing reflexes may have given the impression of the typical mammal's behavioural control system as being akin to a clockwork toy, in fact the picture is far from one of a rigid control system.

The CNS selects responses which, although reflexly organized, are open to a central motivational influence. Insight into the role of the hypothalamus in making behaviour available was provided by an analysis of lordosis. Here, rather than acting to initiate behaviour as such, the hypothalamus was seen to act as a kind of switch which made particular sets of reflexes available. In this way, behaviour is elicited and sequenced under the immediate control of external stimuli. Through extrapolation, the kind of explanation given for lordosis might also account for the selection of a wider range of behaviour patterns.

Experiments in which stimulation of different regions of the hypothalamus played a role in the appearance of different behaviour patterns were described. These were interpreted in terms of the hypothalamus acting to prime different sets of reflexes, depending on the way that the hypothalamus itself is influenced by other systems such as other regions of the limbic system. Experiments where stimulation of the lateral and medial hypothalamus modified the behaviour of a cat towards a rat support the idea of the hypothalamus sensitizing different sets of reflexes. Similarly, it was proposed that, by monitoring body nutrient levels, information about a state of depletion causes the hypothalamus to make feeding-related reflexes available. At the same time as sensitizing reflexes, the hypothalamus plays a role in preparing the body for action in different ways via the ANS.

The picture that emerges of the hypothalamus is of a brain region that is monitoring the physiological state of the organism and making available appropriate reflexes. The hypothalamus also influences the basal ganglia via the medial forebrain bundle and the substantia nigra. In a similar way that the hypothalamus activates reflexly organized behaviour mediated by the brain stem, it was proposed that the hypothalamus activates appetitive behaviour, mediated through the basal ganglia. In this way the hypothalamus influences the selection of more 'free form' behaviour patterns that place the animal in a situation appropriate for consummatory behaviour such as eating, drinking or mating.

A link in the explanatory chain was the identification of hypothalamic involvement in the learning of appropriate appetitive behaviour patterns through the phenomenon of self-stimulation. Finally, the information about the role of the hippocampus as a spatial map points to the possibility of learning 'where' to do things as well as 'what' to do.

Discussions of the complexity of neural organization and consciousness are the subject of the next and final chapter in this book. The problem of how brain mechanisms resolve the problems of conflicting needs, for example, a hungry or thirsty animal being confronted with a sexual partner, will be discussed in Book 5.

# Objectives for Chapter 10

When you have completed this chapter, you should be able to:

10.1   Define and use, or recognize definitions and applications of each of the terms printed in **bold** in the text.

10.2   Describe ways in which sexual and defensive behaviour in response to a given stimulus can vary and relate this variation to the role of the hypothalamus. (*Questions 10.1 and 10.2*)

10.3   Give an outline of the lordosis reflex, relating its causation to its function. (*Questions 10.1 and 10.2*)

10.4   Compare behaviour rewarded by electrical stimulation of the brain with behaviour learned and maintained by conventional reinforcement (e.g. food). (*Question 10.3*)

10.5   Relate the results of experiments recording from single neurons in the hippocampus to the concept of a cognitive map and thereby explain what is meant by place learning. (*Question 10.4*)

# Questions for Chapter 10

**Question 10.1** (*Objectives 10.2 and 10.3*)
What is the main difference between the lordosis reflex and the protective reflexes described in Chapter 9? What is the functional significance of this difference?

**Question 10.2** (*Objectives 10.2 and 10.3*)
Briefly compare and contrast the lordosis reflex and the defensive reflexes discussed in Section 10.3.3. In your account, describe both causal and functional aspects.

**Question 10.3** (*Objective 10.4*)
How would you try to extinguish the behaviour of electrical self-stimulation shown by a rat in a Skinner box?

**Question 10.4** (*Objective 10.5*)
Book 1, Chapter 8 described the outcome of an experiment in which Richard Morris removed the platform from the tank and observed what happened when the rat was placed in the tank. The experiment is summarized in Figure 10.11. In terms of place cells and place learning, describe the relevance of this experiment.

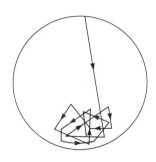

**Figure 10.11**   The path followed by a rat in the tank when the platform is removed.

# Further reading

Gallistel, C. R. (1980) *The Organization of Action—A New Synthesis*, Lawrence Erlbaum Associates.

# CHAPTER 11
## MINDING THE BRAIN

## 11.1   Introduction

The preceding chapters presented an account of the way that brain systems 'work' to analyse sensory information, to control the muscles and thereby to allow the production of appropriate physiological and behavioural responses. These descriptions were intended to give a very general picture of the functional organization of the 'typical' mammalian brain, based on 'bottom-up' neurophysiological investigations. As such, they skirted around discussions of 'higher-order' features of the more complex mammals, such as consciousness and thought. In contrast, this chapter now approaches these phenomena through descriptions of the specializations of the human brain that have been associated with the capacity to use an abstract symbolic language for communication and thought. In keeping with the general approach of this book, it takes a bottom-up approach by describing brain structures and systems that have been implicated in the human capacity to use language. However, the descriptions of the functions served by such structures, as revealed by, for example, the after-effects of damage, lead inevitably to discussion of aspects of human cognition such as memory and consciousness.

In what follows you should not worry about trying to remember all of the details of each experiment or example of brain damage. Rather, it is important to extract an appreciation of the ways in which scientists go about trying to gain an understanding of how the brain functions. For example, you need to be familiar with how brain damage arising from accidents can provide insight into how the intact brain functions, and you should come to appreciate the kinds of problems that scientists encounter in trying to define the deficits in intellectual ability that arise in this way.

In the final section of this chapter, you will also gain some familiarity with how questions on the origins of human consciousness are posed. This section describes material that spans, on the one hand, the behavioural and brain sciences and, on the other, philosophy. Do not worry if you find the style of the argument rather different from those you have met so far. You are not expected to remember all of the details. What is important is to gain some appreciation for the relevance of a 'brain and behavioural perspective' on the issue and how one prominent theorist has set about tackling it.

Chapter 11 begins in more familiar territory by considering, in terms of identifiable anatomical parts, how the brain processes information. It looks at an example where accidents causing damage to the brain have yielded insight into how the brain handles information, which led theorists to an explanatory model. The section goes on to show how the model was then refined in the light of further experience.

# 11.2   The cerebral cortex and speech

The 'classic' picture of the human cognitive ability to communicate through speech, that is to say the ability to translate ideas into words and to comprehend written or spoken communication, suggests that these capacities are uniquely dependent on the cerebral cortex. The localization of speech functions in discrete cortical regions has a relatively long history with the first accounts attributed to Dax, a French physician, in 1836. However, Dax's accounts were 'lost' and the major revival of interest in the localization of speech functions is usually attributed to another French physician, Paul Broca.

## 11.2.1   Broca's area

In the 1860s, Broca studied a number of patients who suffered from disturbances of speech and who, on post-mortem investigation, turned out to have damage to a region of the frontal lobe on the left side of the brain. The location of this area, usually called Broca's area, is shown in Figure 11.1.

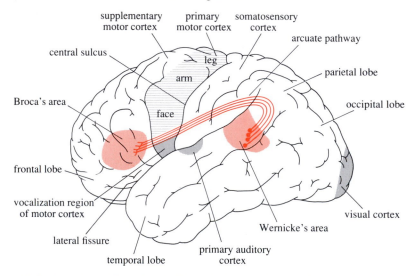

**Figure 11.1**   Location of Broca's and Wernicke's areas in the left cerebral hemisphere, and the positions of the motor, somatosensory, auditory and visual cortical regions.

Typically, patients with damage in the region of Broca's area do not lose the ability to speak but have a characteristic deficit; while they can understand speech and written instructions, their production of speech is impaired. Broca patients use only key words in a slow deliberate speech and employ very simple grammatical structures. They usually use only singular nouns and eliminate articles, adjectives and adverbs, the result being a very restricted communication. A Broca patient asked to repeat a sentence such as 'the large shiny car' may just respond 'car'. Also, the Broca patient speaks hesitantly and gropingly and is aware of his or her problems in communication. The following is a transcript of a description of the plot of a film given by a Broca patient: 'Ah!...Policeman...ah...I know!... cashier!...Money...ah!...cigarettes...I know...this guy...beer...moustache...'

The general medical term used to describe a disturbance in the use of speech is **aphasia**. Strictly speaking, the term aphasia should be used to describe an absence of speech. In such terms, disturbed speech should be described as *dysphasia*, but this course will follow the common usage and use aphasia to denote a disturbance, as well as an absence, of speech.

Disturbances usually associated with damage to Broca's area are described as non-fluent aphasias. Non-fluent aphasias are distinguished from other conditions of poorly articulated language such as those arising from uncoordination of the muscles involved in speaking, called *dysarthrias*, and those arising from weakness of the vocal apparatus, called *dysphonias*. A dysarthria can arise from localized damage to the cerebellum while a dysphonia can accompany other symptoms of Parkinson's disease. Since damage to Broca's area is characterized by difficulty in expression, the disorder is sometimes described as an *expressive aphasia*.

Another feature of Broca's aphasia is that patients usually have a reduced ability to express themselves in writing while showing no deficits in muscular coordination of the hands: that is, they can form letters and words normally. Two major implications follow from looking at the deficits in patients showing Broca's aphasia: (1) the wide range of normal motor activities is not disrupted in Broca's aphasia, so Broca's area is not directly involved in motor control, and (2) the loss of fluency in speech and writing, with no loss of comprehension, shows that Broca's area is not involved with sensory processing. The function of Broca's area in the pathway between sensory input and motor output will become clearer when other brain regions are considered.

## 11.2.2 Wernicke's area

In 1876, Carl Wernicke, a young German neurologist, reported another cortical region where localized damage also produced disorders of speech. Again, this region was located in the left hemisphere of the brain. This region, now called Wernicke's area, lies in the superior margin of the temporal lobe, as shown in Figure 11.1. Damage to Wernicke's area, however, results in a radically different form of aphasia from that described by Broca. In contrast to the Broca patient, the verbal output of a Wernicke patient has normal rate, rhythm and melody. However, they frequently use wrong words or combinations of words and add additional syllables to words and additional words to phrases. The result is that Wernicke patients fail to convey their ideas, or at least they fail to convey any meaning to their listeners. They also have problems in comprehension, both of the spoken and written word, and in writing.

The speech of a Wernicke patient has been likened to a presidential press conference: a lot of words but little meaning. An example that shows the 'grammatical' structure but opacity of meaning in speech produced by a Wernicke patient is 'And I said, this is wrong. I'm going out and doing things and getting ukuleles taken every time and I think I'm doing wrong because I'm supposed to take everything down from the top so that we do four flashes of four volumes before we get down low...' The problem of the patient with damage to Wernicke's area is sometimes described as a *receptive aphasia*.

### 11.2.3 The Wernicke–Geschwind model of language

In 1876, Wernicke published an analysis of the differences between the aphasia reported by Broca and the variety he himself discovered. He argued that the Broca patient showed a disturbance in expression or execution of language whereas Wernicke patients showed an impairment in comprehension. As an explanation of the difference, Wernicke pointed out that the two areas were connected by a pathway, the arcuate pathway, shown in Figure 11.1. He argued that the two different sets of symptoms were caused by different *patterns of disconnection* within this pathway. A Broca patient suffers from a lesion (damage) which disconnects the language system from the surrounding motor structures. The rest of the language system, including Wernicke's area, remains intact. In contrast, in a Wernicke patient, the pathways to the motor systems subserving speech are intact but the damage to Wernicke's area prevents it communicating with Broca's area via the arcuate pathway.

Wernicke proposed that the two areas play radically different roles in language functions, with the Wernicke area being involved in comprehension and the Broca area making the transformation from the internal representation of a communication to the spoken (or written) language.

The century or so following Wernicke's discovery saw many attempts to explain the localization of function in the human brain. However, it took a combination of factors for a coherent theory to emerge. Broadly, these were: (1) the view of the brain as an 'information processing device' that followed in the wake of computers and 'intelligent' machines, and (2) the availability of patients with penetrating injuries to the head as the tragic consequences of World War II and the Korean war. In this context, Wernicke's ideas of the neural basis for speech were developed further by the American neurologist Norman Geschwind, who re-awakened interest in explanations of deficits following brain injury in terms of the disconnections of brain regions. Geschwind's model is shown in Figure 11.2 and is known as the *Wernicke–Geschwind model* for language.

As an example of the type of explanation provided by the Wernicke–Geschwind model, Geschwind describes the 'route' along which information flows in the left hemisphere during the process of seeing an object and naming it. (See Figure 11.2 and the videocassette *The Human Brain* for the visual pathways.) In the first stage of the pathway, the image of an object on the retina is coded into neural activity in the optic nerve. The next stage in the pathway is the lateral geniculate nucleus (LGN), which is a nucleus in the thalamus (arrow 1). The LGN is the visual equivalent of the ventrobasal nucleus that relays and transforms information in the touch pathway (as described in Chapter 8). Early cortical processing of visual information takes place in the primary visual cortex, located in the posterior region of the occipital cortex (arrow 2). Here, several adjacent regions receive input from the LGN.

The next stage in the pathway involves a cortical region surrounding the visual areas whose name, the parietal–temporal–occipital association cortex, indicates that it is a region of cortex that encroaches into several cortical lobes (arrow 3). Since it is 'association cortex', it does not receive input directly from sensory pathways or participate directly in motor systems; rather, it is involved in bringing together information from several sensory modalities. The parietal–temporal–

occipital cortex receives input from the visual, auditory and touch systems. The implication of this is that in this region the representation of an object becomes more specific as neural activity relating to its various sensory qualities converges upon small groups of neurons.

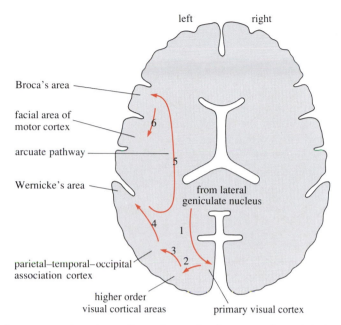

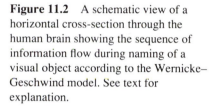

**Figure 11.2**   A schematic view of a horizontal cross-section through the human brain showing the sequence of information flow during naming of a visual object according to the Wernicke–Geschwind model. See text for explanation.

Wernicke's area receives input from the parietal–temporal–occipital association cortex (arrow 4). In this way, it receives information about the sensory qualities of an object. Wernicke proposed that a function of this area was categorization of sensory information in the internal 'codes' appropriate to the language system. Axons from Wernicke's area travel as the arcuate pathway (arrow 5) to synapse in Broca's area. In turn, Broca's area connects with regions of the motor cortex that control muscles in the facial region, including the speech apparatus (arrow 6).

Geschwind proposed that this 'model' of information flow during the activity of naming a visual object is able to account for the effects of a lesion in Wernicke's or Broca's areas. With damage to Wernicke's area, visual images (or spoken words) which would normally be categorized and 'coded' appropriately for the language system, fail to be processed in a language-related way and so do not enter subsequent stages in the language system or are only partially processed. Thus, a lesion to Wernicke's area leaves the language system with no, or incomplete, information and results in a lack of comprehension of sensory information. With such a lesion, while sensory processing itself is not affected, a Wernicke patient is unable to recognize objects or to respond to written and verbal instructions.

Geschwind proposed that Broca's area has two major roles. First, it translates the perceptual aspects of language into a grammatical structure and, second, it translates the grammatical structure of a phrase into 'instructions' for the motor cortex to produce the appropriate sounds (or writing movements).

☐   What predictions does the Wernicke–Geschwind model for language make about the effects of a lesion to Broca's area.

■ First, the connections that Wernicke's area makes with the rest of the brain will be intact so that a Broca patient will have good comprehension of spoken and written language (and his or her own performance problems). Second, and crucial to the disorder, is that the capacity to translate a communication into plans for either appropriate patterns of movement of the muscles of the vocal apparatus, or for writing movements, will be abolished or restricted.

In this way, the Wernicke–Geschwind model of language accounts for the differences between the symptoms of Wernicke's and Broca's aphasia. The value of Geschwind's analysis is that, by focusing on disconnections within pathways, it provides an intuitively plausible understanding of the effects of damage to regions of the left hemisphere in terms of interruption of the flow of information. Furthermore, while acknowledging that different regions of the cortex have different functions, it provides an account of the flow of information between regions of the cortex without requiring the nature of the information passed or the nature of the processing that is carried out within brain regions to be described in more than very general terms.

## 11.2.4 Contemporary views on the localization of language functions

Based on evidence of the effects of localized damage to the human cortex described previously, the following picture emerges. The ability to speak, i.e. to translate thoughts into spoken words and to comprehend spoken and written language, depends on the integrity of a relatively circumscribed pathway that includes Broca's and Wernicke's areas in the left hemisphere connected by the arcuate pathway. This position, encapsulated in the Wernicke–Geschwind model discussed previously, presents a highly localized view of language processing.

More recently, studies of the way that electrical stimulation of the brain produces disturbances of language, and also of the activity of brain regions during speech and thought, has produced evidence for a wider involvement of brain structures in language processing than that suggested by the Wernicke–Geschwind model. Also, while confirming that Broca's and Wernicke's areas are important for speech, these studies indicate that the 'division of labour' between Broca's and Wernicke's areas is not as clear cut as suggested by the Wernicke–Geschwind model.

Figure 11.3 shows regions in which electrical stimulation of the cortex has been found to interfere with speech in conscious patients who were undergoing exploratory investigations prior to surgery. These regions include the primary somatosensory and motor regions for the face located on either side of the central sulcus, Broca's area, Wernicke's area and an extensive region surrounding it. Wernicke's area and the surrounding region are known collectively as the posterior speech zone. There is also a further area of cortex 'tucked' down into the central fissure that separates the two areas of cortex at the midline. This region, which is anterior to the primary motor cortex, is called the supplementary motor region. Electrical stimulation of cortical regions outside these areas was not found to interfere with speech.

The evidence that stimulation of some regions of the cortex produces disturbances of speech, while others do not, is taken as evidence for their involvement in language functions.

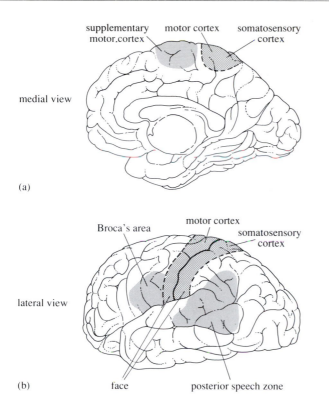

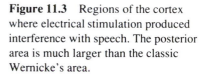

**Figure 11.3**   Regions of the cortex where electrical stimulation produced interference with speech. The posterior area is much larger than the classic Wernicke's area.

☐   What is a possible objection to this interpretation?

■   The stimulation of a particular brain site (call it 'B') might excite fibres *en route* between two other areas, 'A' and 'C', so that the anatomical connections activated would not necessarily have originated in the area (B) in which the electrical stimulation was found to be effective.

One counter to this objection is that in the cortex there is a high degree of local connectivity between cortical regions, but connections with sub-cortical structures travel 'downwards' rather than 'across'. This suggests that the picture of connectivity gained from electrical stimulation of the cortex will be reliable, particularly in defining the boundaries of the regions of cortex in which electrical stimulation interferes with speech.

Another recent approach to mapping cortical regions involved in language uses Positron Emission Tomography (PET scanning) to look at local changes in blood flow in the cerebral cortex that occur during the performance of language-related tasks (see Box 11.1, *overleaf*). Modern sophisticated PET scanners can take almost instantaneous measurements of a large number of cortical regions simultaneously. This information can then be presented as a picture of the surface of the brain broken down into adjacent sections, showing the blood flow in each.

☐ Scanning is used to investigate the functioning of the cortex. What basic assumption must be made in order to do this?

■ That changes in blood flow in a certain cortical region correlate with changes in the activity of the neurons in that region.

In practice, during the performance of sensory and motor tasks, the expected regions of sensory and motor cortex do show an increase in blood flow, confirming that this basic assumption about the relationship between blood flow and neuronal activity is a valid one.

---

### Box 11.1   Positron Emission Tomography (PET)

This is a technique which measures the regional distribution of a previously administered radioactive element that emits positively charged particles called positrons. Positron-emitting elements have been incorporated into naturally-occurring compounds such as water or oxygen for administration to patients who are placed in a PET scanning apparatus. This enables factors such as blood flow, neuroreceptor activity and neurotransmitter metabolism to be measured quantitatively *in vivo* (that is, in a living subject). Mathematical calculations convert the PET data into relevant physiological measures of brain processes that are active during particular functions of the brain. Computer-generated images of these measures can then be displayed on a TV screen. Comparisons can be made of low and high levels of activity between normal control subjects and patients or animals treated in different ways.

---

In 1988, Petersen and colleagues working at Washington University in the USA produced evidence, using the PET scan technique, to show that wider regions of the brain, other than sensory and motor regions, are active during language-related tasks (Petersen *et al.*, 1988). Petersen presented his subjects with words under three conditions. In the first, they were required just to listen to, or look at, the word. In the second, they had to repeat the word. And, in the third condition, called the association task, they had to think of, and speak a use for, the word presented. For example, if the word presented was 'bread', the output might be 'eat'.

Petersen suggested that PET scanning while the first task was being carried out would show which regions were involved in basic sensory processing. The second would show which regions were involved in sensory and motor processing. The third would show which regions were involved in sensory, motor and cognitive processing. He then argued that by subtracting the first PET picture from the second, the result would show which regions were involved in the motor functions of speech. Further, by subtracting the second picture from the third, he argued that the cortical regions involved in cognitive processing would emerge.

As a start, Petersen's results confirmed the findings from electrical stimulation: that primary motor and sensory cortex, the supplementary motor area and Broca's and Wernicke's areas are involved in the production of speech. Figure 11.4 shows the activity in cortical regions attributable to each of the three conditions: sensory, motor and association.

Two features of the distributions of activity are interesting and provide evidence for the involvement of cortical regions outside Broca's and Wernicke's areas in language processing. The first relates to the regions that are active during the sensory processing of the language stimuli. Look at the four triangles in Figure 11.4. The solid triangle shows the region active during visual presentation and the open triangles the regions active during auditory presentation. The most anterior open triangle corresponds to activation of that region of cortex known to process auditory stimuli. Similarly, the single solid triangle occurs in the region of cortex known to process visual information.

With the identification of two of the four triangles as indicating activity in sensory processing regions, this leaves just the remaining two open triangles, indicating activity in Wernicke's area.

☐   What do these triangles 'say' about the function of Wernicke's area?

■   These two open triangles indicate that Wernicke's area is active during auditory presentation of language. The absence of any solid triangles in this region suggests that Wernicke's area is not involved in processing language presented in written form.

☐   What will be the disabilities in understanding spoken and written language following a lesion to Wernicke's area predicted by the Wernicke–Geschwind model and on the basis of Petersen's findings?

■   The Wernicke–Geschwind model predicts that there will be impairment of comprehension of both written and spoken language.  On the basis of Petersen's findings only an impairment in comprehension of speech is expected, not of written communication.

Studies of patients with language difficulties following brain damage support the Petersen prediction that there can be a dissociation of impairment of comprehension between spoken and written language. There are numbers of clinical reports on patients who are able to understand speech but not writing, and on patients who are able to understand written but not spoken instructions. In most of these patients, the precise locations and extents of any brain lesions are not known, so that anatomical evidence for the brain systems mediating these different language functions is not available. However, this evidence of the dissociation of disabilities for comprehension of spoken and written material indicates that the processing of the auditory and visual components of language information occurs in systems that are functionally more separated than the Wernicke–Geschwind model suggests.

The second interesting feature of Petersen's findings concerns the areas of cortex that it shows to be involved in the associative or cognitive elements of the tasks. The regions of activity attributed to the generation of a word related to the stimulus are indicated in Figure 11.4 by the squares.  The most anterior pair of squares, one solid and the other open, lies well outside Broca's area in the frontal lobes of the cortex.

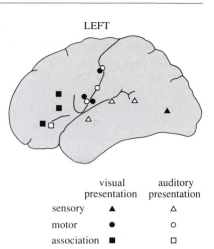

LEFT

|  | visual presentation | auditory presentation |
|---|---|---|
| sensory | ▲ | △ |
| motor | ● | ○ |
| association | ■ | □ |

**Figure 11.4**   The results of Petersen's experiment—see text for details. Solid symbols (▲, ●, ■) show areas of cortex that were active when the word was presented visually. Open symbols (△, ○, □) show areas of cortex that were active when the presentation was auditory (spoken).

Thus, Petersen's findings can be seen not to fit the Wernicke–Geschwind model. First, cortical areas outside the pathway consisting of Wernicke's area, the arcuate pathway and Broca's area are involved in language. Secondly, Wernicke's area does not play a 'universal' role in the comprehension of language. While Wernicke's area is involved in comprehension of spoken language, other structures are involved in the comprehension of written language. There are also other aspects of the Wernicke–Geschwind model that are controversial. It is now commonly accepted that lesions in Broca's area can produce deficits in comprehension and that lesions in the posterior speech region, which includes Wernicke's area, can also produce expressive aphasias that were originally thought to result only from lesions in Broca's area.

The Wernicke–Geschwind model of language summarized information about those regions of the brain that are concerned with the production of speech, which in the majority of people is organized on the left side of the brain. The equivalent regions to Broca's and Wernicke's areas in the right hemisphere have also been implicated in language functions. Localized damage to the right-side regions leave cognitive aspects of language intact but impair the comprehension of affective (emotional) aspects.

Along with the verbal content of spoken language, the melody and intonation of speech and the accompanying movements of the hands and face also convey affect. That is, they provide the emotional overtones of the communication. To an extent, similar receptive and expressive changes to those seen after damage in the left hemisphere are also seen after damage to the right cortex. Damage to posterior regions of the right hemisphere (Wernicke equivalent) produces impairments in comprehending the non-verbal affective components accompanying spoken language. Damage to anterior regions in the right cortex (Broca equivalent) produces impairments in the expression of emotional aspects; typically there is a reduction in facial and bodily expression.

## Summary of Section 11.2

The work of Norman Geschwind in the 1950s and 60s was a turning point in the development of a theoretical understanding of the neural bases of language. From this starting point, a better understanding of the way that the brain processes language has developed. The Wernicke–Geschwind model for language is now seen to be not wrong but rather an oversimplification of the processes that contribute to language and thinking. While the involvement of Broca's and Wernicke's areas is not disputed, they are now seen to be just two regions of the cortex among several that are implicated in language functions. The model provided an organizing framework for subsequent research and development of models. It enabled the distinction between expressive aphasia and receptive aphasia to be drawn and was a stimulus in the search for brain structures underlying language. Perhaps the greatest oversimplification of the Wernicke–Geschwind model lies in its identification of the arcuate pathway as *the* channel conveying information 'comprehended' by Wernicke's area for output via Broca's area. The findings of Petersen indicate that while Wernicke's area is involved in processing auditory information, it is not involved in reading. The implications of Petersen's findings are that different language sub-systems are used to process speech and written information.

The fact that numerous patients have been studied in whom the ability to comprehend spoken instructions remains intact while the ability to comprehend written instructions is impaired, or vice versa, suggests that the anatomical bases for these sub-systems are also distinct. The contemporary view of brain regions involved in language processing is then not of a system organized as a series of stages, in which there is a flow of information down a central 'channel'. Rather, language processing is seen to be carried out simultaneously in parallel by separate channels that process spoken and written information independently. This topic will be revisited in Book 6 in this course.

Another aspect of the Wernicke–Geschwind model that has come under criticism is its sharply-defined division of function between Broca's and Wernicke's areas. Contrary to the Wernicke–Geschwind model, expressive aphasias can result from lesions in Wernicke's area and receptive aphasias from lesions in Broca's area. The full implications of these findings are not clear. They could be explained by variation between individuals in the roles that individual brain structures play, possibly as a result of different developmental pressures on the individual. Or they may indicate that the functions of Broca's and Wernicke's areas are even more complex than previously suggested and that sophisticated modern tests for disturbance of language have shown up complexity of function which earlier, less sophisticated tests did not reveal.

For the purposes of this discussion, which has been to introduce evidence for the specialization of the human brain for language, the Wernicke–Geschwind model provided a good stepping-off point. Damage to the central nervous system as a result of strokes, tumours or penetrating missile injuries very rarely produces a lesion affecting only a specific area of the brain as defined in terms of the brain sciences. What the Wernicke–Geschwind model did was to help to bring together descriptions of differences in speech-related deficits with descriptions of human neuroanatomy. Geschwind gave neurologists and scientists interested in the structure of human cognition a framework, albeit a crude one, for understanding how the human brain organizes its cognitive functions at a neuroanatomical level.

# 11.3  Lateralization of brain structure and cognitive functions

The previous section looked at the localization of structures that are involved in the control of speech in the human brain. The ability to use language is one aspect of human cognitive ability, the capacity to think and reason that everyone takes for granted. Next, the discussions will introduce evidence for the localization of other aspects of the cognitive functions of the human brain that have emerged from studies of the effects of damage to the brain. These studies show that the two hemispheres of the brain are not usually *equally* involved in performing the processes that underlie such skills as writing and speaking. One hemisphere might have sole responsibility or at least the dominant responsibility for a particular skill. This asymmetrical distribution of function in the brain is termed **lateralization**.

## 11.3.1  Verbal and non-verbal components of intelligence

In most right-handed people, the brain structures that are implicated in language are located in the left hemisphere. There is thus an asymmetry in the functions of the two hemispheres. Evidence for such functional asymmetry comes from studies of the effects of general damage to either left or right hemispheres which shows up as characteristic differences in standard tests of human performance. Standard tests of intelligence result in a score called the **intelligence quotient (IQ)**. The Wechsler intelligence test is an example of an intelligence test which distinguishes between verbal and spatial abilities by having two components, one a set of conventional written questions and the other a set of questions involving the manipulation of spatial relationships, such as those shown in Figure 11.5.

As expected, damage to the left hemisphere impairs tasks that depend upon verbal ability, e.g. written questions. In contrast, damage to the right hemisphere has little effect on scores in verbal tests but impairs performance on tasks that depend on an ability to comprehend spatial relationships.

## 11.3.2  Development of cognitive functions

A study by Hans Teuber (1975), working in the USA, shed light on the development of cognitive structures in the human brain. Teuber carried out a longitudinal study (following subjects for long periods of time) investigating the consequences of brain damage at different ages. His population included 34 subjects who had suffered brain damage during the immediate post-natal period, whom he studied when they were adolescents. One index used was verbal and spatial performance scores, obtained from the Wechsler IQ test, which has adult and child scales.

A feature of Teuber's results is that individuals who suffered brain damage in infancy did show evidence of recovery but in ways that were initially unexpected. In contrast, individuals who suffered brain damage as adults showed very little evidence for recovery of function.

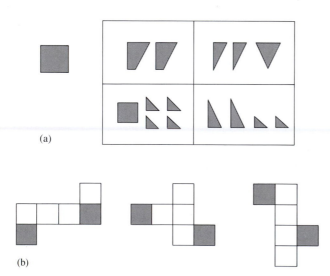

**Figure 11.5**  Examples of visuo-spatial tasks. (a) Which boxed set(s) can form the square on the outside? (b) If you fold these patterns into cubes, in which cube(s) will the dark sides meet at one edge?

Figure 11.6a shows Wechsler IQ test data from 21 subjects, adolescents who had suffered severe damage to the left hemisphere during infancy. It shows the averaged scores of these 21 subjects along with the scores obtained by 21 controls (normal siblings of the patients) on the overall IQ score and on the verbal and spatial performance components.

☐   What interpretation can be made of the differences in the scores of the subjects who suffered early left hemisphere damage and controls shown in Figure11.6a?

■   The difference in scores indicates that both aspects of intelligence, verbal and spatial performance are depressed by early damage to the left hemisphere.

Normally, the right hemisphere is predominantly involved in aspects of spatial performance and the left in verbal performance. However, unexpectedly, Figure 11.6a shows that subjects with damage to the left hemisphere performed equally well on verbal tasks as on spatial tasks. In fact, even subjects who suffered left hemisphere damage in *adulthood* did not show a marked reduction in spatial performance scores compared with their performance on verbal tasks.

Figure 11.6b shows the scores on the same tests obtained by 13 adolescents who had suffered damage to the right hemisphere during infancy, along with the scores of 13 controls (normal siblings).

☐   How do you interpret the differences in the scores between patients who suffered early right hemisphere damage and normal controls, as shown in Figure 11.6b?

■   The reduction in scores shown by the patients in Figure 11.6b compared with controls is in line with the conventional wisdom about localization of speech and visuo-spatial functions in left and right hemispheres, respectively. Damage to the right hemisphere produces a drop in spatial performance but does not markedly affect verbal performance.

Teuber concluded that the left and right hemispheres become committed to their functions at different times. He argued:

1   that the time course for the development of language structures differs from the time course(s) of development of structures that contribute to performance on non-verbal IQ scores and

2   that the language system becomes committed early while the right hemisphere still remains 'flexible'.

A consequence of this plasticity is that, after early left hemisphere damage, language functions can develop in the right hemisphere. However, this reduces the 'space' available for the development of non-verbal functions, so there is a reduction in both verbal and spatial performance. Where there is early damage to the right hemisphere, the left hemisphere is already committed to language functions, and the spatial functions cannot find enough uncommitted neural tissue in the left hemisphere in which to develop fully. The result is a marked reduction in non-verbal performance with no comparable drop in verbal performance, which is in line with the pattern of verbal and non-verbal deficits seen after damage to the right hemisphere.

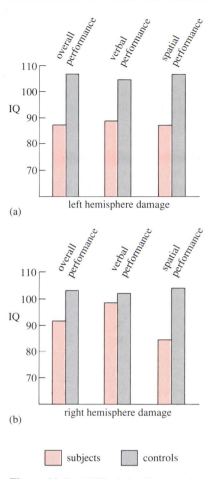

**Figure 11.6**   (a) Wechsler IQ score for 21 adolescent subjects who had suffered severe damage to the left hemisphere during infancy are compared with scores of 21 controls (normal siblings). (b) Wechsler IQ scores for 13 adolescent subjects who had suffered severe damage to the right hemisphere during infancy are compared with the scores of 13 controls (normal siblings). Differences between subjects and controls are significant except for verbal performance associated with right-hemisphere damage.

### 11.3.3 Structural correlates of language functions—comparative aspects

The use of an abstract symbolic language to communicate by means of speech is one characteristic that distinguishes humans from other primates. There is evidence that non-human primates such as chimpanzees use sounds and gestures for communication that share features of language. Chimpanzees have also been trained to use a vocal or gestural language (such as the sign language used by deaf people) that follows the structure of human language. However, they learn this kind of language very slowly and only to a limited extent. Following a massive review of the literature, the UK psychologist Euan Macphail concluded in 1982 that 'humans acquire language (and non-humans do not), not because humans are more intelligent (*per se*), but because humans possess some species-specific mechanism which is a prerequisite of language-acquisition'. In this context, in 1968, Norman Geschwind and Walter Levitsky published the results of a study in which they systematically investigated the anatomical correlates of language functions in the human brain by measuring brain regions. They measured the left and right hemispheres in 100 human brains post-mortem. The feature that they measured was the planum temporale, which lies in the temporal gyrus, and on the left side contains the posterior speech area which includes Wernicke's area (Figure 11.7).

In 65% of the brains they found that the left planum temporale was larger than the right; in 24% they were approximately equal in size; and only in 11% was the right larger than the left. Later work using non-invasive scanning procedures confirmed these observations in adults and also in human fetuses. While left/right asymmetries are reported to occur between brain regions in non-human animals such as chickens and frogs and are not exclusive to the human brain, it is significant that left/right asymmetries are not reported to occur in the planum temporale in non-human primates.

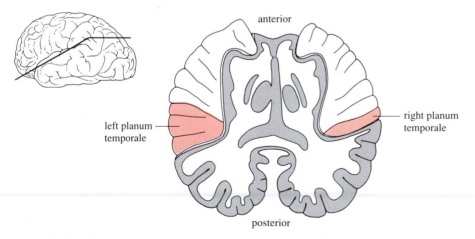
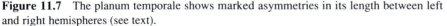

**Figure 11.7** The planum temporale shows marked asymmetries in its length between left and right hemispheres (see text).

An implication of Geschwind and Levitsky's finding is that language functions do not necessarily develop in the left hemisphere. They suggest that, as indicated by the enlargement of the planum temporale, language functions develop in the right hemisphere in a proportion of the population. There is a further suggestion that, in some individuals, language functions are not lateralized. These predictions, based on anatomical structure, have been confirmed to some extent by a behavioural study of the lateralization of language functions. Here, a fast acting barbiturate anaesthetic was injected into either the left or right carotid arteries in conscious subjects. The left and right carotid arteries supply blood to the left and right hemispheres, respectively. The subjects were either left-handed, right-handed, or ambidextrous. As the anaesthetic was injected, the subjects were instructed to count out loud. If the barbiturate reached the hemisphere containing language functions, the counting stopped. The results of the investigation are shown in Table 11.1. These results confirm that language is not exclusively lateralized in the left hemisphere but that the right hemisphere can also be dominant for language, that is to say it can have sole control of speech.

**Table 11.1**  Percentages of subjects for whom language was found to be dominant in the left hemisphere, dominant in the right hemisphere, or dominant in neither.

|  | Left | No apparent dominance | Right |
|---|---|---|---|
| Language dominance | 83% | 9.5% | 7.5% |

Table 11.1 shows that, for most people, the left hemisphere exerts a dominant control over speech. For some people though, either the right hemisphere is dominant or there is no apparent hemispheric dominance.

## 11.3.4  Development of cognitive structures and recovery from brain damage

The picture of the development of the CNS that emerges from mammalian studies is of a system resulting from a complex interaction between genetic and environmental factors. The development of the mammalian CNS will be discussed in detail in Book 4 in this course. During development the genetic 'program', which (except in the case of identical twins) is unique to the individual, unfolds but not in an absolute way. That is to say, at each stage, its expression is influenced not only by the individual's current environment but by all the interactions that have already taken place between the genotype and the environment. That is, at any stage, the genetic program is expressed within a developmental state that is unique to that individual.

On the one hand, there is a progressive unfolding of genetic factors that specify features of the brain's structure. On the other, these genetic factors unfold within the context of the specific nervous system structures and environmental influences that act at that time. You will remember from Book 1, Chapters 3 and 5, that the genotype is not a blue-print that specifies precisely how structures develop, but rather that their specification is more fluid, allowing for variability in the developing brain structure within which they operate.

A conclusion from the Teuber study described previously (Section 11.3.2) on the consequences of damage to the region in the left cortex that would normally develop language systems, is that the continuing expression of genetic factors that influence the development of language structures results in the 'colonization' of other cortical areas. The evidence that, in some 20% of the population, speech is represented in the right hemisphere or in both left and right hemispheres (Table 11.1) also indicates that the development of language systems is not specified in an absolute or rigid way. Rather, under situations where there is no abnormality in development, the right cortex also has the capacity to develop structures that support language.

It is a reasonable hypothesis that recovery from the effects of damage to the left cortex takes advantage of this ability of the normal right cortex to develop language structures. It is possible that language functions develop in regions of the temporal lobes either because: (1) these regions have some intrinsic structure required for the development of language, or (2) other regions of the cortex such as the primary and secondary sensory regions and the motor regions become committed to their functions and mature earlier than regions of association cortex such as the temporal lobes. However, both possibilities remain speculative suggestions.

Teuber's study of damaged brains shows that compensation can occur if the damage is to the very young brain. In contrast, after damage to the language structures in the adult brain, there is little compensation. Cases of extensive damage to the cortex confirm the general picture of lateralization of speech in the left hemisphere. In some rare cases, the entire left cortex has been removed in individuals who were left-dominant for speech. The speech that such individuals have left is reported to be restricted to very limited utterances such as the swearing that often spontaneously accompanies emotional stress.

While Teuber's evidence is indirect, it does suggest that the ability of the human brain to recover from the effects of damage depends upon its ability to develop or modify its micro-structure. That is, recovery of language functions after damage depends on the ability to form or reform the pathways and connections that bring different sources of 'information' together in ways that enable language to be used. The strong implication of Teuber's studies is that recovery of language functions is not possible to any significant extent outside the period when the human brain is normally developing its language structures.

Evidence cited in this chapter about: (1) the effects of damage to Broca's and Wernicke's areas or the arcuate pathway, (2) the studies of the regions of the brain that are active during speech, (3) the asymmetry in the human planum temporale, and (4) the evidence for a restricted period for the development of language, all point to a predisposition of the human brain to develop structures specific for language in which, in the majority of individuals, control of speech is on the left hand side of the brain.

The ability of humans to communicate using a symbolic language distinguishes us from most animals, except closely related primates such as chimpanzees. Even here, there is an obvious difference in the degree to which language can be acquired and used. Studies in which infant chimps have been raised either as members of human families or with intensive coaching in the use of speech indicate that the abilities, even of chimps, are extremely limited and acquired with only very great difficulty. In contrast, human children acquire language very easily. In the relatively short period of four years after birth, a child picks up the complexities of spoken language, regardless of what its native tongue and cultural environment actually are. A child hears language from its parents, siblings and others in an informal way. No-one has to teach a child the formalities of sentence construction. Studies of language development indicate that when children first start to form sentences it is not done in an haphazard or random way. It is accepted that children extract the rules of grammar and syntax and put them to use without being consciously aware of them.

The linguist Noam Chomsky, working in Cambridge, Massachusetts, argues that humans inherit a specific process which he calls the *language acquisition device*, which gives us 'universal rules of grammar'. These universal rules give a child the ability to recognize the structure of his or her native language. Then, what has to be learned is the particular language, for example French or English, embedded in a specific dialect and accent. Another view is that language learning is just a specific instance of a more general cognitive ability, in the same way that humans do not, for example, have to learn consciously to distinguish objects from their backgrounds or to infer causality from temporally related sequences of experiences. It is argued that thought, and so language, are similar in this respect.

## Summary of Section 11.3

Section 11.3 has presented further evidence that the human cerebral cortex, far from being symmetrical, is highly asymmetrical in both structure and function. The most striking anatomical difference lies in the development of the planum temporale, a region which includes Wernicke's area, which in most people is greatly enlarged on the left side of the brain. Evidence from damage to the left and right hemispheres in humans shows that the anatomical asymmetries are parallelled by functional asymmetries. In the majority of people the left hemisphere is dominant for the production of speech.

Damage to the left hemisphere produces deficits in receptive or expressive aspects of spoken or written language, also called receptive and expressive aphasias, depending on the regions suffering the damage.

The difference in the ability of human and non-human primates to acquire and use language has been interpreted as being due to a species-specific human neurological structure that allows the acquisition of language. Anatomical evidence indicates that, in the majority of humans, the planum temporale on the left side is enlarged relative to the right. The fact that a significant proportion of brains examined post-mortem have either a reversed asymmetry or no asymmetry suggests that a proportion of the normal population have speech controlled from the right hemisphere or show bilateral control. This prediction is borne out by behavioural studies which show that significant proportions of normal humans have speech controlled from the right hemisphere or from both hemispheres.

Damage to the infant brain can be followed by some recovery of language and non-verbal cognitive functions, as measured by IQ tests. The capacity of the adult to recover from damage is more restricted. The patterns of recovery of verbal and non-verbal functions seen after damage to the infant brain suggest that the systems that contribute to verbal cognitive functions mature earlier than those contributing to non-verbal cognitive functions. Furthermore, the ability to recover from the effects of brain damage depends on the availability of the normal processes of development, which are not available in the adult brain. The ability of the normal right hemisphere to develop control over language suggests that the process of development of any species-specific neurological structures that contribute to the acquisition and use of language in humans is not the result of a highly specific genetic blueprint but is 'programmed' in a more flexible way.

# 11.4 Memory, amnesia and consciousness

In this section, information about memory systems in the brain that has emerged largely through studies of the after-effects of brain damage will be described. The biochemical and structural correlates of memory stores will be discussed in detail in Book 4 in this course.

As well as being involved in the comprehension and production of language, the human temporal lobes have also been implicated in long-term memory functions. The human brain is able to store information for very long periods of time. In the study of human memory, it is conventional to distinguish between **working memory** (sometimes also called **short-term memory**) and **long-term memory** storage. Our experience of only being able to remember unfamiliar phone numbers for short periods (seconds rather than minutes) unless repeated to ourselves is an example of the transient nature of working memory.

Long-term memory has different characteristics from working memory, as evidenced by our ability to remember frequently used phone numbers. Evidence for the involvement of the temporal lobes in long-term memory functions comes from patients who have had accidental damage to regions of the temporal lobes or who have had temporal lobe tissue removed surgically.

## 11.4.1 Temporal lobes and epilepsy

The temporal lobes are large regions of the cortex that curve down and under towards the midline of the brain. The area of temporal lobe immediately beneath the parietal lobe is the lateral region. As this structure folds down and around, it becomes the medial region of the temporal lobes, which form the underside of the cortex, as shown in Figure 11.8. The medial temporal lobe merges with the entorhinal cortex which, in turn provides a major input to the hippocampus, via the subiculum.

The lateral temporal lobes are sites that are vulnerable to damage and damaged temporal lobe tissue is often the source of epileptic activity. Activity occurring simultaneously in many neurons in a damaged region can spread to other, normally functioning, regions of the brain causing an epileptic seizure. In some epileptic patients where anti-convulsive drugs do not control the condition, damaged temporal lobe tissue is removed to reduce the incidence of seizures.

Damage to the temporal lobes results in very little impairment, if any, to someone's working memory but can have quite dramatic effects on long-term memory. Brenda Milner, working at McGill University in Montreal in 1966, carried out a study of the deficits of people who had lost left or right lateral temporal lobe tissue. She found that right-sided lateral temporal lobe lesions produced deficits in memory for non-verbal material. Non-verbal material is material that is difficult to classify verbally, such as abstract patterns. Milner found deficits whether the material was presented visually or aurally.

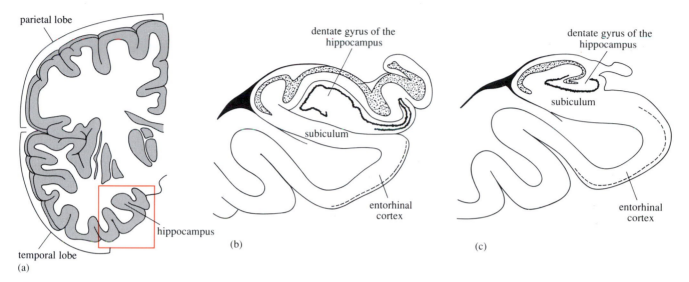

**Figure 11.8**   (a) A coronal section through the left side of the brain showing the temporal and parietal lobes of the brain and the hippocampus. (b) Enlargement of the hippocampal area of (a), showing the entorhinal cortex, subiculum and dentate gyrus. (c) A more posterior section of the area shown in (b).

On the one hand, Milner's subjects with right temporal lobe lesions did not show significant impairment in learning verbal material. Her subjects with left temporal lobe lesions showed quite the opposite impairments. They showed little impairment in non-verbal learning tasks, such as those requiring manipulation of the relationships of objects to each other or in remembering sequences of movements, but were significantly impaired in verbal learning tasks.

This pattern of relationship between the site of a lesion and the effects on behaviour where (1) a lesion at site A produces disturbances only in function X and (2) a lesion in site B produces a disturbance in function Y but not X, is called a **double dissociation**. It is taken as strong evidence for the localization of function X in site A and function Y in site B.

☐   Given the double dissociation between functions affected by right- and left-side damage to the lateral temporal lobes, what can be concluded about the functions of the left and right lateral temporal lobes?

■   The double dissociation shows that the left lateral temporal lobe plays a role in the processing and/or storage of verbal material while the right lateral lobe plays a role in the processing and/or storage of material that is not classified verbally.

## 11.4.2  Temporal lobes and the amnesic syndrome

The single most influential study of memory impairments following damage to the temporal lobes was carried out by Milner in the 1950s and 60s on a subject called H.M. H.M. had had temporal lobe tissue removed on both sides of his brain (a bilateral lesion) to alleviate severe epilepsy. As well as removing localized regions of lateral and medial temporal lobe tissue, the lesion encroached through the entorhinal cortex and subiculum into the hippocampus and also into the amygdala, on both sides of the brain (see Figure 11.9).

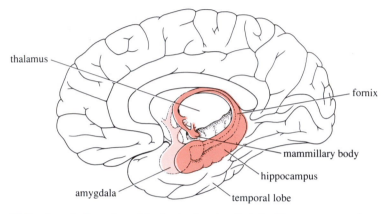

**Figure 11.9**   A sagittal section of the brain showing that the hippocampus and amygdala are sub-cortical structures underlying the temporal lobe.

After the operation, H.M. was left with a profound **anterograde amnesia**, that is, an inability to remember anything new for any length of time. For example, on each occasion H.M. met a person, such as his hospital physicians whom he saw regularly, he had to be re-introduced. Also, he could not remember what had been said or what had been done on previous examinations. Milner's testing showed that H.M.'s working (short-term) memory was normal. His digit span, i.e. his ability to repeat back lists of random digits in the correct order as soon as they had been spoken, was normal. Also, H.M.'s ability to use language and to know the meanings of words remained intact.

Subsequent testing revealed that H.M. also had a **retrograde amnesia**, that is his memory for events that occurred before his operation was also impaired. One method that gives a good measure of retrograde amnesia is to ask the patient to name photographs of the politicians, statesmen, pop stars, film stars and other celebrities who were prominent in particular periods or to give information about what they were or what they did. H.M. was unable to recall events that had occurred less than twelve years before his operation. While he was apparently able to recall events from his childhood, there has subsequently been controversy as to whether this evidence is reliable. His apparent recall may have been influenced by the way that questions about his childhood memories were asked; the mode of asking might have cued him into making responses that suggested a capacity for recall.

One area where H.M. was able to acquire information was in his development of new motor skills. Day-by-day, with practice, he was able to improve his performance on tasks classed as motor learning, such as learning to navigate his way through a finger maze, even though he was not able to recall having practiced on the maze.

H.M.'s symptoms following his operation provide the classic description of the *amnesic syndrome*:

1   a profound anterograde amnesia,

2   a less profound retrograde amnesia,

3   a preserved capability to use and understand spoken and written language, and

4   a preserved capacity for motor learning.

H.M.'s symptoms provided a powerful impetus to research into the neurophysiological basis of human memory. Although data from a single subject must be interpreted with caution, H.M. provided evidence for the existence of at least three memory systems in the human brain. The effect of the bilateral temporal lobe lesion dissociated working memory from long-term memory for events. However, not all aspects of long-term memory were disrupted, suggesting that the long-term memory for events was mediated by different systems from those for the long-term memory for language and motor skills.

Some subjects displaying disturbances of memory other than the global deficit shown by H.M. also show difficulties in remembering the order in which recent events have taken place and in remembering when and where information was acquired. There are suggestions that these deficits are separable from the amnesic syndrome and are attributable to damage to the medial thalamus and to the mammillary bodies of the hypothalamus or to regions of the frontal cortex. Damage to these structures, as well as more diffuse degeneration throughout the cortex, is seen in patients suffering from Korsakoff's syndrome. This results from a thiamine deficiency caused by chronic alcohol abuse. As well as showing amnesia, Korsakoff patients show marked problems in remembering the order of events and sources of information.

## 11.4.3   Amnesia and the localization of memory functions

The problems of determining which brain structures are involved with which aspects of memory disorders are acute because 'Mother Nature' rarely carries out well controlled 'experiments'. The poor lifestyle of individuals who become Korsakoff syndrome patients generally results in more brain damage than just to the medial thalamus, mammillary bodies and frontal cortex. Similarly, victims of stroke or other accidents that result in loss of brain cells, such as carbon monoxide poisoning, rarely have localized brain damage. Also, in the classic case of H.M., the bilateral damage caused by his operation was widespread and encroached on the amygdala and extensive regions of the temporal lobes as well as the hippocampus. While H.M. and similar cases were originally cited as evidence for the involvement of the whole temporal lobes in memory functions, now the evidence points more specifically to the medial temporal lobe and hippocampus being the structures in which damage will result in amnesia.

Recent evidence for the involvement of the hippocampus comes from a subject, known as R.B., first reported in 1985 by Larry Squire and Stuart Zola-Morgan working in San Diego, California (Squire and Zola-Morgan, 1988). R.B. was a postal worker suffering from heart disease, who at the age of 52, underwent a coronary artery by-pass operation. During the operation he suffered a heart attack with temporary loss of blood supply to the brain. R.B. was later found to have a profound anterograde amnesia similar to that shown by H.M. One difference was that R.B. did not show as extensive a retrograde amnesia and, in fact, for events immediately preceding his operations he had better than average recall.

R.B. died just five years after his operation. On post-mortem examination, the damage to his brain was found to be restricted to a small localized region in both hippocampi. There was no evidence of damage in the temporal lobes, amygdala, mammillary bodies, medial thalamus or frontal lobes. While this important case does not deny that damage to other brain structures can produce disturbances in memory, it points to the focal nature of the hippocampus in human memory systems and illustrates how memory is susceptible to very small bilateral lesions in this structure.

The previous section described Brenda Milner's finding that damage to the left lateral temporal lobe interfered with memory for language-related functions and damage to the right with memory for spatial tasks. An implication of this is that the left and right medial temporal lobes and hippocampi are also specialized for processing verbal and spatial information. Table 11.2 shows an analysis of the effects of damage to either the left or right hippocampus on memory tests which involve either verbal or spatial information.

In Table 11.2 the first eight tests are spatial in nature and the following six are verbal. The details of the individual tests are not important. What is important is the clear relationship between performance on each type of test, verbal or spatial, and the location of the lesion in either the left or right hippocampus. Damage to the left hippocampus impairs performance on verbal tests but not on tests requiring spatial skills. Damage to the right hippocampus impairs performance on spatial tests but not on verbal tests.

☐ How is such a relationship between site of damage and nature of functional impairment described?

■ There is said to be a double dissociation between the site of the lesion and the nature of impairment similar to that described above for damage to the lateral temporal lobes.

☐ What do the results in Table 11.2 indicate about the specialization of left and right hippocampi?

■ There is a clear pattern of interaction between the nature of the test material and the effect of the side of the hippocampal lesion. Damage to the right hippocampus has no effect on performance on verbal tasks but impairs spatial tasks. For left hippocampal lesions, the reverse is true. The results indicate that the left human hippocampus is specialized to process verbal information and the right to process spatial information.

**Table 11.2**   Analysis of effects of damage to the hippocampus.

| Test | Site of lesion | |
|------|:----------------:|:----------------:|
| | Left hippocampus | Right hippocampus |
| Tactile maze learning | – | × |
| Visual maze learning | – | × |
| Facial recognition | – | × |
| Spatial block span + 1 | – | × |
| Spatial position | – | × |
| Spatial association | – | × |
| Spatial memory | – | × |
| Self-ordered design recall | – | × |
| | | |
| Recall of nonsense syllables | × | – |
| Recall of word lists | × | – |
| Digit span + 1 | × | – |
| Non-spatial association | × | – |
| Self-ordered word recall | × | – |
| Recall of consonant trigrams | × | – |

Note: × = significant impairment; – = normal performance.

Thus a consistent picture has emerged of the roles of the lateral and medial temporal lobes and the left and right hippocampi in memory function, with the evidence from R.B. indicating the focal nature of the hippocampus itself in producing anterograde amnesia.

☐ R.B. and H.M. showed comparable magnitudes of anterograde amnesia. However, R.B. showed a relatively short period of retrograde amnesia (about one year) compared with the much longer period shown by H.M. (about twelve years). What does a comparison of these times, in relation to the extensiveness of their bilateral lesions within the brain, suggest about the structures implicated in retrograde amnesia?

■ First, the comparison suggests that, while damage to the hippocampus itself produces anterograde amnesia, it does not produce such a profound retrograde amnesia. The comparison suggests that it is damage to structures such as the lateral or medial temporal lobes or amygdala that produces the retrograde amnesia.

The phenomenon of retrograde amnesia is a puzzle. The loss of memory of events prior to the amnesia-provoking incident suggests that the damaged structures outside the hippocampus play a role in either the retrieval or storage of memory.

☐ For those neural structures where damage results in retrograde amnesia, what aspect of the amnesia suggests that the structures are not involved in memory retrieval functions?

■ The fact that retrograde amnesia is not absolute. Subjects such as R.B. were able to recall events going back from a year before the amnesic incident. Therefore, such subjects were able to recall stored information. The implication was that memory retrieval mechanisms were intact.

One possible explanation for the variability of retrograde amnesia and the fact that it is rarely complete is that memory traces move in the brain over time. Older memories move to different sites outside those where damage results in retrograde amnesia. Another possibility is that memories are in fact stored at sites outside the areas where damage produces retrograde amnesia but that retrieval processes change after a period of time. According to this hypothesis, as a result of rehearsal (repetition) or encounters with similar material, a recategorization of the existing memory occurs with the formation of additional representations, which are then independent of the structures in which damage results in retrograde amnesia.

Analysis of the after-effects of brain damage on memory is continuing to uncover quite unexpected phenomena suggesting that memory processes are much more dynamic than originally suspected. That is to say, a memory might be laid down in one location but over time transfer to a different location. Such phenomena will keep theorists and experimenters busy for the foreseeable future. Book 6 in this course will return to this topic.

## 11.4.4  Episodic and semantic memory

The evidence introduced in previous sections indicates that the contents of consciousness could be dramatically restricted by damage to small regions of the brain. Damage to the hippocampus and related structures, resulting in amnesia, prevents the storage or retrieval of information that would normally be available for recall in the future. Also, from the evidence of retrograde amnesia, access is denied to information that would normally be available for recall. However, the inability to retrieve stored information is not absolute. Amnesic subjects show different periods of retrograde amnesia. More significantly, there is an entire class of stored information that is unaffected by lesions that result in retrograde amnesia. An amnesic person is able to converse normally and fluently and is able to understand spoken and written instructions. By implication, the amnesic person is able to 'remember' the meanings of words and the structure of language and what the person they are talking to has just said, long enough at least to reply and thus hold a conversation.

Psychologists distinguish between memory systems for events and memory that is evidenced by the ability to use language. In 1972, the American psychologist Endel Tulving proposed a distinction between **episodic memory** and **semantic memory** systems, which, in behavioural studies, show different characteristics.

In Tulving's scheme, semantic memory includes memory for general knowledge of the world. For example, semantic memory includes the knowledge of words and how to use them, such as the French or English words for white grains of sodium chloride (sel or salt). Semantic memory also provides a working knowledge of the regularities of the world, such as the number of inches in a foot. In contrast, episodic memory is more about what has been done or what has happened to us, for example what you had for breakfast or whether you have met someone recently.

At first sight, the amnesia displayed by H.M., R.B. and others conforms with a distinction between episodic and semantic memory. Both H.M. and R.B. displayed a working knowledge of the world; they could converse, read, and carry out their normal daily activities, such as dressing, using knives, forks and other utensils. This indication of the sparing of semantic memory contrasted with their inability to recall episodic events once they had 'dropped-out' from consciousness, suggesting different and independent neural bases for semantic and episodic memory.

As well as giving the ability to understand the meanings of words, semantic memory is thought to provide information about the 'structural' features of the environment such as giving familiarity with the home and the neighbourhood and with the 'currency' of day-to-day experience. However, testing showed that, as well as being impaired in episodic memory, H.M. and R.B. were also impaired in their abilities to update their semantic memory. One test of the integrity of semantic memory is the ability to remember the names of politicians such as presidents or prime ministers. Over many years of testing, H.M. showed little evidence of updating his semantic memory. For example, when asked to name the current president, he still gave the name of the encumbent of that office at the time of his operation. The impairment of both semantic and episodic memory in H.M. and R.B. suggests then that these two aspects of memory are not as independent as first thought, at least at a neural level.

☐ Bearing in mind the previous discussion of retrograde amnesia, what other explanation is there for the apparent sparing of semantic memory?

■ It could be that semantic memory is 'older' memory that has been spared because it has become independent of the structures where damage produces retrograde amnesia.

## 11.4.5   Conscious involvement and the amnesic syndrome

☐ How does the distinction between episodic and semantic memory help in understanding the amnesic syndrome?

■ It reflects the observation that amnesics are not able to remember events that occur after the amnesia-provoking event but are able to speak and converse normally and show an understanding of the structure of the world.

However, as described previously, the ability of the amnesic to remember both new episodic and new semantic information is impaired. The fact that both semantic and episodic memory are impaired by the damage that produces amnesia indicates that they are not necessarily as independent at a neural level as implied by the distinction between episodic and semantic memory made as a result of behavioural observations.

Another attempt at a classification of memory systems, suggested by the amnesic's ability to learn motor skills, was proposed by Neal Cohen and Larry Squire, working at the Veteran's Administration Hospital, San Diego, California. They distinguished between declarative memory and procedural memory. You first encountered this distinction in Book 1, Chapter 8, in the context of animals learning in mazes and Skinner boxes. The distinction proposed by Cohen and

Squire has important features in common with the earlier one but does not necessarily match it exactly.

In the present context, declarative memory allows information to be stored in a way that is later available as conscious recollection and can be expressed as verbal declarative statements such as "I read a fascinating book called … last week which said '…' " or in non-verbal acts such as calling to mind the images of a remembered episode. Examples of procedural memory are riding a bike or playing a musical instrument, skills that can be performed without conscious recollection. The distinction between declarative and procedural memory is likened to 'knowing what' and 'knowing how'.

Central to Squire's description of the distinction between declarative and procedural memory is that, with use, declarative learning is transformed into procedural memory. He cites the example of learning to ride a bike or drive a car. At first, there is a lot of cognitive involvement but, with practice, driving or riding becomes automatic and places much less of a load on consciousness.

☐ Can you see how Squire's description of declarative and procedural learning fits with the phenomenon of retrograde amnesia?

■ With use, declarative learning becomes transformed into procedural learning and thus may have a dual representation in the brain, i.e. in the structures in which damage produces retrograde amnesia and elsewhere.

For a long time, H.M.'s ability to learn motor skills was an interesting anomaly pointing to a separate neural basis for the learning of motor skills, possibly involving the cerebellum. With years of painstaking investigation of the amnesic syndrome, though, other 'anomalies' became apparent. Now, the list of memories spared in the amnesic syndrome includes not only learning of motor skills, but also the ability to develop new perceptual and cognitive skills such as learning to solve the Towers of Hanoi puzzle (see Figure 11.10).

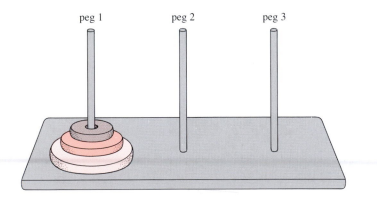

**Figure 11.10** The Towers of Hanoi puzzle. The task is to move the rings from peg 1 to peg 3, with the rings ending up in the same relationship of smallest on the top and largest on the bottom. The restrictions are that only one ring can be moved at a time and that a larger ring cannot be placed on top of a smaller one.

Figure 11.11 shows Squire's classification of memory types, in which the list of memory 'types' that are not disturbed in the amnesic syndrome are grouped as non-declarative memory. Amnesics lose the ability to update their episodic and semantic memories, and so these two memory types are included under the declarative memory category.

As well as the examples of procedural memory, the list of non-declarative memory also includes classical conditioning (Book 1, Chapter 6) and a phenomenon called *priming* first reported by Elizabeth Warrington of the National Hospital for Nervous Diseases in London and Laurence Weiskrantz of the University of Oxford.

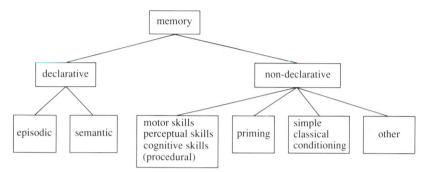

**Figure 11.11**   The classification of memory based on investigations of the amnesic syndrome.

Warrington and Weiskrantz demonstrated that amnesics were able to recognize previously presented words and pictures under conditions where they were primed, i.e. they were given a cue consisting of a fragment of the original and asked to complete it. Warrington and Weiskrantz's finding that learning can be demonstrated when the amnesic is cued about the properties of the item to be recalled provided a clue about the nature of the deficit underlying the amnesic syndrome. The cueing process is thought to act to bring information into consciousness and to act as a replacement for processes lost after the damage resulting in amnesia. In this way, the amnesic deficit can be explained, not by an inability to learn in itself, but by the loss of the ability to access learned information in consciousness.

Another distinction that is currently providing a focus for investigation into the causes of amnesia is between explicit and implicit memory tasks. This distinction focuses on the amnesic's difficulty with accessing information consciously. Typically, such deficits are seen when the amnesic patient has to remember where or when a stimulus was seen before. The retrieval of such information is an example of explicit memory access and is contrasted with tasks in which memory is accessed implicitly, such as when naming an object. The distinction between explicit and implicit memory access was proposed in 1987 by Daniel Schachter, a psychologist working at the University of Arizona. Schachter proposes that 'Explicit memory is revealed when performance on a task requires conscious recollection of previous experiences'. He defines implicit memory in a very opaque way as 'Implicit memory is revealed when performance on a task is facilitated in the absence of conscious recollection'.

An example of a task that taps memory explicitly is where a subject has to remember whether a word or a picture has been seen previously. Typically, amnesic subjects do very badly on such tasks. However, on tasks such as learning motor skills, where they do not have to remember explicitly what they did before, their performance is much more like non-amnesic subjects.

A classic experiment that is taken to show the difference in ability of amnesic and non-amnesic subjects to access information explicitly was carried out by P. Graf, L. Squire and G. Mandler in 1984 and published in a paper entitled 'The information that amnesic patients do not forget'. In this experiment, amnesic and non-amnesic subjects were each given a list of words and asked to decide how much they liked each word. In this way, each subject was exposed to every word on their list but without instructions to remember them.

This exposure to a list was then followed by one of four tests. Three of the four tests involved the subjects deciding whether they could remember the words occurring in the list. These tasks were:

1   free recall—tell me what words you can remember?

2   cued recall—tell me if this word was on the list?

3   recognition—were any of these words in the list?

4   word completion

The fourth test, word completion, did not require the subjects to determine whether they had seen a word before. In this test the subjects were presented with a three letter word fragment such as BAR and asked to write down the first word they thought of, e.g. BARTER, BARGAIN and so on. The score was the number of words that were elicited that had appeared on the list previously presented.

The results of this experiment are shown in Figure 11.12. In this figure the differences between the scores of the amnesic and non-amnesic subjects on the first three tasks, tests of free recall, cued recall and recognition memory, are significantly different. Amnesics do worse. The scores on the fourth task, word completion, are not significantly different and are taken as evidence for no difference in performance. An interpretation of these results is that where amnesic subjects have to use conscious recollection of a previous episode they perform worse than non-amnesics. However, where the task does not involve conscious recollection they are able to perform normally.

☐   Consider the distinctions between, on the one hand, explicit and implicit memory and, on the other hand, declarative and non-declarative memory. At first sight, are there any similarities between these distinctions?

■   A common factor between the two distinctions is the identification that amnesics are not impaired in performing those tasks that do not involve conscious processing of information.

Although the declarative/non-declarative and explicit/implicit distinctions are descriptive and do not explain the causes of the memory deficits that are apparent in the behaviour of amnesics, they do point to a deficit in some aspect of the thought processes involved in normal memory.

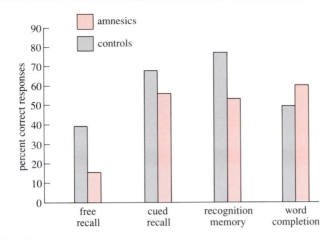

**Figure 11.12** Free recall, cued recall, recognition memory and word completion scores for amnesic and non-amnesic subjects—see text for details.

In a recent analysis of the amnesic deficit, Alan Baddeley, a prominent memory researcher working at the Applied Psychology Unit, Cambridge, points out that the unimpaired capacity of the amnesic to recall normally events that occurred prior to the onset of the amnesia indicates that the memory recall processes are themselves functioning normally. This points to some deficit in long-term storage processes rather than a deficit in recall underlying the amnesic syndrome. Here, Baddeley's suggestion is that the amnesic deficit lies in an inability to store associations between events that were previously separate. Without these links, the contents of consciousness fail to form and/or trigger the associations that normally provide the richness of our mental lives and leave the amnesic trapped in a world which virtually stopped at the time of the onset of the amnesia.

### 11.4.6 Amnesia and intelligence

Brain damage that produces the amnesic syndrome is not, in itself, thought to impair measures of cognitive ability as measured by standard verbal and non-verbal tests of intelligence. The evidence here comes from several people whose IQs remained relatively unchanged after localized brain damage which produced severe amnesia. In other people, reductions in verbal or non-verbal IQ scores are attributed to the effects of more widespread brain damage. For example, such damage is seen following long-term alcohol abuse leading to Korsakoff's syndrome, which is characterized by amnesia accompanied by personality and intelligence changes.

### Summary of Section 11.4

The analysis of amnesias has had a profound influence on the understanding of the organization of memory within the brain. Studies of amnesia have identified brain structures such as the temporal lobes, hippocampus, amygdala, mammillary bodies and frontal lobes as being involved in memory. The last decade or so has seen a dramatic change in the understanding of amnesia. Early studies of patients such as H.M. suggested that damage to the temporal lobes and associated structures interfered with the ability to transfer information from working memory into a long-term store while leaving the patient able to use language-related memory. These early studies supported the distinction between episodic and semantic memory as reflecting the existence of independent neural systems for each.

The demonstration of the ability of amnesics to acquire manual skills then added a further memory category, procedural memory, to be accounted for. The implications drawn from early studies of amnesia were that four independent brain systems were involved in memory: systems for working (short term), episodic, semantic and procedural memory. The discovery that the ability to update both semantic memory and episodic memory was impaired led to the acceptance that these two categories of memory were not necessarily distinct at a neural level.

The amnesic patient, R.B., who, at post-mortem, was found to have bilateral lesions localized within the same region of each hippocampus, helped clarify the role of the temporal lobes and hippocampus as the sources of amnesia. In R.B., bilateral damage to the hippocampus alone was sufficient to produce anterograde amnesia. In comparison with H.M.'s retrograde amnesia of twelve years or more, R.B.'s retrograde amnesia was limited to about a year. A comparison of the two cases suggests that damage outside the hippocampus, to the medial and lateral temporal lobes and to the amygdala, contributes to the retrograde amnesia.

One suggestion for memories that are spared from retrograde amnesia is that, as a result of rehearsal or episodes with similar material, recategorization of existing episodic memory takes place. This recategorization then results in the formation of additional representations of the memory in locations which are independent of the structures where damage results in retrograde amnesia.

More exciting has been the recognition that amnesic deficits occur under particular testing conditions, i.e. those where the tasks require the subject to access information consciously. The suggestion here is that the amnesic syndrome results from an inability for conscious processes to access information via the associative links that normally contribute to the contents of the flow of consciousness. The fact that recall of events prior to the amnesia-provoking event is possible has led to the suggestion that the amnesic is unable to form such associative links normally and that this is the primary deficit underlying the amnesic syndrome.

Section 11.4 introduced several categorizations of memory: episodic / semantic, declarative / procedural and explicit / implicit. The difficulties in working with such categories and trying to form a picture of the way that the different categories relate to one another are two-fold. First, as categories, they are not exhaustive. That is to say, they describe restricted aspects of the phenomena of long-term memory and such categorization usually originated because it helped highlight some aspect of the amnesic syndrome. For example, the declarative/ procedural distinction neglects a much wider range of long-term memory phenomena described all-encompassingly as non-declarative memory.

Secondly, these different categorizations are overlapping and not mutually exclusive. That is, (1) episodic / semantic, (2) declarative / procedural, and (3) explicit / implicit do not represent three distinct and mutually exclusive subclasses of memory. Thus such categorization must be contrasted with the rigour and exclusivity whereby, for example, dogs and cats are classed as different mammals, which in turn are different from seagulls and buzzards, these being different birds.

The value of these three distinctions is that they help understanding of particular phenomena that arise under specific testing conditions rather than suggesting separate and independent memory systems with distinct neuroanatomical bases.

# 11.5   Consciousness in an evolutionary context

## 11.5.1   Introduction

Damage to such structures as Wernicke's area and the hippocampus causes deficits in the affected individual's cognitive processes, leaving them unable to function normally. For example, damage to Wernicke's area can produce impairments in the ability to comprehend information and to communicate, i.e. disorders in thinking. The 'word-salad' speech of a Wernicke patient suggests that some fundamental feature within the thought processes normally called consciousness has been damaged. Or, to take another example, the analysis of the effects of bilateral damage to the hippocampus suggests that there is an impairment in the ability to bring information into consciousness.

Talking generally, both impairments result in alterations in consciousness. The major difficulty in describing the nature of such deficits is that the single term 'consciousness', in common with the expression 'personal experience', implies some single process. However, the different symptoms that result from damage to Wernicke's area and to the hippocampus show that consciousness is not best described as a single process. An alternative position is that consciousness may be the result of the operation of a number of different brain systems, involving memory and language, and that the phenomenon called consciousness is the result of their interactions. According to this view, consciousness is a property of the systems of the brain that mediate our cognitive processes, i.e. it is a *system property* (Chapter 1).

## 11.5.2   Consciousness, modularity and cognitive science

Cognitive neuropsychology attempts to describe the structure of human cognition and relate it to the structures of the brain. That is to say, it is the discipline concerned with the processes that underlie consciousness. Investigations, mainly with brain-damaged subjects, have produced a picture of human cognition as something with a *modular* structure. A cognitive module is a 'unit' which processes its information independently of other modules. Cognitive neuropsychology can be seen as an extension of the endeavour to describe the localization of function within the brain. Its goal is to describe the characteristics of the cognitive processes that are localized within the brain, without particular concern for the details of their underlying physiology.

A study by Elizabeth Warrington, carried out in 1982, gives an example of the way that evidence for modularity has been obtained. A month after suffering a minor stroke, D.R.C. reported difficulty with elementary arithmetic. His scores on the sub-tests of the Wechsler Adult Intelligence Scale (WAIS) are shown in Table 11.3 (*overleaf*).

**Table 11.3**  D.R.C.'s scores on the sub-components of the WAIS.

| | | | |
|---|---|---|---|
| Arithmetic | 4 | Picture completion | 10 |
| Similarities | 11 | Block design | 12 |
| Digit span | 14 | Picture arrangement | 12 |
| Vocabulary | 14 | | |

On all the sub-component tests of the WAIS except for the arithmetic test, D.R.C.'s scores were normal. On the arithmetic test, however, he was significantly impaired relative to his other scores. The WAIS test indicated that, while D.R.C.'s ability to use language and read and his memory were normal, he was unable to carry out elementary arithmetic. On simple arithmetic tests, such as 4 add 2, 6 take away 3, 5 multiplied by 8, D.R.C. performed very poorly. For example, when asked to add 7 and 5, his solution was 'about 13'. However, he was able to estimate accurately the numbers of dots presented in a two-second exposure, and could estimate the distance from London to New York.

D.R.C.'s cognitive deficit is called *acalculia*. It is often seen associated with aphasia, alexia and agraphia (disturbances of speech, reading and writing, respectively) but rarely in such a 'pure' form as displayed by D.R.C.. Although, again, results from a single subject must be interpreted with caution, D.R.C.'s acalculia, in the absence of any other measurable cognitive deficit, is a good example of the modularity in human cognitive processes, with the implication that such modules have localized neuroanatomical bases.

The idea of modularity of cognition was first formally proposed by an American cognitive psychologist, Jerry Fodor, working at Cambridge, Massachusetts, in the 1970s. Among other criteria, Fodor proposed that cognitive modules should show *informational encapsulation* and *domain specificity*. By 'informational encapsulation' he meant that a module carries out its processing in complete 'ignorance' of, and isolation from, processing going on elsewhere in the brain, and that it can only accept one type of input. D.R.C.'s symptoms imply informational encapsulation because other cognitive functions were apparently unimpaired. For D.R.C.'s disorder to have occurred in such a 'clean' way, the region of brain destroyed also meets the criteria of domain specificity, which means that other regions of the brain were unable to replace the lost functions.

Book 6 will return to descriptions of the modular structure of human cognition. For the present, the example of acalculia has served to illustrate the way that contemporary cognitive neuroscience attempts to describe the structure of human cognition. From a close analysis of the cognitive deficits shown by people who have suffered brain damage, cognitive neuropsychology then attempts to identify the modular structures contributing to consciousness.

While it is generally acknowledged that consciousness is an important phenomenon to be explained, cognitive neuroscience is far from having developed appropriate concepts with which to attack the problem. In fact there is healthy disagreement over whether consciousness can be described as the *input* to a specific cognitive module, such as a module mediating short-term memory, or whether consciousness will be what is 'left' when all the cognitive modules have been described. In the latter case, it would constitute a non-modular system that 'supervises' the work of the 'lower-level' cognitive modules. Some cognitive neuropsychologists hold the view that analysis of cognitive deficits is inappropriate to the study of consciousness.

### 11.5.3   Biological and evolutionary bases of cognition and consciousness

So far, human cognition has been portrayed as being built up from modular structures and also closely related to the capacity to use language. Chomsky's proposition that humans inherited a 'language acquisition device' was introduced, and anatomical evidence for an enlargement of the human brain in the region of Wernicke's area relative to other primates was described. While this may be more than circumstantial evidence for an inherited neurological basis for language acquisition, it is difficult to extend this line of argument to cover the inheritance of neurological structures described previously as cognitive modules.

The most powerful arguments against any proposal that human cognitive modules as such are inherited arise from consideration of the historical time span of some of the cognitive processes that have been described as having a modular basis, such as arithmetic ability, reading and writing. All these have been shown to be individually and independently disturbed after brain damage.

☐    What is the argument against each such cognitive skill having an independent inherited basis?

■    The argument against these processes being inherited is that until about 100 years ago, most people were not literate or numerate and did not possess the reading, writing and arithmetical skills for which cognitive modules have been described. Thus, it is difficult to see how selection for specific cognitive skills and specific cognitive modules could have occurred.

Nevertheless, human cognition with its reliance on language does seem to mark a qualitative difference between humans and other animals. This difference is sufficiently great for some scientists still to adhere to the position of Rene Descartes, the 17th century French philosopher and researcher, who said that mind and matter are qualitatively different and that mind (or soul) is a phenomenon peculiar to humans. This position of **Cartesian dualism** holds that, in principle, mind is not open to scientific investigation since it operates outside the domain of science and the laws of physics.

A basic thread running throughout this book is that any understanding of the brain must acknowledge its evolutionary history. Previous discussions have indicated that the phenomenon referred to as consciousness or mind can be shown to depend upon brain structures, e.g. Wernicke's area and the hippocampus. Though cognitive modules may not be localizable in the same way, the method of their discovery implies a physical basis within the brain.

While distinct structures underlying specific individual cognitive modules are not inherited in the sense that arms and legs or our eye or hair colour are inherited, a *capacity to develop* cognitive structures is part of each individual's inheritance. The question, though, is one of the uniqueness of the structures that support human cognition: are the structures that mediate cognitive processes qualitatively different from brain structures in non-human animals or are the differences merely quantitative? That is, are the differences one of kind or of degree?

Similar discussions have already been aired in this book, albeit from a different perspective.

☐ Can you recollect the discussion of the human capacity for control over individual fingers and its neuroanatomical basis (Chapter 9) ?

■ This capacity is related to the termination of a large number of pyramidal tract axons directly upon α motor neurons in the region of the spinal cord concerned with control over the hands.

In other primates, a smaller proportion of the pyramidal tract axons terminate directly upon α motor neurons. Thus, manual dexterity through independent control of the fingers, a feature strongly developed only in humans, can be seen to be dependent upon the further evolution of a structure that is found in related species. From this evolutionary perspective, the phenomena of mind and consciousness might be seen as being different, not in kind but in degree, from related species. That is, in this evolutionary perspective, the brain structures that give humans the capacity for thought and consciousness can be seen to be developments of structures possessed by closely related species. These structures, in turn, have their origins in structures possessed by some more distant ancestor.

As a conclusion to this book, the views of Gerald Edelman, a Nobel prize-winning American immunologist now working in New York, will be described (Edelman, 1989). Edelman has tried to describe the nature of the processes that evolved in mammals that are the antecedents of cognition in humans. Edelman's views on consciousness are a blend of philosophy and neuroscience, and the style of the following discussion will be markedly different from previous sections.

*The Remembered Present* by Gerald Edelman is a noteworthy recent attempt to put the phenomena of consciousness in a neurophysiological context that also takes the brain's evolutionary history into account. In this conceptually very dense and difficult book for which we provide only a conceptually dense and difficult summary here, Edelman proposes that consciousness is the result of an evolutionary 'strategy' that required the integration of a number of lines of evolutionary development. He proposes that four conditions were necessary for consciousness to arise:

1   The organism's nervous system must have developed the ability to divide perceptions into categories (perceptual categorization).

2   The organism's nervous system must be structured so that it can discriminate between self and non-self events.

3   The organism's nervous system must be capable of learning, that is to say, of changing its behaviour as the result of relating its present state to its past states.

4   The organism must possess a memory system capable of continual recategorization through the process of associating new events with previously stored information.

In Edelman's scheme, all these four necessary requirements for the existence of consciousness operate prior to and independently of consciousness. They provide a functional 'platform' from which consciousness can develop. In these propositions, Edelman encapsulates information that has been presented in various places and forms in this book.

## Proposition 1

Here, Edelman proposes that potentially conscious organisms must have developed the capacity for perceptual categorization.

☐ From your recollection of the preceding chapters, what neurophysiological mechanisms were described which indicate that mammals have this capacity?

■ Several examples are available. For instance, the hierarchical structure in the touch pathway gives the capability of representing different classes of touch to the skin, such as a touch stimulus moving in different directions within the same region of skin (Chapter 9).

As another example, the hierarchical arrangement by which receptive fields are 'linked' through inhibitory interneurons in the process called lateral inhibition is a fundamental process within sensory systems which allows 'higher order' stimulus features (such as direction of movement) to be extracted. Lateral inhibition and feature extraction will be discussed further in Chapter 4 of Book 3.

Part of Edelman's criterion of perceptual categorization is that the supposedly conscious organism has developed the capacity for a rich representation of its environment, via a system of parallel sensory channels of different modalities. Here, Edelman is alluding to the pattern of evolution seen in mammals where the cortex has enlarged relative to sub-cortical structures, with the development of multiple 'maps' of sensory information accompanied by expansion of association cortex. It is the development of both processes, enabling sensory feature extraction and systems for association of different modalities, that provides the basis for a rich representation of the environment.

## Proposition 2

By the distinction between self and non-self, Edelman is not using the term 'self' in its common usage to refer to a conscious entity. Rather he uses the term to describe a more fundamental capacity for the organism to distinguish between external and internal stimuli. In Edelman's usage, the ability to distinguish self relies on the ability of an organism's nervous system to represent external and internal events independently. At one end of the biological spectrum there are single-celled organisms such as the amoebae which do not have a differentiated nervous system capable of distinctions between self and non-self events. At the other end, in mammals, complex systems have evolved which permit such distinctions and which, according to Edelman, have further evolved to allow a conscious representation of the self.

☐ What mammalian brain systems 'manage' the distinction of the 'self'?

■ The limbic system and hypothalamus constitute a system that has evolved to control homeostatic and endocrine functions that monitor the 'self' and which acts to select adaptive behaviour relating to maintenance of the self.

## Propositions 3 and 4

In propositions 3 and 4, Edelman suggests that supposedly conscious organisms must have developed a memory system that not only has the capacity to store information about actual stimulus qualities but that it must be capable of recategorizing stored information as a result of its experience. In recategorization, Edelman proposes that 'values' are associated with the categorization of stimuli. In this way, future behaviour in response to environmental stimuli will depend upon the associations formed through recategorization, and thus on previous experience.

As an interpretation of Edelman's use of the term 'values', consider the discussions of motivation presented in Book 1, Chapter 7. Motivational control systems were described as changing the significance of stimuli according to the internal condition of the animal. For example, a food-related stimulus takes on a 'positive' value when the animal is energy deficient. This principle is equally applicable to the reactions to a temperature stimulus as a function of internal body temperature. Expressed in other words, when something becomes a positive reinforcer it acquires a value.

What Edelman then proposes is that a supposedly conscious organism must have evolved a way of storing information about the nature of its responses to stimuli, along with the information about their perceptual categories.

Classical and instrumental conditioning (Book 1, Chapter 6) are two ways through which the behaviour of animals is modified. The view of some behaviourists is that, in such conditioning, the learning organism plays a passive role in the learning process; it is the environmental contingencies that determine the animal's future behaviour. While not denying the existence or contributions of classical and operant conditioning, Edelman's pre-condition for the development of consciousness is that the organism does not simply depend upon automatically formed links between events, e.g. stimuli and responses, to determine its behaviour. Rather, Edelman sees a conscious animal as playing a more active role, and that a cornerstone of consciousness is the ability to represent the external world within the nervous system and to use those representations and their associations to determine behaviour.

According to Edelman, as well as having to meet his four *necessary* conditions outlined previously, that is to possess neural systems for perceptual recategorization, learning, memory and self/non-self discrimination, two further evolutionary events were required to create the *sufficient* conditions for consciousness to emerge.

The first event was the evolution of memory systems that are able to represent information 'conceptually'. In Edelman's scheme a concept at its minimal level of representation relies on an ability to distinguish objects from actions. Concepts are representations of the animal's world that evolved prior to language and provide the evolutionary basis for human language. Edelman speculates that if any animal with this conceptual capacity could speak, it would reveal its concepts as things, motions and classes. Edelman sees the evolution of a representation in terms of concepts as being essential for an animal to identify a particular thing or action and to control its future behaviour in a more or less general way.

The second sufficient evolutionary event depended upon the first and was the evolution of memory systems that link on-going perceptual categorization by the sensory systems, with the stored representation of perceptual categories and their associated values. In the absence of such associative memory mechanisms, the behaviour of an animal would be determined solely by the dominance of one external event over others. To escape this domination Edelman believes that an animal must have the capacity to represent external events; to link those events with their consequences; to store the information about events and consequences and to use the stored information to determine behaviour.

The consciousness that Edelman proposes can result from these necessary and sufficient conditions is not necessarily synonymous with the understanding of consciousness gained from our own experience. Edelman proposes that consciousness is an evolutionary strategy that frees its possessor from the dominance of an immediately driven response and is not a uniquely human phenomenon. Here, Edelman distinguishes between *primary* and *higher-order consciousness*.

According to Edelman, animal species whose nervous systems meet the necessary and sufficient conditions have the capacity for primary consciousness. Here, Edelman acknowledges that consciousness is not a uniquely human phenomenon and suggests that humans and perhaps some other non-human primates have evolved processes that superimpose higher-order consciousness upon primary consciousness. Edelman's schematic representation of the relationships between the 'components' of primary consciousness and the neuroanatomy of the mammalian brain is shown in Figure 11.13. You do not need to remember the details of this figure.

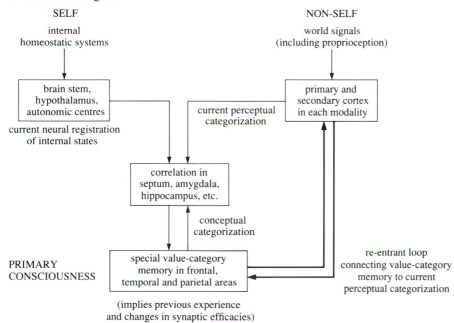

**Figure 11.13**   Edelman's necessary and sufficient elements for primary consciousness. Primary consciousness requires: (1) perceptual categorization by selective cortical systems for each modality, (2) memory, (3) learning, and (4) a biological self–non-self distinction.

Through primary consciousness, an animal generates a 'mental image' of events and their consequences. In this way, primary consciousness permits the formation

325

of 'concepts' of the external world. A concept is the amalgam of the representation of an environmental event and the internal consequences or value it achieved. He proposes that higher-order consciousness requires the ability, not only to form concepts but also to 'think', that is to order and otherwise manipulate concepts. A schematic representation of the brain systems that Edelman proposes as supporting higher-order consciousness is shown in Figure 11.14. Again, you do not need to remember the details of this figure.

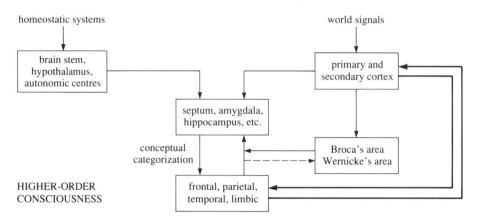

**Figure 11.14**   A schematic representation of the brain systems involved in higher-order consciousness.

In Edelman's scheme, during evolution and in the development of individual thought, the concepts that are the markers of primary consciousness precede language and meaning. Further, the emergence of the ability to form concepts provides the gateway to higher-order consciousness, both in evolution and in the individual. Concepts are driven by the perceptual apparatus and require memory and, Edelman proposes, structure the world into things, motions and classes. Thought, Edelman proposes, requires a further evolutionary development, a new kind of memory that can place concepts in an ordered relationship. It is this memory, according to Edelman, that imposes order on the world, by requiring that concepts relating to objects and concepts relating to actions be linked in specific ways. In this way, thought is given a structure which, to distinguish it from the syntactical structure of spoken language, Edelman describes as pre-syntactic.

As an example of pre-syntactic thought, Edelman cites the ability of 18-month-old chimpanzees to recognize that two objects belong to the same category, and also that two different objects are organized in the same relation. That is, they can decide on sameness or difference, make analogies and also assess intentions and guide their actions by such processes.

Higher-order consciousness, according to Edelman, does not require 'true' language and is not a uniquely human phenomenon. It does, however, require the evolution of the structures that supported primary-order consciousness to allow a symbolic modelling of the distinction between self and non-self to the extent that the possessor can be 'conscious of consciousness'.

What is the adaptive value of consciousness? In the evolution of the mammalian brain, primary consciousness is seen to have conferred selective advantage on its possessors and to have been subject to evolutionary development in much the same way as other mammalian features such as the development of the pyramidal tract and manual dexterity discussed in Chapter 9. The proposed adaptive functions of consciousness are shown in Table 11.4.

Humans and higher primates such as chimpanzees show forms of higher-order consciousness that extend primary consciousness through the mediation of language. Chimpanzees appear to use individual symbols with some degree of meaning and not just as simple signs, and also show evidence of self awareness. The evolution of language is seen to require the continuing evolution of the memory system giving presyntactic organization of thought, together with the associated development of cortical regions (Broca's and Wernicke's areas and the arcuate pathway) with connection to areas responsible for planning motor sequences and for acoustic perception. Edelman suggests that such evolutionary developments could have been gradual. Any slight selective advantage that accrued from the emerging ability to represent even a small set of signs and symbols by vocal utterances would then set the stage for mutations enhancing appropriate structural changes in the brain, vocal tract or in emotional expression. These would have enhanced the capability for hunting, mating or the rearing of young, and so would have increased fitness.

**Table 11.4** Edelman's proposed adaptive functions of primary and higher-order consciousness.

| Proposed adaptive functions of consciousness | Primary | Higher order |
|---|---|---|
| Provides explicit means for relating an individual to its acts and rewards | y | y |
| Helps in abstracting, organizing and lending salience to complex changes in the environment marked by stimuli affecting several senses | y | y |
| Provides a coherent aid for attention in sequencing complex learning tasks and in correcting errors in automatic actions (learned motor skills) during changing conditions | n | y |
| Allows long range anticipation of events and their relation to the past by means of explicit connections to long term memory | n | y |
| Enhances adaptability by permitting planning or 'modelling the world' outside real time (e.g. events can be remembered or imagined as taking place during 'imaginary time', which is not related to the 'real time' of the outside world) | n | y |
| Permits explicit comparison of outcomes on the basis of individual values and previous choices | n | y |
| Allows re-organization of memories and plans | n | y |
| Necessary for linguistic communication | y | y |

y = process plays a role; n = process does not play a role.

Edelman's approach follows on from, and is embedded in, a sea of philosophical debate about the nature of consciousness and the relationships between matter and mind. As you progress through this course, you will encounter other examples that are central to an understanding of the relationships between brain and behaviour. In the context of this book, which has provided an introduction to brain structures and functions, Edelman's approach is appropriate because it attempts to provide an account for the phenomenon of consciousness in a wider evolutionary context which emphasizes the importance of brain structure without unduly emphasizing the human brain.

# Summary of Chapter 11

The discussions in this chapter moved from the descriptions of structure and associated explanations of function in the mammalian brain to consider structures and functions that are specific to the human brain, especially those implicated in the human ability to think, reason, and communicate using language. These abilities provide strong evidence for lateralization of cognitive functions in the human brain.

The analysis of the roles of Wernicke's and Broca's areas, both of which are regions of association cortex, indicate that the term 'association' is not appropriate to describe their functions. A better way of describing what these regions do is to say they are *active elements* in a system which both transmits and processes information. Early studies of the consequences of damage to these regions suggested that Wernicke's area functions to translate visual and auditory sensory information into appropriate internal 'codes', while Broca's area translates internal codes, or 'thought', into forms appropriate for output via the speech apparatus and through the musculature of the hand as writing. The Wernicke–Geschwind model described the consequences of damage to Wernicke's or Broca's areas in terms of the disconnection of its input and outputs.

Subsequent investigation revealed that the components of the language system are not as restricted as indicated by the Wernicke–Geschwind model, nor are they arranged in such a conveniently serial fashion. There is evidence that comprehension of spoken and written language is carried out simultaneously by separate 'channels'. The consequences of localized lesions, where channels or sub-components of channels are selectively damaged, can still be analysed in terms of disconnections between the various parts of the language system.

Damage to the temporal lobes of the cortex and to some sub-cortical structures can have a profound effect on memory functions that are intimately related to thought and language. Human memory has been shown to depend on an extensive system involving the temporal lobes, hippocampus, amygdala, mammillary bodies, regions of the thalamus and frontal cortex. Bilateral damage to the hippocampus alone has been shown to contribute to the profound anterograde amnesia that characterizes the amnesic syndrome. Amnesia resulting from damage to these structures cannot be explained in terms of a simple disconnection analysis, such as the disconnection of a short-term memory store from a long-term store which depended on the short-term store for its input.

Attempts to characterize the loss of ability to store new memory and to update old memories, found after bilateral damage to the hippocampus and temporal lobes, revealed that the amnesia is not as total as originally described. These attempts have resulted in a variety of overlapping categorizations of memory.

Amnesia is not a result of a disconnection of stored information in itself. In the amnesic syndrome, older memories 'escape' the retrograde amnesia, so amnesia is not the result of a global disconnection of stored memories. Here, the suggestion is that, in amnesia, information becomes 'disconnected' because damage to the hippocampus and other structures in some way prevents 'links' being established between new information and already-stored information. In the absence of such links, the associative processes that normally act to bring information into consciousness do not have information upon which to work. The deficiency then leaves the individual with access to the current events in working memory or to information stored prior to the amnesic event.

According to this explanation, the paradox of retrograde amnesia is resolved by the hypothesis that, as memories are accessed, they are recategorized and given 'new' storage 'locations' in systems that are not affected by the hippocampal damage.

The human facility for language appears to depend upon species-specific neurological structures, with regions of the temporal lobes such as the planum temporale, which contains Wernicke's area, being specifically implicated.

A theory of the evolution of human consciousness and language has been proposed by Edelman. His approach offers a contrast to the bottom-up approach of the preceding chapters. Rather than starting with the individual structures of the brain and asking what they do, Edelman starts from an analysis of the way that human behaviour is regulated through consciousness. He then asks such questions as: What must the brain structures be doing in support of consciousness? How could such functions have evolved and what are the implications for non-human animals? The result is a speculative but provocative account of brain structures and relationships that are necessary and sufficient for consciousness to evolve in animal species. The account provides a basis for understanding, in a general way, the differences between human and non-human consciousness.

# Objectives for Chapter 11

After completing this chapter, you should be able to:

11.1   Define and use definitions and applications of each of the terms printed in **bold** in the text.

11.2   Recognize and distinguish between descriptions of Broca's and Wernicke's aphasia. (*Question 11.1*)

11.3   Distinguish between receptive and expressive disorders and relate them to brain anatomy. (*Question 11.1*)

11.4   Describe or recognize an explanation of the effects of brain damage in terms of patterns of disconnection. (*Question 11.1*)

11.5   Give an account of the Wernicke–Geschwind model of language. (*Question 11.1*)

11.6   Describe relationships between brain structure, brain damage and measures of IQ. (*Question 11.2*)

11.7    Describe the distinctions between working, episodic, semantic and procedural memory. (*Question 11.3*)

11.8    Describe the symptoms of the amnesic syndrome. (*Questions 11.4 and 11.5*)

11.9    Describe current views on the implications of amnesic deficits for the categorization of human memory stores. (*Questions 11.4 and 11.5*)

11.10   Describe Edelman's four necessary conditions and two sufficient conditions for the existence of consciousness. (*Question 11.6*)

11.11   Describe Edelman's distinctions between primary and higher order consciousness. (*Question 11.7*)

# Questions for Chapter 11

### Question 11.1 (*Objectives 11.2–11.5*)
In the context of the Wernicke–Geschwind model of language, which of the following statements are correct?

(a) Wernicke's area is involved in the translation of the internal representation of speech into speech forms.

(b) Wernicke's area plays a central role in the comprehension of auditory and visual information.

(c) Damage to Wernicke's area results in an inability to hear spoken instructions or to see written instructions.

(d) Damage to Broca's area results in a non-fluent aphasia.

(e) Damage to Wernicke's area results in an expressive aphasia.

(f) Damage to Broca's area disconnects the language system of the brain from its output via the speech apparatus.

### Question 11.2 (*Objective 11.6*)
Which of the following statements are correct?

(a) IQ tests show that the left side of the brain is specialized for processing visuo-spatial information.

(b) Damage to the left side of the brain during infancy affects the development of language functions while sparing non-verbal functions.

(c) Receptive and expressive language disorders can result from damage to the left or right hemispheres.

(d) It is likely that recovery of function can occur if the damage takes place during the period of infancy when the brain is developing its structure.

### Question 11.3 (*Objective 11.7*)
Which sort of memory—procedural, episodic, semantic or working—would be involved in the following?

(a) The memory that the French word for house is *maison*.

(b) The memory that allows you to open a tin can with a can opener.

(c) The memory of what you were doing when Margaret Thatcher's resignation was announced.

(d) You want to dial British Rail, Milton Keynes Central. A friend calls out that the number is 370883. You hold the memory long enough to dial and then it is lost.

### Question 11.4 (*Objectives 11.8 and 11.9*)

Suppose you have observed that damage to brain region 'X' impairs a specific cognitive capacity 'A'. The argument is then made that perhaps the disruption is not so specific but that all cognitive capacities are likely to be disrupted by the damage, associated with a general lowering of performance. In this context, explain what is meant by the expression 'double dissociation' and why demonstration of a double dissociation between two regions 'X' and 'Y' would be relevant to the argument.

### Question 11.5 (*Objectives 11.8 and 11.9*)

Which of the following statements are correct?

(a) Damage to the right temporal lobe results in an impairment in tasks which involve memory for verbally encoded material.

(b) The term 'anterograde amnesia' refers to a disruption of memory for events experienced after excision of tissue has been carried out.

(c) Working, episodic, semantic and procedural memory are different long-term memory stores.

(d) H.M.'s symptoms indicate that damage to the temporal lobes, hippocampus and associated structures left semantic and procedural memory systems unimpaired while damaging episodic memory.

(e) It is generally accepted that semantic memory is unimpaired in amnesia, because amnesics such as H.M. and R.B. have the ability to use and comprehend speech.

(f) Some theorists have rejected the proposal that semantic and episodic memory are separate memory systems, because amnesics show deficits in the ability to update semantic memory.

(g) With time and experience some information acquired as declarative learning can be transformed into procedural memories. In some cases, this can place less of a load on consciousness.

(h) Riding a bicycle is a task that depends on implicit memory.

(i) A current description of the amnesic deficit is that amnesics are impaired on tasks which require conscious recollection of previous processing of information.

### Question 11.6 (*Objective 11.10*)

Which of the following is one of Edelman's sufficient conditions for consciousness to emerge?

(a) The animal's nervous system must be capable of learning, that is to say, the animal must be capable of changing its behaviour as a result of relating its present state to its past states.

(b) The nervous system must have developed the ability to carry out perceptual categorization.

(c) The nervous system can monitor the internal state of the animal.

(d) The animal must have evolved memory systems that are able to represent information conceptually.

**Question 11.7** (*Objective 11.11*)
In Edelman's terms, which of the following would you see as evidence for the existence of higher-order consciousness?

(a) the capacity for classical conditioning

(b) the capacity for object recognition

(c) the capacity for complex learning

(d) the capacity to be conscious of being conscious

# References

Edelman, G. M. (1989) *The Remembered Present: A Biological Theory of Consciousness*, Basic Books. (Note this book is difficult reading and is outside the scope of this course.)

Petersen, S. E., Fox, P. T., Posner, M. I., Minton, M. and Raichle, M. E. (1988) Positron Emission Tomographic studies of the cortical anatomy for single word processing, *Nature*, **331**, pp. 585–589.

Squire, L. R. and Zola-Morgan, S. (1988) Memory: brain systems and behaviour, *Trends in Neurosciences*, **11**(4), pp. 170–175.

Teuber, H. L. (1975) Recovery of function after brain injury in man, in *Outcomes of Severe Damage to the Nervous System*, Ciba Foundation, 34, Elsevier/North Holland.

# Further reading

Baddeley, A. (1990) *Human Memory: Theory and Practice*, Lawrence Erlbaum Associates.

Eysenck, M. W. and Keane, M. T. (1990) *Cognitive Psychology: A Student's Handbook*, Lawrence Erlbaum Associates.

# GENERAL FURTHER READING

Jennett, S. (1989) *Human Physiology*, Churchill Livingstone. (The sections on cells, communication and control (Chapters 2–4), and interactions with the outside world (Chapters 12–14) provide a useful extension of the material covered in Book 2.)

Levitan, I. B. and Kaczmarek, L. K. (1991) *The Neuron: Cell and Molecular Biology*, Oxford University Press.

Starr, C. and Taggart, R. (1995) *Biology: The Unity and Diversity of Life,* 7th edn, Wadsworth Publishing Company Inc. (Contains a good general account of nervous systems, the brain and sensory systems.)

*There are a number of advanced texts that contain more detailed information, particularly concerning brain anatomy.*

Carpenter, R. H. S. (1996) *Neurophysiology*, 3rd edn. Physiological Principles of Medicine Series, Oxford University Press Inc. (Edward Arnold UK). (An advanced textbook, containing detailed information on the function of the brain, nervous systems and the senses.)

Diamond, M. C., Scheibel, A. B. and Elson, L. M. (1985) *The Human Brain Coloring Book*, Harper. (The book covers both gross and fine structure of the brain in great detail. A useful (and cheap) reference work on brain anatomy for the enthusiast.)

Kiernan, J. A. (1987) *Introduction to Human Neuroscience*, Lipincott Co. (An advanced textbook, well illustrated but rather densely written, which covers much of the ground that Book 2 does, but in much greater detail.)

Young, D. (1989) *Nerve Cells and Animal Behaviour*, Cambridge University Press. (A very good account of the link between nerve cells and behaviour. Particularly good (although detailed) on locust flight and intraspecific signals.)

*There are a range of human anatomy and physiology books aimed at medical students that provide very detailed anatomical details. They are often beautifully illustrated, but while they cover all the anatomy needed in this course, they go well beyond what is required. For example:*

Nolte, J. (1998) *The Human Brain*, 4th edn, C. Mosby–Year Book Inc.

Prezbindowski, K. S. and Tortora, G. J. (1996) *Principles of Anatomy and Physiology*, 8th edn, Addison-Wesley Educational Publishers Inc.

# ANSWERS TO QUESTIONS

## Chapter 1

### Question 1.1
The optic nerve is made up millions of *axons*, each of which is able to transmit *action potentials*. Each action potential consists of a change in voltage across the *membrane* of the axon.

### Question 1.2
Neuron A *excites* neuron C, whereas neuron B *inhibits* it.

### Question 1.3
No. There is no reason to expect a little bit of consciousness to reside in each neuron. Rather, the notion of system properties implies that consciousness *only* emerges at a certain level of complexity. It is something that only arises when lots of neurons are connected together to form complex circuits.

## Chapter 2

### Question 2.1
(a) 5; (b) 1; (c) 2; (d) 3; (e) 4.

### Question 2.2
The membrane contains receptors that signal the presence of prey to *Amoeba*, which then moves towards the signal using contractile protein filaments. The prey is engulfed and enclosed within a vacuole into which enzymes are secreted and the prey is digested.

### Question 2.3
Check your labels with Figure 2.18.

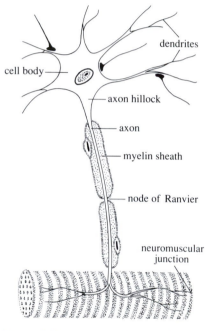

**Figure 2.18** Answer to Question 2.3

### Question 2.4
The nervous system relies on the conduction of electrical signals to perform its role in coordinating and controlling the activity of cells in the body. The electrical property of the neuronal membrane, i.e. the membrane potentials created by its selective permeability, allows these electrical signals to be generated.

### Question 2.5
The synaptic potential (either excitatory or inhibitory) is a graded potential, the action potential is an all-or-none event. The neuron receives thousands of synaptic inputs; the generation of an action potential at the axon hillock depends on the balance of excitatory and inhibitory synaptic potentials arriving at the cell. Once the threshold is reached, an action potential is generated which is conducted unchanged, in some cases over long distances, to other cells. In this way the

neuron acts as a computing device whose output is reliably relayed to other excitable cells.

## Question 2.6

Both membrane and sensory receptors are concerned with detecting events. The membrane receptor signals the presence of a particular transmitter to the cell, the sensory receptor signals an event to the nervous system.

The combination of membrane receptor and transmitter produces a synaptic potential in the postsynaptic cell. The excitation of a sensory receptor also produces a potential in the cell. In both cases activation causes a change in the permeability of the membrane to charged molecules.

## Question 2.7

Not really. The connections between neurons are not simple on-or-off switches. The dendrites receive many hundreds of synapses which produce graded excitatory or inhibitory potentials. The response of an individual neuron depends upon the spatial and temporal activity of the synapses. The behaviour of a network of neurons is consequently far more complex than that of an old-fashioned telephone exchange. Also the connections are not necessarily permanent, but can be changed with use (as will be discussed in Book 4).

## Question 2.8

The glial cells maintain the local environment surrounding neurons in a way that is optimal for their function. The glial cell sheath surrounding the axons in the vertebrate nervous system is important because it increases the rate of conduction of action potentials (and therefore of information transfer).

# Chapter 3

### Question 3.1

(c) is correct.

Figure 3.4 shows that in the neuron there is a high concentration of $K^+$ on the inside of the cell and a low concentration on the outside, a high concentration of $Na^+$ on the outside of the cell and a low concentration on the inside, and a low concentration of $Cl^-$ on the inside of the cell and a high concentration on the outside.

(a) therefore cannot be correct since $Na^+$ concentration is the other way round.

(b) cannot be correct since $Cl^-$ concentration is the other way round.

(c) is correct since it has the relative concentrations of $Na^+$, $K^+$ and $Cl^-$ the right way round, as described above.

### Question 3.2

(a), (b), (c) and (d) are all true.

(a)  See Section 3.4.

(b) The membrane potential is such that the inside of the neuron is negative with respect to the outside. This will attract positive ions (i.e. $Na^+$) into the cell. Since the extracellular concentration of $Na^+$ is high and the intracellular concentration low, the concentration gradient for $Na^+$ also acts so as to move $Na^+$ into the cell.

(c) That this is the mode of operation of the sodium–potassium pump is described in Section 3.4 and shown in Figure 3.5.

(d) This is described in Section 3.2.3.

## Question 3.3

(a), (c) and (e) are true.

(a) That this is the case is described in Section 3.6.

(b) Opening and closing of a population of $K^+$ channels plays a role in the action potential but only in the latter part of it. It is not responsible for the rising (depolarization) phase, which is due to the opening of $Na^+$ channels. Statement (b) is therefore false.

(c) That this is the case is described in Section 3.6.

(d) The repolarizing phase of the action potential is the result of $K^+$ ions leaving the cell; however, this is not the result of the sodium–potassium pump. Rather the sodium–potassium pump moves $K^+$ ions *into* the cell and does so at a steady rate. Statement (d) is therefore false.

(e) That this is the case is described in Section 3.6.

## Question 3.4

(a), (b), (c), (d) and (f) are true.

(a) That this is the case is described in Section 3.9.

(b) That this is the case is described in Section 3.9.

(c) If you got this wrong, look back at Section 3.9. If positive ions move into the cell, the membrane potential becomes less negative. This constitutes an EPSP, so statement (c) is true.

(d) That this is the case is described in Section 3.9. If negative ions flow out of the cell, the membrane potential becomes less negative. This constitutes an EPSP.

(e) If negative ions flow into the cell, this will make the inside more negative with respect to the outside. This would constitute an IPSP rather than an EPSP, so statement (e) is false.

(f) That this is the case is described in Section 3.9. If positive ions flow out of the cell, this will move the membrane potential to a value more negative than the resting potential. This constitutes an IPSP.

## Question 3.5

The statement is fine apart from the last sentence, which is wrong. The sodium–potassium pump 'ticks-over' at a fairly steady rate. It does not fluctuate during the action potential.

## Question 3.6

(b) and (c).

(a) If you thought this statement was true, you might be confusing speed of conduction with whether or not an action potential will arise. Whether or not an action potential has recently been generated can influence whether a second action potential will arise; a refractory period follows an action potential. However, should a second action potential arise, its *speed of conduction* does not depend upon whether another action potential has recently been transmitted.

(b) The diameter of an axon is one factor determining the speed of transmission of an action potential (Section 3.8).

(c) The myelin sheath, and the gaps in the sheath (nodes of Ranvier) provide a considerable increase in speed of transmission of an action potential compared with an unmyelinated axon of the same diameter.

(d) The action of the sodium–potassium pump is to exchange ions across the membrane at a fairly steady, 'background' rate. Its activity does not fluctuate instant by instant and in any case has no effect on the *speed* of conduction of an action potential.

(e) For a given set of axon properties (e.g. diameter, presence or absence of myelination), the action potential travels at a constant speed, irrespective of the length of the axon.

(f) If you thought this statement was true, you might be confusing two things here. The balance of EPSPs and IPSPs will determine whether or not an action potential *arises* in the first place. Once initiated, the action potential will travel at a speed determined by the diameter of the axon and whether or not it is myelinated.

## Question 3.7

If an action potential has travelled along a portion of axon, the voltage-gated channels in the membrane of that region need to reassume a form that allows them to open again. In other words, a refractory period must elapse. If the action potential is stimulated somewhere midway along the axon, the region to either side has not been stimulated and so an action potential can spread out to either side. In nerve cells, the generation of an action potential at one end of the axon, the axon hillock, means that the action potentials will travel in one direction only.

# Chapter 4

## Question 4.1

The correct answer is (d).

(a) See Section 4.1. At the chemical synapse there is a small gap between the presynaptic membrane and the postsynaptic membrane. In the electrical synapse, the membranes make direct contact.

(b) See Section 4.1, where the greater possibilities afforded by the chemical synapse are described.

(c) See Section 4.2.1, where the delay in the chemical synapse is contrasted with the lack of delay at the electrical synapse.

(d) That this is the case is described in Section 4.2.1.

## Question 4.2

1 Axon (or more specifically axon terminal)

2 Synaptic vesicle

3 Presynaptic membrane

4 Synaptic cleft

5 Transmitter molecule

6 Postsynaptic membrane

## Question 4.3

Action potentials arriving at the presynaptic terminal increase the permeability of the membrane to $Ca^{2+}$ ions. The resulting increased intracellular $Ca^{2+}$ ion concentration causes neurotransmitter-filled synaptic vesicles to fuse with the presynaptic membrane and, by the process of exocytosis, to release their contents into the synaptic cleft. The transmitter molecules then diffuse across the cleft and become attached to postsynaptic membrane receptors. The binding of transmitter to the receptors alters the permeability of the postsynaptic membrane which, in turn, changes the membrane potential. Depending on the type of neurotransmitter–receptor connection, these changes can produce EPSPs or IPSPs.

## Question 4.4

Their effects would cancel out, leaving little or no change in membrane potential. The tendency of 1 to depolarize is cancelled by the tendency of 3 to hyperpolarize.

## Question 4.5

1 The substance must be synthesized in neurons and stored at their axon terminals.

2 The substance must be released into the synaptic cleft when the neuron is stimulated.

3 Receptors must be present on the postsynaptic membrane that are capable of being activated by the substance.

4 There must be a specific inactivation process for the elimination of the substance from the synaptic cleft.

## Question 4.6

(c) is the correct answer. If you had any other answers, look back at Section 4.5.8, where the action of curare at the ACh synapse is described.

# Chapter 5

### Question 5.1

It is legitimate to describe an animal as having an immunological memory of past encounters with infectious organisms because the immune system 'remembers' infectious organisms it has met before, greeting them rapidly with a series of cellular and biochemical defences, unlike its slow response to new infections. This is analogous to the precise memory humans form of each face that they meet, and the different responses they show to old and new acquaintances.

However, the analogy should not be stretched too far. Memories held in the nervous system can be recalled and reinterpreted and they are subject to many kinds of modification by experience—a far richer and more complex set of processes than that displayed in immunological memory.

### Question 5.2

You should recall from Chapters 2 and 4 that the same transmitter molecule can have either an excitatory or an inhibitory action depending on the nature of the receptor that it binds to. It is therefore entirely possible that noradrenalin enhances the immune response by simultaneously activating helper T cells and inhibiting suppressor T cells because they have (respectively) excitatory or inhibitory receptors for this neurotransmitter.

### Question 5.3

The experiment shown in Figure 5.10 demonstrates that, between the first and the twenty-fifth week, symptoms appear in *fewer* animals given paired cyclo-phosphamide and saccharin and then reinforced with saccharin in 50% of the study weeks (the $CS_{50\%}$ group) than in animals that received the same doses of drug and saccharin without pairing the two stimuli (the $NC_{50\%}$ group). Thus more of the conditioned animals remained well than of the unconditioned. However, there are serious limitations to this therapeutic method. The delay in onset of symptoms in the conditioned animals compared with the unconditioned animals was only evident for those that became ill before the 25th week—thereafter there was no difference between the conditioned and the unconditioned groups. Moreover, symptoms eventually developed even in animals that were given cyclophosphamide *every* week (the $CS_{100\%}$ group), showing that immuno-suppression with this drug was not sufficient to cure this autoimmune disease.

# Chapter 6

### Question 6.1

The projections from sensory receptors (light, vibration or touch) are topographically arranged, i.e. neighbouring receptors project to neighbouring areas of the brain.

### Question 6.2

The nerve net, like the neurons in more complex animals, acts as a communication system, coordinating the activities of different parts of the animal in response to changes in the external environment. The capacity of these electrically excitable cells to transmit information is fundamental to neural function.

### Question 6.3

The sea-anemone is a sedentary animal, while jellyfish actively swim to catch food; the latter therefore need additional sensory information provided by the simple eye and balance organs. The coordination of muscular activity during swimming requires a rather more sophisticated nervous system, e.g. the fast conducting rings around the base of the bell.

### Question 6.4

Habituation (the waning of a response to repeated stimulation) prevents the animal responding repeatedly to harmless stimuli that are repeated. Rhythm generation by neuron networks is the basis for some types of animal movement. Both these functions depend on synaptic interactions between groups of neurons.

### Question 6.5

In vertebrates the speed of action potential conduction is mainly enhanced by the presence of a coating of myelin on the axons. In invertebrates the conduction speed is enhanced by the larger diameter of some of the axons.

### Question 6.6

The squid is an active hunter, with its swimming prowess depending on the fast, synchronous contraction of muscles innervated by large diameter axons. These are large enough for electrical probes to be inserted to observe the changes in potential and ion movements accompanying the action potential.

# Chapter 7

### Question 7.1

Option (d) is false. The muscle action potential is much longer than the nerve action potential (compare Figure 7.17 with Figure 3.11).

### Question 7.2

(a) True. There is a latent period between the stimulus and the onset of contraction (Figure 7.17).

(b) False. Muscles cannot actively relax. Relaxation is a passive phase. Lengthening is produced by the action of antagonistic muscles.

(c) False. The tension produced depends on the intensity of the stimulus (Figure 7.19). Also, the muscle may contain more than one motor unit with different thresholds for each.

(d) True. The relaxation phase lasts longer than the contraction phase.

(e) True. Active contraction lasts much longer than the action potential that produced it.

(f) False. There may be more than one motor unit in the muscle so although this may be true for some muscle twitches it is not a true statement in general.

(g)  False. Successive twitches may produce the same force, but if the size of the stimulation varies then larger or smaller twitches might be observed due to the capacity of muscles with multiple motor units to give an apparent graded response.

## Question 7.3

(a)  False. In tetanus successive muscle contractions *do* fuse.

(b)  True. Tetanus is a smooth contraction in which individual twitches cannot be distinguished.

(c)  False. Muscles may not work at their maximum capacity in tetanus as not all motor units may be active.

(d)  False. Tetanus can be produced by excitation of a single motor unit.

(e)  False. Unusually strong contractions of a muscle are not necessarily produced by tetanus.

## Question 7.4

If you can be sure that each cycle is almost exactly like the next, as you often can be with locomotory rhythms, then all the measurements necessary to build up a complete picture of the behaviour pattern can be accumulated over many cycles and need not be made all at the same time.

## Question 7.5

If the rhythm in a flight interneuron is changed by artificial stimulation with a rhythmic stimulus, the flight muscle rhythm then follows the new one. If it resets itself when the stimulation is removed, it is reasonable to assume that the interneuron is rhythmically active.

## Question 7.6

A completed diagram is given in Figure 7.30.

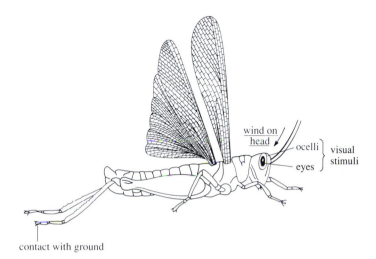

**Figure 7.30**    Answer to Question 7.6.

# Chapter 8

## Question 8.1

Check your labelling with Figure 8.14. The small olfactory bulbs together with the large cerebellum and optic tectum suggest that this fish relies much more on vision than on smell. In fact, it was the brain of a cod, which is a predatory fish living in open water.

## Question 8.2

Check your labels with Figure 8.35. The presence of the sympathetic ganglia means this must be a thoracic segment. Grey matter contains the neuron cell bodies, while the white matter contains many myelinated axons. The motor neurons are the neurons with the largest cell bodies in the spinal cord; they innervate muscles.

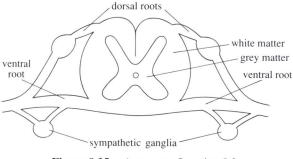

**Figure 8.35**   Answer to Question 8.2.

## Question 8.3

(c)

The central region of the spinal cord contains numbers of cell bodies and their processes. It is grey matter. The myelinated axons which connect the spinal cord with the brain travel in pathways surrounding the central regions and have a whitish appearance because of the myelin sheaths.

## Question 8.4

The optic input to the tectum and thalamus is arranged topographically, i.e. neighbouring areas of retina project to neighbouring areas of these structures. This provides the animal with an internal representation of the external world.

## Question 8.5

No, the mammalian cerebral cortex has taken over the role of visual analysis: the optic tectum (superior colliculi) in mammals controls eye movements and orientation responses.

## Question 8.6

The sympathetic division of the ANS, together with the adrenal glands, are responsible for preparing the body for an emergency, when the heart beats faster and sweat glands are activated. The adrenal gland releases the hormone adrenalin which has a widespread and relatively long lasting action on target organs. What is interesting is that the symptoms were the result of what the person *thought* was a dangerous situation, illustrating the control of autonomic function by the cortex.

## Question 8.7

All sensory information (except olfactory input from the nose) passes through the thalamus on its way to the cortex. The thalamic nuclei receive inputs also from the cortex and other areas of the brain. The thalamus therefore is much more like a controlled gateway to the cortex than a simple passage.

## Question 8.8

The inputs from the thalamus relaying specific sensory information to the primary sensory cortical areas have compact terminals in layer 4: other thalamic inputs and those from association axons are more diffuse.

## Question 8.9

The importance of tactile information from the lips and fingers in primate life is reflected in their larger representation on the somatosensory cortex. The whiskers play an important role in the control of behaviour in the mainly nocturnal rat and, consequently, they have a specialized region of cortex to which they project (the barrel fields). The importance of the trunk in elephants is likely to be reflected in its large representation on the cortex.

## Question 8.10

Rats, with their laterally placed eyes, have only 10% binocular overlap, so that most optic axons cross to the contralateral side of the brain. Humans have much greater binocular overlap and so fewer axons cross over.

## Question 8.11

The cerebral cortex serves the function of both processing sensory information and forming motor commands, both functions being essential in movement. A high proportion of the behavioural patterns of mammals with large cerebral cortices is learnt, allowing such animals to adapt to environmental changes quickly and efficiently. The cerebellum is involved in controlling skilled movements; many of these movements are also learnt and the cerebellum probably plays a role in this activity. In primates both cerebral and cerebellar cortices are enlarged, compared with other animals.

# Chapter 9

## Question 9.1

(d)

A dermatome is the 'collection' of receptive fields of touch-sensitive neurons whose axons enter the spinal cord via the dorsal root ganglia in a single segment of the spinal cord.

## Question 9.2

(a), (c) and (d)

The structure of the muscle spindle and its relationship with working muscle is shown in Figure 9.6. While this muscle spindle can contract, it does not generate any significant force and does not contribute to movement of joints.

## Question 9.3

(a), (c), (f) and (g)

The cell bodies of sensory neurons are located in the dorsal ganglia, outside the spinal cord grey matter, while motor neurons are located in ventral regions. By definition, a polysynaptic reflex has more than one synapse in its control pathway.

## Question 9.4

(b)

By definition, a ballistic movement occurs too rapidly for feedback to interfere in its execution.

## Question 9.5

(b), (d), (f) and (h)

(a)  The pyramidal tract  descends to the spinal cord motor neurons—there are no motor neurons in the brain stem.

(c)  The pyramidal tract makes direct connections with $\alpha$ motor neurons in humans, not $\gamma$ motor neurons.

(e)  The pathways cross at the level of the brain stem in the structure called the medulla.

(g)  In Parkinson's disease the pathway to the basal ganglia degenerates.

## Question 9.6

(a), (b), (c), (e), (f), (h) and (i)

(d)  Ventrobasal neurons have receptive fields with a concentric organization, their outer areas being inhibitory and their inner areas excitatory.

(g)  The outer region will inhibit the effect of the centre region.

# Chapter 10

## Question 10.1

The protective reflexes are available all of the time, except in abnormal conditions (e.g. pathological) states. Their availability does not fluctuate as a function of some internal state of the animal. By contrast, the availability of the lordosis reflex fluctuates as a function of the internal state of the animal, i.e. the degree of sensitization of the hypothalamus by oestrogen.

The functional significance of this difference is that at all times reflexes must be available to protect the animal from noxious stimuli. By contrast, it is only of adaptive value for the female rat to display lordosis at times when fertilization is possible.

## Question 10.2

A similarity is that in both cases, the response to a given stimulus can be shown not to be constant. In the case of lordosis, the tactile stimulus is associated with lordosis if the hypothalamus has been sensitized by oestrogen. It is not shown when the hypothalamus is not sensitized. In the case of tactile stimulation of the cat's face, this is normally associated with turning the head away. If the hypothalamus is electrically stimulated at the same time as the tactile stimulus is applied, an attack response is evoked.

The difference between the two is that, whereas the central change that underlies the difference in response is hormonally mediated in the case of lordosis, it is not assumed to be mediated by hormones in the case of the defensive behaviour. This would make good sense in functional terms. Lordosis would be expected to reflect the hormonal state of the animal concerning the chances of fertilization. There is no cost attached to a relatively slow change between a state of receptivity and non-receptivity. By contrast, in the case of defensive behaviours the cat would need to change behaviour almost instantaneously, between withdrawal and attack, according to the second-by-second context in which it finds itself.

## Question 10.3

Disconnect the electric current.

## Question 10.4

As Figure 10.11 shows, the rat with prior experience in this environment makes a beeline for where the platform was located. This is true no matter where in the tank the rat is placed. Therefore the rat shows evidence of having performed place learning. At a neural level it would be assumed that there are place cells corresponding to features of the environment: there would be place cells corresponding to the location of the platform (even though it is no longer present). These place cells play a role in maintaining the rat's swimming behaviour in the vicinity of where the platform used to be located.

# Chapter 11

## Question 11.1

(b), (d) and (f)

(a) is not true since, in the Wernicke–Geschwind model, Wernicke's area is concerned with comprehension of speech rather than the production of speech.

(c) is not true. The perceptual processes as such are not disrupted. Comprehension based upon the perceptions is disrupted.

(e) is not true. Damage to Wernicke's area results in a receptive aphasia.

## Question 11.2

(c) and (d)

(a) is not correct. It is normally the right side of the brain that is specialized for processing visuo-spatial information.

(b) is not correct. It is true that damage to the left side of the brain during infancy affects the development of language functions. It is also true that the left hemisphere tends to be specialized for language and the right hemisphere for visuo-spatial tasks. However, if you look at Figure 11.6, you will see that left-hemisphere damage during infancy has not spared spatial performance (i.e. a non-verbal performance).

## Question 11.3

(a)  semantic

(b)  procedural

(c)  episodic

(d)  working

## Question 11.4

A double dissociation is where both (1) damage to region X disrupts cognitive skill A but leaves B intact, and (2) damage to region Y disrupts cognitive skill B but leaves A intact. The fact that X leaves skill B intact is an argument against the damage to X having a general effect on all cognitive skills.

## Question 11.5

(b), (f), (g), (h) and (i)

(a) is not correct. Look at Section 11.4.1. You will see that damage to the right temporal lobe does not cause a disruption of memory for verbal material.

(c) is not correct. Episodic, semantic and procedural memories are long-term memories but working memory is not. Rather, it is something held briefly, for instance, a telephone number that is dialled and then forgotten.

(d) is not correct. Look at Section 11.4.4. H.M. was disrupted in his ability to update semantic memory.

(e) is not correct. Look at Section 11.4.4. H.M. was disrupted in his ability to update semantic memory.

## Question 11.6

(d)

(a), (b) and (c) are not correct. According to Edelman, the capacities for learning, perceptual categorization, and monitoring the internal state are *necessary* but not *sufficient* conditions for consciousness to emerge. They are capacities possessed by species to which consciousness would not normally be attributed.

## Question 11.7

(d)

(a), (b) and (c) are not correct. According to Edelman, a capacity for classical conditioning, object recognition, and complex learning are *necessary* conditions. However, these are also associated with species that one would not normally describe as conscious.

# GLOSSARY

**absolute refractory period**   The time throughout the repolarization phase of the action potential during which no amount of externally applied depolarization can initiate another action potential. (Section 3.8)

**action potential**   A momentary and localized change in electrical potential across the membrane of a neuron or muscle cell caused by a rapid change in the membrane's permeability to $Na^+$. (Section 2.3.2)

**afferent**   Carrying information *to* a particular group of neurons. (Section 6.3.1)

**agonist**   A chemical substance capable of mimicking the physiological effect of a transmitter by specifically interacting with its natural receptors. An agonist is usually very similar in shape and chemical structure to the natural transmitter and has the same effect on the postsynaptic cell. (Section 4.2.5)

**antagonist**   A chemical substance that may totally block or reduce the intensity of the physiological response evoked by a neurotransmitter. Antagonists may bind to the transmitter itself, rendering it unable to combine with its natural receptor; or they may resemble the transmitter and bind with the receptor site (without producing the same response in the postsynaptic cell as the natural transmitter), thereby blocking the receptor site. (Section 4.2.5)

**antagonistic**   Refers to groups of muscle that produce opposing effects. (Section 7.5)

**anterior**   Towards the front; used when referring to a part of the body, such as the human brain. (Section 8.1.1)

**anterograde amnesia**   An inability to remember new information for any length of time. (Section 11.4.2)

**anterograde transport**   Transport of material along the axon which proceeds in the same direction as action potentials. (Section 8.7.1)

**antibody**   Simple protein molecule synthesized by white cells as part of the immune defence system; a Y-shaped molecule with a binding site at the tip of each arm that can bind a specific antigen. (Section 5.3)

**antigen**   Strictly speaking, any cell or molecule to which an antibody can bind, but often used as shorthand for 'any foreign cell or molecule'. (Section 5.2.1)

**aphasia**   General medical term used to describe a disturbance of speech; strictly, an absence of speech. (Section 11.2.1)

**appetitive behaviour**   Relatively flexible behaviour based on locomotion, leading to such things as food, water or a mate; it is terminated by consummatory behaviour. (Section 10.1)

**association axon**   Axon which links two areas of the cerebral cortex. (Section 8.8.1)

**association cortex**    Areas of the cerebral cortex which are involved in higher processing of sensory information; they integrate incoming sensory information with that stored in the memory. (Section 8.4.3)

**autoimmune disease**    A type of disease in which the immune system of an organism attacks normal, healthy body tissue of that same organism. (Section 5.6.2)

**autonomic nervous system (ANS)**    The part of the nervous system concerned with regulating the activity of the internal organs. It is composed of groups of neurons which innervate the muscles of the gut, heart, and glands. (Section 5.6.1)

**axon hillock**    The region of the cell body from which the axon emerges, and where the action potential is first generated. (Section 2.3.1)

**axon terminal**    Small terminal expansion of the axon at the synapse where neurotransmitter molecules are stored and released. (Section 2.3.1)

**axon**    The extension of a neuron that conducts action potentials away from the cell body. (Sections  1.2 and 2.3.1)

**bilateral symmetry**    The condition where an animal can be divided into mirror-image right and left halves by a vertical plane running along its midline from head to toe. (Section 6.3)

**binocular vision**    The condition where the two eyes receive inputs from an overlapping region of visual space; it is present to a greater or lesser extent in most mammals. (Section 8.8.3)

**blood–brain barrier**    A barrier formed by special cells, with tight seals between them, that line the blood vessels of the brain; it regulates the movements of chemicals from the blood to the fluid that bathes the neurons of the brain. (Section 2.4.4)

**brain stem**    The collective name for the midbrain and the pons and medulla of the hindbrain. (Section 8.4.1)

**Cartesian dualism**    The principle, based on the theory of Rene Descartes, that mind and matter are qualitatively different, and that because the mind does not operate within the laws of physics it cannot be investigated scientifically. Descartes also postulated that the mind (or soul) was unique to humans. (Section 11.5.3)

**caudal**    Towards the tail end of an animal. (Section 8.1.1)

**cell membrane**    Extremely thin layer (about 8–10 nm thick) which forms the external surface of all cells; it regulates the passage of substances into and out of the cell. (Section 2.2.1)

**central nervous system (CNS)**    The brain and spinal cord. (Section 1.2)

**cephalization**    The enlargement of the ganglia towards the head end of the central nervous system. (Section 6.3.1)

**cervical**    Relating to the neck, e.g. the cervical segments of the spinal cord are located in the neck region and innervate the forelimbs. (Section 8.3)

**chemoreceptors**   Sensory neurons which respond to chemical stimuli. (Section 2.4.1)

**commissure**   Bundle of axons connecting the ganglia of one segment across the midline in the invertebrate nervous system (Section 6.3.1), or connecting the two halves of the brain across the midline in the vertebrate nervous system.

**compound eye**   The type of eye found in insects and crustaceans; it consists of a collection of individual units, each of which has its own lens and photoreceptors. (Section 6.3.3)

**concentration gradient**   A difference in the concentration of a particular substance between two regions. (Section 3.2.2)

**conduction velocity**   The speed at which an action potential travels along an axon. (Section 3.8)

**connective**   Bundle of axons connecting the ganglia of adjacent segments on the same side of the midline in the invertebrate nervous system. (Section 6.3.1)

**consummatory behaviour**   Reflexive, species-typical behaviour which is the termination of appetitive behaviour. (Section 10.1)

**contralateral**   Structures located on opposite sides of the midline of an animal. (Section 8.1.1)

**convergent inputs**   Axons from many neurons which all synapse on a single cell. (Section 2.3.3)

**cytoplasm**   The contents of a cell, excluding the nucleus. Within the cytoplasm are the cell organelles. (Section 2.2.1)

**cytotoxic contact**   Killing of infectious organisms by contact with white cells, which secrete specialized cytotoxic (cell-killing) chemicals. (Section 5.3)

**dendrite**   Extension of a neuron that receives many synapses from other neurons; it does not usually conduct action potentials. (Section 2.3.1)

**dendritic spines**   Small protrusions on the surface of dendrites which are contacted by, usually, one presynaptic terminal. (Section 2.3.3)

**dermatome**   The area of skin whose sensory receptors are connected with sensory neurons that lie in a single dorsal root ganglion. (Section 9.3)

**divergent outputs**   The outputs of one neuron that form the inputs to a number of other neurons. (Section 2.3.3)

**dorsal**   Towards an animal's back. (Section 6.3)

**double dissociation**   The situation where a lesion at site A produces a disturbance in function X but not Y, and a lesion at site B produces a disturbance in function Y but not X. (Section 11.4.1)

**effector cells**   Cells that bring about action outside the nervous system; e.g. muscle cells, or the hormone-releasing cells of the endocrine system. (Section 2.4.2)

**efferent**   Carrying information *away from* a particular group of neurons. (Section 6.3.1)

**electrical self-stimulation**   The phenomenon whereby an animal with an electrode implanted in certain regions of its brain (e.g. hypothalamus) will learn to press a bar in a Skinner box to receive an electrical shock to its brain. (Section 10.5)

**end plate potential**   Depolarization at the end plate due to release of transmitter by the axon terminal of the motor neuron; if large enough this change in potential leads to muscle contraction. (Section 2.4.2)

**end plate**   The postsynaptic area of vertebrate skeletal muscle. (Section 2.4.2)

**endocytosis**   A process by which the cell takes in substances or particles by surrounding them with part of the cell membrane, which then becomes detached to form a 'bubble' (vacuole) within the cell. The opposite process is exocytosis. Endocytosis is important in the re-uptake of neurotransmitter molecules into the presynaptic cell or into glial cells. (Section 4.2.3)

**endorphins**   A group of opioid transmitters which are synthesized by the body and which reduce the perception of pain. (Section 4.5.6)

**enkephalins**   A group of opioid transmitters which are synthesized by the body and which reduce the perception of pain. (Section 4.5.6)

**episodic memory**   Memory about things an individual has done, or events which have affected that individual. (Section 11.4.4)

**equilibrium**   A state of dynamic balance in which movement of molecules between different regions (e.g. on either side of the cell membrane) is the same in both directions, so that there is no net movement between the regions. (Section 3.2.2)

**excitation**   An influence of one neuron on another which increases the probability that the second neuron will produce an action potential. (Section 1.2)

**excitatory postsynaptic potential (EPSP)**   A change in local potential occurring at the synapse which depolarizes the postsynaptic cell and thus makes an action potential more likely. (Section 2.3.3)

**forebrain**   The most rostral part of the brain; involved in analysing olfactory information. (Section 8.4.1)

**ganglion**   A collection of neuronal cell bodies. (Section 6.3.1)

**grey matter**   The central region of the spinal cord and brain stem and the outer layer of the cerebral hemispheres, which consist mainly of neuronal cell bodies. (Section 8.2)

**hindbrain**   The most caudal part of the brain; involved in processing information about vibration and orientation. (Section 8.4.1)

**humoral factors**   Molecules circulating freely in the body fluids. In modern immunology, the term is used for molecules synthesized by particular white cells after contact with a pathogen, for example antibodies. (Section 5.3)

**hyperpolarization**   A change in the membrane potential to a value more *negative* than the resting value. (Section 3.6)

**immune system** A collection of cells and their secreted products responsible for protecting the body against invasion by pathogens such as bacteria or parasites. (Section 2.1)

**immunological memory** The capacity of the immune system to recognize which pathogens it has encountered before. It involves the proliferation of white cells after first contact with a specific pathogen. Subsequent encounters are dealt with more effectively by a greater number of white cells. (Section 5.2.2)

**inferior** Towards the lower, or ventral, part of the human brain. (Section 8.1.1)

**inflammation** Local rapid response characterized by swelling, redness, heat and pain around the site of an infection or allergic reaction. The response is generated by chemicals released by white cells. These chemicals cause leakage and dilation of blood vessels. (Section 5.3)

**inhibition** An influence of one neuron on another which decreases the probability that the second neuron will produce an action potential. (Section 1.2)

**inhibitory postsynaptic potential (IPSP)** A change in the membrane potential of a neuron produced by synaptic activity that decreases the overall depolarization of the postsynaptic cell and makes the neuron less likely to generate an action potential. (Section 2.3.3)

**intelligence quotient (IQ)** The score which is the result of a standard intelligence test. (Section 11.3.1)

**intrinsic neurons** Neurons whose axons remain within the area where their cell bodies are located, e.g. in the cerebral cortex. (Section 8.8.1)

**invertebrates** Multicellular animals without a backbone e.g. insects, snails, worms, jellyfish. (Section 6.1)

**ipsilateral** Structures which are located on the same side of the midline of an animal. (Section 8.1.1)

**lateral** Away from the midline of an animal in a horizontal plane. (Section 8.1.1)

**lateral inhibition** An antagonistic relationship between two areas of a receptive field, e.g. the inner and outer parts of a concentrically organized receptive field. (Section 9.5.3)

**lateralization** The asymmetrical distribution of function between the two hemispheres of the brain, e.g. localization of language in the left hemisphere. (Section 11.3)

**levels of explanation** Explanations within the brain and behavioural sciences can be couched in various ways, using the concepts and terms of various disciplines. These disciplines may range from explanations in terms of interactions between molecules to interactions within societies, or anywhere in between. (Section 1.3)

**long-term memory** Memory which is stored by the brain for extremely long periods of time. (Section 11.4)

**lumbar** Relating to the lower back, e.g. the lumbar segments of the spinal cord are located in the lower back region and innervate the hind limbs. (Section 8.3)

**lymphokines**   Signalling molecules secreted by helper and suppressor T cells which either promote or inhibit the activity of other white cells in response to an infection. (Section 5.4.2)

**mechanoreceptors**   Sensory receptors that produce action potentials in sensory neurons as a result of deformation of their cell membrane. These include touch receptors and hair cells as well as proprioceptors. ( Section 2.4.1)

**medial**   Towards the midline of an animal. (Section 8.1.1)

**membrane potential**   Difference in electrical voltage between the inside and outside of a living cell produced by selective permeability of the membrane to ions. (Section 2.3.2)

**midbrain**   The middle part of the brain, involved in analysing visual information and initiating motor activities in response to this information. (Section 8.4.1)

**monosynaptic reflex**   A neural pathway consisting of a sensory neuron connected in the spinal cord directly to a motor neuron. Such a pathway thus only has one synapse. (Section 9.3.1)

**motor neuron**   A neuron with its cell body within the spinal cord or brain stem whose axon innervates a muscle. (Section 2.4.2)

**motor system**   The collective term for the central nervous system structures involved in the control of the skeletal muscles. (Section 9.1)

**motor unit**   The group of muscle fibres which is innervated by a single motor neuron. (Section 7.6.2)

**myelin**   A fatty substance derived from the cell membrane of specialized glial cells which surrounds some axons in vertebrates. It is formed by the glial cells wrapping themselves around the axons, and acts as an electrically insulating sheath, allowing rapid propagation of the action potential over long distances. (Section 2.4.4)

**nerve net**   A 'net' of electrically excitable cells such as that forming the nervous system of sea-anemones and jellyfish. (Section 6.2)

**neuromodulator**   A peptide molecule similar to a neurotransmitter, but which diffuses into groups of neurons and therefore affects large numbers of neurons simultaneously. (Section 4.5.6)

**neuromuscular junction**   The synapse between a motor neuron and a muscle cell. (Section 2.4.2)

**neuron**   A type of cell in the nervous system specialized to receive input in chemical form, and to transmit information along its axon, usually by means of action potentials, to other cells via synaptic connections. (Section 1.1)

**neuropile**   The network of axons and dendrites that forms the centre of a ganglion in the invertebrate nervous system. (Section 6.3.1)

**neurosecretory cells**   Cells forming part of the endocrine system; they release hormones into the bloodstream. (Section 8.6)

**neurotransmitter**   A small molecule released at a synapse, that binds to a specific receptor on the postsynaptic membrane, and changes the local potential of the membrane, making it less likely (if inhibitory) or more likely (if excitatory) that an action potential will be generated in the postsynaptic neuron. (Section 2.3.3)

**nociceptor**   A type of sensory receptor which is found in the skin and internal tissues and which detects stimuli that may lead to tissue damage. (Section 4.5.6)

**node of Ranvier**   A gap between the glial cells that form the myelin sheath around the axons of vertebrates. (Section 2.4.4)

**nucleus**   In the context of the nervous system, an anatomically distinct group of interconnected neurons in the central or autonomic nervous systems, which have a common function. (Section 8.1)

**pacemakers**   Neurons that generate signals (action potentials) at regular intervals. (Section 7.2.2)

**parasympathetic division**   Part of the autonomic nervous system which maintains the normal resting state of the internal organs. It has ganglia situated within the target organs. (Section 8.5)

**pathogen**   Disease-causing organism. (Sections 2.1 and 5.2.1)

**peripheral nervous system (PNS)**   Neural tissue lying outside the brain and spinal cord; it includes the axons of sensory and motor neurons connecting the central nervous system with the periphery. (Section 1.2)

**phagocytosis**   The process by which a cell engulfs food and digests it, or a pathogen and destroys it; a form of endocytosis. (Section 5.3)

**photoreceptor**   Sensory cell sensitive to light. It transduces light energy into electrical energy. (Section 2.4.1)

**place cell**   A neuron in the hippocampus which codes for a particular location in the environment. It transmits action potentials when the animal is in that particular location. (Section 10.6)

**place learning**   The ability of an animal to construct and update a spatial or cognitive map of its environment. (Section 10.6)

**platelet**   Fragment of large cell that develops in the bone marrow. Platelets are released into the bloodstream in very large numbers and are involved in blood-clotting mechanisms. (Section 5.4.1)

**polysynaptic reflex**   A neural pathway consisting of a sensory neuron and a motor neuron, between which there are one or more spinal cord interneurons. Such a pathway thus has more than one synapse. (Section 9.3.1)

**posterior**   Towards the rear; used when referring to a part of the body such as the human brain. (Section 8.1.1)

**postsynaptic membrane**   A region of the membrane of an excitable cell directly adjacent to a presynaptic axon terminal. It is specialized for receiving transmitter molecules. (Section 2.3.1)

**potential difference**   A difference in electrical potential (voltage) between two adjacent regions. (Section 2.3.2)

**presynaptic inhibition**   A relationship between two neurons in which activity in one alters the release of neurotransmitter from the second neuron which results in a decrease in postsynaptic potential such that no action potential is propagated. (Section 4.3)

**presynaptic membrane**   A region of the membrane of the axon terminal of an excitable cell adjacent to the postsynaptic membrane. It is specialized for releasing transmitter molecules. (Section 2.3.1)

**primary motor cortex**   The topographically organised area of the cerebral cortex which sends outputs, via the motor neurons, to the muscles in the opposite side of the body. (Section 8.4.3)

**primary sensory cortex**   The areas of the cerebral cortex which receive incoming sensory information about sensations from the body surface (e.g. touch), vision and hearing. (Section 8.4.3)

**projection neurons**   Neurons in one part of the central nervous system whose axons convey information to another part. (Section 8. 2)

**receptive field**   That part of the sensory field which, when it is stimulated, activates the neuron under study; e.g. the small patch of skin from which a single sensory neuron gets its input. (Section 9.5.2)

**receptor potential**   The electrical signal (change in the membrane potential) produced by appropriate stimulation of a sensory cell. (Section 2.4.1)

**receptor-gated channel**   An ion channel in a membrane that is only open when an associated receptor site is occupied by a specific transmitter molecule. (Section 3.9)

**reciprocal antagonist inhibition**   The spinal cord reflex mechanism that prevents simultaneous contraction of opposing sets of muscles. (Section 9.3.3)

**relative refractory period**   The period of recovery after an action potential, during which action potentials can only be produced by stimulation greater than normal. In sea-anemones, the period of recovery after an action potential during which smaller than normal action potentials are produced. (Section 7.2.2)

**repolarization**   The return of the membrane potential to its resting state during an action potential. (Section 3.6)

**retrograde amnesia**   Impairment of memory for events which happened prior to the event causing the amnesia. (Section 11.4.2)

**retrograde transport**   Transport of material along the axon which is in the opposite direction to the conduction of action potentials. (Section 8.7.1)

**rostral**   Towards the nose of an animal. (Section 8.1.1)

**Schwann cell**   A type of glial cell in the peripheral nervous system that forms a myelin sheath around axons and thereby speeds up the conduction of action potentials. (Section 3.8)

**second messengers**   Molecules within the cell that transmit information between different parts of the cell.   They are responsible for opening receptor-gated channels following the binding of transmitter molecules to receptors. (Section 4.2.5)

**segmentation**   The organization of the bodies of most animals, on the basis of a series of repeated structural units, or segments. (Section 6.3)

**semantic memory**   Memory which includes general knowledge of the world, including the use of language. (Section 11.4.4)

**semipermeable membrane**   A membrane that allows the passage of some substances and not of others; such substances may be solvent molecules or dissolved molecules (solutes). (Section 3.2.2)

**short-term memory**   Memory where information is only stored for the period of time in which it is needed, e.g. an unfamiliar telephone number; also known as working memory. (Section 11.4)

**small lymphocyte**   One of the most numerous types of white cell in the immune system; the only type that synthesizes antibodies, lymphokines or neurotransmitters and which displays immunological memory. (Section 5.4.2)

**smooth muscle**   A type of muscle which does not have striated myofibrils; found in the gut, the walls of blood vessels and in other internal organs. (Section 7.6.1)

**sodium–potassium pump**   The active mechanism in the membrane of a neuron whereby $Na^+$ ions are expelled from the inside of the cell and $K^+$ ions retrieved from the outside. (Section 3.4)

**somatosensory**   Concerned with the sensations from the body surface, e.g. touch, temperature and tissue damage (pain). (Section 8.8.1)

**spatial summation**   The integration of the depolarizing or hyperpolarizing effects occurring at synapses at different locations on the neuron. (Section 4.3)

**species-typical behaviour**   Behaviour shown in an almost identical manner by all members of a particular species (or by all members of one sex of a species, in the case of behaviour specific to one sex). (Section 10.1)

**specific thalamic nuclei**   Groups of neurons within the thalamus that relay touch, visual and auditory information to the primary sensory areas of the cerebral cortex. (Section 8.4.3)

**striated muscle**   A type of muscle which has a striped (or striated) appearance under a microscope using polarized light, due to the repeating units of its myofibrils; found in the skeletal muscles. (Section 7.6.1)

**superior**   Towards the upper, or dorsal, part of the human brain (Section 8.1.1)

**sympathetic division**   Part of the autonomic nervous system which alters the metabolic state of the animal in response to danger. It has pairs of ganglia on each side of the thoracic segments of the spinal cord. (Section 8.5)

**synapse**   The area of close contact between a neuron and another excitable cell (e.g. neuron, muscle fibre or gland cell) with which it communicates. (Section 2.3.1)

**synaptic cleft**   The gap separating the membrane of the presynaptic neuron and that of the postsynaptic neuron or effector cell. (Section 2.3.1)

**synaptic delay**   The time between the arrival of the action potential at the presynaptic axon terminal and any effect that this brings about in the postsynaptic cell; generally of the order of about 0.5 ms. (Section 4.2.1)

**synaptic potential**   The change in the membrane potential of an excitable cell produced when transmitter released by the presynaptic terminal binds with receptors in the postsynaptic membrane. (Section 2.3.3)

**synaptic vesicle**   Membrane-enclosed sac containing neurotransmitter found in the axon terminals of neurons. The contents of the sacs are released into the synaptic cleft upon the arrival of an action potential at the axon terminal. (Section 2.3.1)

**synergistic**   Acting together; in the context of the motor system, groups of muscles that act together to produce the same direction of movement. (Section 7.5)

**system property**   When components are assembled to constitute a system there are certain properties that only occur, and can only be understood, at the level of the whole system. These are termed system properties. (Section 1.3)

**temporal summation**   The integration of the effects of incoming signals on the postsynaptic neuron within the dimension of time. (Section 4.3)

**tetanus**   Sustained contraction of a muscle as a result of a high frequency of stimulation of the motor neurons which innervate it. (Section 7.6.3)

**thermoreceptor**   Sensory cell sensitive to temperature. It transduces heat energy into electrical energy. (Section 2.4.1)

**thoracic**   Relating to the thorax (chest), e.g. the thoracic segments of the spinal cord innervate the chest region and provide the preganglionic fibres of the sympathetic division of the autonomic nervous system. (Section 8.3)

**topographic**   Arranged so that spatial relationships are preserved; in the context of the nervous system arranged so that neighbouring receptors or neurons send their axons to neighbouring neurons in another part of the nervous system. (Section 6.3.2)

**transducer**   Structure that converts one form of energy into another. Sensory receptors convert, for example, light or mechanical energy into electrical energy. (Section 2.4.1)

**transmitter**   See *neurotransmitter*. (Section 2.3.3)

**ventral**   Towards an animal's belly. (Section 6.3)

**vertebrates**   Animals with a vertebral column (backbone), e.g. birds, fish, amphibians, reptiles, mammals. (Section 6.1)

**voltage-gated channel**   Channel in the membrane of an excitable cell that allows the passage of ions; it opens when the membrane potential reaches a particular level. (Section 3.6)

**white cells**   The cells of the immune system responsible for much of the biological response against pathogens. (Section 5.2)

**white matter**    The outer part of the spinal cord and brain stem and the inner part of the cerebral hemispheres, consisting mainly of bundles of myelinated axons. (Section 8.2)

**working memory**    Memory where information is only stored for the period of time in which it is needed, e.g. an unfamiliar telephone number; also known as short-term memory. (Section 11.4)

# ACKNOWLEDGEMENTS

Grateful acknowledgement is made to the following sources for permission to reproduce material in this book:

FIGURES

*Figures 2.1, 2.5, 6.4b, 6.6e, 6.13:* Pearse, V., Pearse, J., Buschbaum, M. and Buschbaum, R. (1987) *Living Invertebrates*, Blackwell Scientific Publications Ltd; *Figure 2.2:* courtesy of Opax Microscopes; *Figure 2.4:* courtesy of Jeol (UK) Ltd; *Figures 2.6a, b, c, 6.3:* Carpenter, R. H. S. (1990) *Neurophysiology*, Edward Arnold Publishers; *Figures 2.6d, 2.16, 6.8b, 6.14c:* Alberts, B., Bray, D., Lewis, J., Ratt, M., Roberts, K. and Watson, J. D. (1989) *Molecular Biology of the Cell*, Garland Publishing Inc.; *Figure 2.8a, b, c*: Photographs courtesy of Dr Vicky Stirling from specimens supplied by Dr Steven Davies, University College, London; *Figures 2.8d, 2.15:* courtesy of Dr Michael Stewart; *Figure 2.10:* Cajal, S. (1960) *Studies on Vertebrate Neurogenesis*, courtesy of Charles C. Thomas (Publisher), Springfield, Illinois; *Figures 2.14, 2.17, 2.18:* Katz, B. (1966) *Nerve, Muscle and Synapse*, McGraw-Hill (reprinted with the permission of McGraw-Hill Inc.); *Figures 3.11, 9.16, 9.17, 9.21, 9.23, 9.26, 9.27, 10.2b, 11.1, 11.2:* Kandel, E. R. and Schwartz, J. H. (1985) *Principles of Neural Science*, Elsevier Science Publishers. Copyright © 1985 by Elsevier Science Publishing Co. Inc.; *Figure 5.1:* from *The Immune System*, by N. K. Jerne. Copyright © 1973 by Scientific American Inc. (all rights reserved); *Figure 5.2:* Hildemann, W. H., Johnson, I. S. and Jokiel, P. L. (1978) *Science*, **204**, pp. 420–422. Copyright © 1978 by the American Association for the Advancement of Science; *Figure 5.8:* Ader, R., Cohen, N. and Borbjerg, D. (1982) *Journal of Comparative and Physiological Psychology*, **96**, pp. 517–521. Copyright © 1982 by the American Psychological Association (adapted with permission); *Figure 5.9:* Ader, R. and Cohen, N. (1981) in Ader, R. (ed.) *Psychoneuroimmunology*, Academic Press Inc.; *Figure 5.10:* Ader, R. and Cohen, N. (1982) *Science*, **215**, pp. 1534–1536. Copyright © 1982 by the American Association for the Advancement of Science; *Figure 6.2b:* Batham, E. J., Pantin, C. F. A. and Robson, E. A. (1960) *Quarterly Journal of Microscopic Science*, **101**, pp. 487–510, Company of Biologists Ltd; *Figure 6.2c, d:* Mackie, G. O. (1960) *Quarterly Journal of Microscopic Science*, **101**, pp. 119–131, Company of Biologists Ltd; *Figure 6.6d:* Bracegirdle, B. and Miles, P. H. (1978) adapted from *An Atlas of Chordate Structure*, Heinemann Educational; *Figure 6.7a:* courtesy of Professor J. G. Nicholls; *Figures 6.8a, 7.22:* Burrows, M. (1975) in Usherwood, P. N. R. and Newth, D. R. (eds) *'Simple' Nervous Systems*, Edward Arnold Publishers; *Figure 6.10a, b, c:* Kandel, E. R. (1976) adapted from *Cellular Basis of Behaviour*. Copyright © 1976 by W. H. Freeman and Co. (reprinted with permission); *Figure 6.14b:* Garland Publishing Inc.; *Figure 7.2:* Kershaw, D. R. (1983) *Animal Diversity*, HarperCollins; *Figure 7.3:* McFarlane, I. D. (1976) *Journal of Experimental Biology*, **64**, pp. 431–436, Company of Biologists Ltd; *Figures 7.4, 7.6:* McFarlane, I. D. (1982) in Shelton, G. A. B. (ed.) *Electrical Conduction and Behaviour in 'Simple' Invertebrates*, Clarendon Press, Oxford; *Figure 7.9:* Ottaway, J. R. (1978) *Australian Journal of*

*Marine* and *Freshwater Research*, **29**, pp. 787–802, CSIRO Editorial Services; *Figures 7.11, 7.19, 7.27, 7.28:* Young, D. (1989) *Nerve Cells and Animal Behaviour*, Cambridge University Press; *Figure 7.12b:* Wilson, D. M. and Weis-Fogh, T. (1962) *Journal of Experimental Biology,* **40**, pp. 643–667, Company of Biologists Ltd; *Figure 7.16:* Pringle, J. (1981) *Journal of Experimental Biology*, **94**, pp. 1–14, Company of Biologists Ltd; *Figure 7.18:* Neville, A. C. and Weis-Fogh, T. (1963) *Journal of Experimental Biology*, **40**, pp. 111–121, Company of Biologists Ltd; *Figure 7.21b:* Hill, R. W. and Wyse, G. A. (1989) *Animal Physiology,* Harper and Row, Inc.; *Figure 7.23a:* Robertson, R. M. and Pearson, K. G. (1982) *Journal of Comparative Physiology A*, **146**, pp. 311–320, Springer-Verlag, Heidelberg; *Figure 7.24:* Robertson, R. M. and Pearson, K. G. (1985) *Journal of Neurophysiology*, **53**, pp. 110–128, American Physiological Society; *Figure 7.27:* Mohl, B. (1985) *Journal of Comparative Physiology A*, **156**, pp. 103–116, Springer-Verlag, Heidelberg; *Figure 8.1d:* courtesy of Dr Robin Orchardson; *Figure 8.10b:* Luciano, D. S., Vander, A. J. and Sherman, J. H. (1978) *Human Function and Structure*, McGraw-Hill Inc.; *Figure 8.12:* Tortora, G. J. and Anagnostakos, N. P. (1990) *Principles of Anatomy and Physiology,* 6th edn, HarperCollins; *Figure 8.16:* Fujisawa, H. (1981) *Brain Research*, **206**, pp. 27–37, Company of Biologists Ltd; *Figure 8.17:* courtesy of Dr Vicky Stirling; *Figure 8.18a:* Cook, J. E. and Beckev, D. L. (1988) *Development*, **64**, pp. 321–329, Company of Biologists Ltd; *Figure 8.24a:* Ranson, S. W. (1959) *The Anatomy of the Nervous System,* Harcourt Brace Jovanovich Inc.; *Figure 8.25:* Walsch, K. (1978) *Neuropsychology: A Clinical Approach,* Churchill Livingstone Ltd; *Figure 8.26:* Marsh, J. T., Worden, F. G. and Hicks, L. (1962) *Science,* **137**, pp. 280–282. Copyright © 1962 American Association for the Advancement of Science; *Figure 8.28:* from *The Development of the Brain*, by W. M. Cowan. Copyright © 1979 by Scientific American Inc. (all rights reserved); *Figure 8.31:* Brodal, A. (1981) *Neurological Anatomy in Relation to Clinical Medicine*, 3rd edn. Copyright © 1969, 1981 by Oxford University Press Inc. (reprinted with permission); *Figure 9.4:* Carola, R., Harley, J. P. and Noback, C. R. (1990) *Human Anatomy and Physiology (International Edition)*, McGraw-Hill; *Figure 9.25:* The Natural History Museum, London; *Figure 10.6:* Pfaff, D. W. (1980) *Estrogens and Brain Function*, Springer-Verlag, Heidelberg; *Figure 10.9:* Bloom, F. E. and Lazerson, A. (1988) *Brain, Mind and Behavior*, 2nd edn. Copyright © 1988 by Educational Broadcasting Corporation (reprinted with permission of W. H. Freeman and Co.); *Figure 11.4:* Petersen, S. E., Fox, P. T., Posner, M. I., Minton, M. and Raichle, M. E. (1988) *Nature*, **331**, pp. 585–589, Macmillan; *Figure 11.5:* Springer, S. P. and Deutsch, G. (1989) *Left Brain, Right Brain*, 3rd edn. Copyright © 1989 by Springer and Deutsch (reprinted by permission of W. H. Freeman and Co.); *Figures 11.7, 11.8, 11.9:* Kolb, B. and Whishaw, I. Q. (1990) *Fundamentals of Human Neuropsychology*. Copyright © 1990 by W. H. Freeman and Co. (reprinted with permission).

# INDEX